Get the most out of your book, access your included ancillaries today!

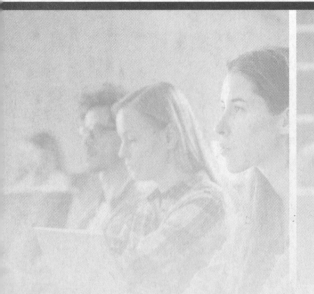

For Students & Instructors:

✔ **The Affordable Care Act:** An Update

✔ **The Affordable Care Act:** A Brief History, Assessment, and Future Challenges

✔ **Provisions of the Patient Protection and Affordable Care Act of 2010**

✔ **eChapter:** A Visual Overview of Health Care Delivery in the United States

✔ **Case Exercises for Nurses**

✔ **Audio podcasts** provide summaries for each chapter with real-world context of topics featured in the news

Access these materials by visiting:
http://connect.springerpub.com/content/book/978-0-8261-7273-0

Instructor's Materials:

✔ **Instructor's Manual:** 9780826172914

✔ **PowerPoints:** 9780826172747

✔ **Test Bank:** 9780826172761

✔ **Transition Guide for the 12th Edition:** 9780826172785

✔ **Image Bank:** 9780826172778

✔ **Syllabus for Public Health and Health Care Administration:** 9780826172938

✔ **Syllabus for Nursing:** 9780826172945

Qualified instructors may request these materials by emailing:
textbook@springerpub.com

Jonas & Kovner's

HEALTH CARE DELIVERY IN THE UNITED STATES

James R. Knickman, PhD, is the Robert Derzon Chair in Public and Health Affairs at New York University with joint appointments at the NYU Wagner School of Public Service and at NYU Langone Medical School's Department of Population Health. He has spent four decades splitting his time between academe and the philanthropic sector. His work focuses on health policy and he has played many roles both as a researcher and a leader in philanthropy to advance the use of public policy to improve the American health care system. He was a Vice President at the Robert Wood Johnson Foundation and President of the New York State Health Foundation. He has a PhD in Public Policy Analysis from the University of Pennsylvania and did his undergraduate work at Fordham University. He serves on the Board of Directors at three non-profit organizations, including chairing the National Council on Aging.

Brian Elbel, PhD, MPH, is an associate professor of Population Health and Health Policy at the New York University School of Medicine, where he heads the Section on Health Choice, Policy and Evaluation within the Department of Population Health, and at the NYU Wagner Graduate School of Public Service. He is the Assistant Dean for Strategic Initiatives in the Office of Science and Research of NYU Langone Health and the Director of the NYU Langone Comprehensive Program on Obesity. He studies how individuals make decisions that influence their health, with a particular emphasis on evaluation, obesity, and food choice. His work uses behavioral economics to understand health decision-making among vulnerable groups, and the role and influence of public policy on these decisions. His research has been funded by the National Institutes of Health, Centers for Disease Control and Prevention, the National Science Foundation and the Robert Wood Johnson Foundation and has been featured in national television, radio, and print media. Dr. Elbel earned his bachelor's degree from The University of Texas at Austin and his master's and doctorate in Health Policy/Health Economics from Yale University.

Jonas & Kovner's

HEALTH CARE DELIVERY IN THE UNITED STATES

12th Edition

EDITORS
JAMES R. KNICKMAN, PhD
BRIAN ELBEL, PhD, MPH

FOUNDING EDITOR
STEVEN JONAS, MD, MPH, MS, FNYAS

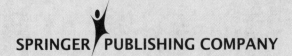
SPRINGER PUBLISHING COMPANY

Springer Publishing Company, LLC
11 West 42nd Street
New York, NY 10036
www.springerpub.com
connect.springerpub.com

Acquisitions Editor: David D'Addona
Compositor: Integra

ISBN: 9780826172723
ebook ISBN: 9780826172730
DOI: 10.1891/9780826172730

INSTRUCTOR'S MATERIALS: Qualified instructors may request supplements by emailing textbook@springerpub.com:
Instructor's Manual: 9780826172914
PowerPoints: 9780826172747
Test Bank: 9780826172761
Transition Guide for the 12th Edition: 9780826172785
Image Bank: 9780826172778
Syllabus for Public Health: 9780826172938
Syllabus for Nursing: 9780826172945
Supplementary materials are available from http://connect.springerpub.com/content/book/978-0-8261-7273-0
The Affordable Care Act: An Update
The Affordable Care Act: A Brief History, Assessment, and Future Challenges
Provisions of the Patient Protection and Affordable Care Act of 2010
eChapter: A Visual Overview of Health Care Delivery in the United States
Case Exercises for Nurses
For Students and Instructors: Visit ushealthcaredelivery.com for additional materials including an update on the Affordable Care Act.

19 20 21 22/5 4 3

Library of Congress Cataloging-in-Publication Data

Names: Knickman, James, editor. | Elbel, Brian, [date] editor.
Title: Jonas & Kovner's health care delivery in the United States / [edited by] James R. Knickman, Brian Elbel.
Other titles: Jonas and Kovner's health care delivery in the United States |
   Health care delivery in the United States
Description: 12th edition. | New York : Springer Publishing Company, [2019] |
   Includes bibliographical references and index.
Identifiers: LCCN 2018048861 (print) | LCCN 2018049494 (ebook) | ISBN
   9780826172730 | ISBN 9780826172723 (alk. paper) | ISBN 0826172725 (alk.paper)
Subjects: | MESH: Delivery of Health Care | Health Services | Health Policy |
   Quality of Health Care | United States
Classification: LCC RA395.A3 (ebook) | LCC RA395.A3 (print) | NLM W 84 AA1 |
   DDC 362.10973—dc23   LC record available at https://lccn.loc.gov/2018048861

Contact us to receive discount rates on bulk purchases.
We can also customize our books to meet your needs.
For more information please contact: sales@springerpub.com

CONTENTS

PART I HEALTH POLICY

PART IV FUTURE OF U.S. HEALTH CARE

LIST OF FEATURES

SUPPLEMENTARY MATERIAL

The Affordable Care Act: An Update
The Affordable Care Act: A Brief History, Assessment, and Future Challenges
Provisions of the Patient Protection and Affordable Care Act of 2010
eChapter: A Visual Overview of Health Care Delivery in the United States
Case Exercises for Nurses

indicates a podcast is available for the chapter.

LIST OF PODCASTS

Chapter 1
The Challenge of Health Care Delivery and Health Policy

Chapter 2
Organization of Care

Chapter 3
The Politics of Health Care in the United States

Chapter 4
Comparative Health Systems

Chapter 5
Population Health

Chapter 6
Public Health: A Transformation in the 21st Century

Chapter 7
Health and Behavior

Chapter 8
Vulnerable Populations: Meeting the Health Needs of Populations Facing Health Inequities

Chapter 9
The Health Workforce

Chapter 10
Health Care Financing

Chapter 11
Health Care Costs and Value

Chapter 12
High-Quality Health Care

Chapter 13
Health Care Management

Chapter 14
Health Information Technology

Chapter 15
The Future of Health Care Delivery and Health Policy

FOREWORD

According to Russo and Gourevitch (Chapter 5), Americans' chances for living long and healthy lives are not improving, despite ever-greater spending on health care itself. The United States spends more and its residents are in worse health than nearly all other developed economies. This is one of the main issues that health care leaders and managers need to address in the coming years. Can we get more value for the money we are spending on health care? Besides being a local matter, whose delivery differs in each community, health care presents national economic and political challenges to us all. Many principles of improving health-care, such as ensuring better access to care, higher quality care, and controlling costs and spending are held by a spectrum of "tribes" within the major political parties. But there seem to be a few differing principles, such as requiring Americans to buy mandatory health insurance or pay a tax penalty, that hurt the ability to create a more stable system and provide more value to Americans.

This book provides evidence based on history and context to draw your own conclusions rather than playing to existing views and biases. For example, one part of the solution to our delivery problems may be to have health workers work more effectively in interdisciplinary teams. Insights into some of the consequences of this kind of solution can be found in a number of chapters in this book: Organization of Care (how is care organized?), Politics of Healthcare (how do political choices impact how it is governed and how care is paid for?), Comparative Health Systems (how is care organized in other countries?), The Health Workforce (who is in the workforce and what do they do?), and also in chapters about what health care costs and what value do we get for our money, how is quality health care assured, and what are the various futures of health care delivery.

Over 500,000 readers of this book in its previous editions have been introduced to the issues facing our nation in delivering health care and striving to keep people healthy. The book lays out the evidence of what has and has not worked in health care, and where the challenges lie ahead. A strength of the book is that it both helps readers become more knowledgeable about how the health system works and explains why it is so complicated to make the system work better. A few notable examples discussed in Chapter 15 of the 12th edition include the challenges of privately sharing "big data" across health care organizations to achieve secured and accurate interoperability, of addressing the high costs of prescription drugs causing financial toxicity, of creating a more vibrant culture of health, of meeting the demands of an increasing aging population, and of addressing the health care workforce shortages which impact the occupations of those who use this book, such as managers, nurses, physicians, and public health workers. This book has been in the making for over 40 years and 12 editions. NYU Dean Sherry Glied said about the 11th edition that it demonstrates once again why this

volume has come to be so prized—it helps readers of different health care professions chart a middle course to a swinging pendulum of health system reform and
prepares them to take a long view to cope with challenges that affect health care
delivery in the United States. I predict the 12th edition will be equally prized.
Health Care Delivery in the United States gives the reader what he or she needs
to understand and form opinions about the issues, to understand which factors
cause which results, and to better understand what we know about health care
and what we don't know, what we can fix in the short run, and what we can't fix
without making changes which are politically unacceptable to those who have the
votes or the dollars.

   Health Care Delivery in the United States benefits from the talents and experience of James R. Knickman and Brian Elbel who now succeed me as editors of
this text. I have worked with both of these NYU faculty for many years and they
are wise and good friends. Jim started his career as a faculty member at NYU,
where he has returned. He is best known for his many years as a leading grant-
maker supporting health services research and innovation as head of research
and evaluation at the Robert Wood Johnson Foundation. He also spent 10 years
building the New York State Health Foundation which, under his stewardship,
has been an important contributor to health system improvements in New York
State. Brian Elbel is a professor both at NYU School of Medicine and NYU Wagner's Health Policy and Management program. His research focuses on how public policy, environmental factors, and community initiatives can influence the
choices people make, particularly on food policy. Jim and Brian bring disciplin-
ary perspectives of policy and economics to delivering a textbook that effectively
introduces learners to the complex worlds of American health care.

Anthony R. Kovner, PhD
Professor Emeritus, New York University
Robert F. Wagner School of Public Service
New York, New York

ACKNOWLEDGMENTS

The editors would like to express deep appreciation to the team of people who made this book possible. First, we thank our 28 authors of the 15 chapters that comprise the book. They are all noted experts in their fields, and we appreciate their willingness to translate their knowledge into chapters that introduce future leaders to the workings of the U.S. health system. Second, we wish to acknowledge the superb editorial role played by David D'Addona and Jaclyn Shultz as well as the quality control of production under Joanne Jay's direction at Springer Publishing Company. We appreciate David's insights about how to publish a textbook that is current to the digital landscape and have benefited from Joanne's keeping the process moving in creating an effective and enjoyable learning experience for HCDUS readers. We thank Natalie Covill and Allison Mercurio who each provided valued assistance gathering current data to update the book. We value the sage advice and assistance of our colleague and friend, Anthony Kovner, who helped to set the bar high for this book over many years. Finally, we would like to acknowledge Steve Jonas, who originated this book 12 editions ago.

ORGANIZATION
OF THIS BOOK

This is the 12th edition of *Jonas & Kovner's Health Care Delivery in the United States*, which, although its title has evolved in the last 40 years, has stayed true to its original purpose: helping instructors and students better understand the complicated, expensive, and ever-changing U.S. health care delivery system, public health system, and health policy. It is a privilege to be able to work with instructors around the world to introduce the leaders of tomorrow to the health field.

Our nation has embarked on an ambitious attempt to reshape how we go about taking care of the health concerns of our population and, with a new administration, faces scrutiny and attempts to dismantle and defund the Patient Protection and Affordable Care Act (ACA). On the one hand, there is a renewed energy to develop initiatives that focus on keeping people healthy. On the other hand, there is a great deal of experimenting with the organization of the care system that addresses the needs of people who have medical problems associated with injuries and disease. The aim of this experimentation is to improve the quality of health and medical care and to bring costs in line with what Americans can afford and want to spend on the health sector. Inefficient and inconsistent quality and value of care have led to political posturing and efforts to reduce the ACA's influence on the health care delivery system.

This text begins by describing the current status of the U.S. health care system and explaining the complicated public policy process that has so much influence on the way health care is delivered and financed in this country (Part One). Following Part One, we address both the challenge of keeping people healthy (Part Two) and the challenge of delivering efficient medical care that helps people recover from medical conditions that do occur (Part Three). The text ends with a consideration of where the health system might be headed in the years to come and what forces will shape it over time (Part Four).

Each chapter starts with a list of the learning objectives addressed by the chapter, a list of key terms that are central to the chapter's focus, and an outline of what is to come. Each chapter ends with a list of discussion questions and a case exercise encouraging the reader to apply the ideas of the chapter to real-life issues and challenges that face health care leaders focused on management issues and policy issues. For nursing instructors, there are additional case exercises available online that add a specific nursing context for students.

In addition to this text, an online Instructor's Manual, which includes a variety of background materials that teachers will find useful in guiding class discussion, is available. It also offers additional resources and class projects that are useful to students and the learning process. There are also several online supplements, including four eChapters: covering the Provisions of the Patient Protection and Affordable Care Act of 2010, A Visual Overview of Health Care Delivery in the

United States, The Affordable Care Act: A Brief History, Assessment, and Future Challenges and an annual ACA Update. Additionally, PowerPoints, Syllabi, a Test Bank, and a Transition Guide are available to instructors via textbook@springerpub.com. New to the 12th edition are audio podcast chapter summaries that can be accessed in print, ebook, and online versions of the text by students and instructors alike.

Students and instructors are encouraged to visit Springer Publishing Connect™ for all additional materials pertaining to the text by using the access code on the inside front cover.

We encourage instructors and students to communicate with us about this edition, so that we may make the 13th edition even more useful to you. Please submit any comments or questions to us at james.knickman@nyu.edu and brian.elbel@nyulangone.org, and we will get back to you. As always, we appreciate your suggestions.

James R. Knickman, PhD
Brian Elbel, PhD, MPH

CONTRIBUTORS

Elaine F. Cassidy, PhD, is a senior consultant in research and evaluation at consulting firm Equal Measure, where she manages projects related to health promotion, particularly among underprivileged populations. Before joining Equal Measure, Dr. Cassidy served as a program officer in research and evaluation at the Robert Wood Johnson Foundation, where she oversaw research and evaluation activities for the Vulnerable Populations portfolio. Her work and professional interests focus primarily on child and adolescent health and risk behavior, violence prevention, and school-based interventions, primarily for young people living in low-income, urban environments. She is a trained school psychologist and mental health clinician who has provided therapeutic care to children and families in school, outpatient, and acute partial hospitalization settings. She holds an MSEd in psychological services from the University of Pennsylvania and a PhD in school, community, and child-clinical psychology from the University of Pennsylvania.

Susan A. Chapman, PhD, RN, FAAN, is a professor in the Department of Social and Behavioral Sciences, University of California, San Francisco School of Nursing, and faculty at Healthforce Center at UCSF and the Philip R. Lee Institute for Health Policy Studies. She is co-director of the UCSF Health Workforce Research Center on Long-Term Care. She is co-director of the master's and doctoral programs in health policy at the UCSF School of Nursing. Her scholarly work focuses on health workforce research, health policy analysis, and program evaluation. Susan's workforce research focuses on transforming models of primary care to address new and expanded roles for the health care workforce and addressing workforce needs in behavioral health and long-term care.

Carolyn M. Clancy, MD, MACP, serves as the Executive in Charge, Veterans Health Administration (VHA), with the authority to perform the functions and duties of the Under Secretary for Health. She was previously the Interim Under Secretary for Health from 2014–2015. She is a highly experienced and nationally recognized physician executive. Prior to her current position, she served as the Deputy Under Secretary for Health for Organizational Excellence overseeing VHA's performance, quality, safety, risk management, systems engineering, auditing, oversight, ethics and accreditation programs, as well as ten years as the Director, Agency for Healthcare Research and Quality. In 2015, Dr. Clancy was selected as the Outstanding Federal Executive of the Year by Disabled American Veterans. Dr. Clancy has contributed to eight academic textbooks and authored, co-authored and provided invited commentary in more than 225 scholarly journal articles. An elected member of the National Academy of Medicine, Dr. Clancy was most recently presented with the 2014 Quality Champion Award, National

Committee for Quality Assurance and was also named as Honorary Fellow, American Academy of Nursing.

Karen B. DeSalvo, MD, MPH, MSc, is professor of Medicine and Population Health at the University of Texas at Austin Dell Medical School. She is a graduate of Tulane University Schools of Medicine and Public Health and the Harvard School of Public Health, was an Robert Wood Johnson Generalist Faculty Scholar, and is board-certified in Internal Medicine. Dr. DeSalvo has been an attending physician at Charity Hospital in New Orleans, professor and vice dean for Community Affairs and Health Policy at Tulane School of Medicine. She was Health Commissioner for the City of New Orleans. Most recently, she served in the Obama Administration at the U.S. Department of Health and Human Services as National Coordinator for Health Information Technology and Assistant Secretary for Health (Acting). Dr. DeSalvo is an elected member of the Institute of Medicine of the National Academy of Sciences and is a nationally recognized thought leader in public health, health information technology, social determinants of health, and the strategies required to transition to value-based care.

Cathleen O. Erwin, PhD, MBA, is an associate professor and health services administration program director in the Department of Political Science at Auburn University. Dr. Erwin received her doctoral degree in administration-health services from the University of Alabama at Birmingham. Her research primarily revolves around strategic management, organizational performance, and governance in health care organizations. Dr. Erwin's teaching portfolio includes courses in health care delivery systems, insurance and reimbursement, quality management, strategic management, health information technology, and fundraising. She is a past president of the Alabama chapter of the American College of Healthcare Executives (ACHE) and is an appointed member of the board for the Health Care Management Division of the Academy of Management.

Irene Fraser, PhD, is a political scientist who has specialized in research on health care access (Medicaid, private health insurance, uncompensated care), and the measurement, reporting and improvement of health care safety, quality, and value. She is a senior fellow at NORC at the University of Chicago. She serves on the Board of The Leapfrog Group, a national nonprofit organization that promotes improvements in the safety of health care by giving consumers data to make more informed hospital choices and also serves on the Board of The Villages at Rockville, a Continuing Care Community. She is also active in AcademyHealth, where she serves on the Nominating Committee. From 1996 to 2015, she was director of the Center for Delivery, Organization, and Markets at the Agency for Healthcare Research and Quality (AHRQ). Dr. Fraser also spent eight years at the American Hospital Association, as senior policy manager on indigent care, Medicaid, and health care reform, and Director of Ambulatory Care. Before that, Dr. Fraser was associate professor of Political Science and Director of the Public Policy program at Barat College, and adjunct faculty to the Institute for Health

Law at Loyola School of Law. Dr. Fraser's work has appeared in *Health Affairs, Inquiry, Health Care Financing Review, Medical Care Research and Review, Journal of Healthcare Management, Journal of Ambulatory Care Management, Health Services Research,* and *Journal of Health Politics, Policy and Law.*

Jacqueline Martinez Garcel, MPH, is the CEO of the Latino Community Foundation (LCF)—the only statewide foundation solely focused on investing in Latino leaders. The mission of LCF is to unleash the power of Latinos in California. LCF leads one of the largest networks of civically engaged Latino philanthropists in the country. Jacqueline is driven by a sense of urgency, justice, and determination to create opportunities for Latinos to thrive economically and engage politically. Previously, she served as vice president at the New York State Health Foundation (NYSHealth) where she helped establish the foundation as a resource for policy-makers and community leaders across the state. Prior to joining NYSHealth, she was the executive director for the Northern Manhattan Community Voices Collaborative (Community Voices), an initiative funded by the W.K. Kellogg Foundation to improve access and quality of care for vulnerable populations. Jacqueline worked with Dr. H. Jack Geiger at the City University of New York to complete an analysis of racial and ethnic disparities in diagnosis and treatment in the U.S. health care system. Jacqueline has been appointed to several boards, including the Institute for Civic Leadership, NAMI-NYC Metro, and Grantmakers in Health. She currently serves on the KQED Community Advisory Panel and co-chairs the National Latino Funds Alliance (NLFA). She holds a MPH from Columbia University and a BS from Cornell University.

Marc N. Gourevitch, MD, MPH, is the Muriel G. and George W. Singer Professor and founding chair of the Department of Population Health at NYU Langone Medical Center. The focus of Dr. Gourevitch's work is on developing approaches that leverage both health care delivery and policy- and community-level interventions to advance the health of populations. Dr. Gourevitch leads the City Health Dashboard initiative, funded by the Robert Wood Johnson Foundation, which aims to equip city and community leaders with an accurate understanding of the health of their urban populations, including social, economic, and environmental drivers, to support population health improvement initiatives. Dr. Gourevitch previously served as founding director of NYU Langone's Division of General Internal Medicine and led NYU Langone's CDC-funded Fellowship in Medicine and Public Health Research. A graduate of Harvard College and Harvard Medical School, he trained in primary care/internal medicine at NYU and Bellevue Hospital and received his MPH from Columbia University's Mailman School of Public Health.

Michael K. Gusmano, PhD, is an associate professor, director of the concentration in health systems and policy, and director of the doctoral program at the Rutgers University School of Public Health. He is also a research scholar at the Hastings Center and a visiting fellow at the Nelson A. Rockefeller Institute of Government of the State University of New York. Dr. Gusmano serves as the International

Editor of the *Journal of Aging and Social Policy*, Associate Editor for *Health Economics, Policy and Law*, and is on the board of editors of the *Journal of Health Politics, Policy and Law* and *World Medical and Health Policy*, and on the editorial committee of the *Hastings Center Report*. He has published six books and more than 100 scholarly articles.

Rogan Kersh, PhD, is provost and professor of political science at Wake Forest University. He has published three books, on American political history and on health policy; a fourth edition of *By the People: Debating American Government* (with James Morone) will be published in 2019 by Oxford University Press. His current book project is on "Millennials, Politics, and Culture"; he has given dozens of talks on the millennial generation to audiences across the United States and Europe, including at TEDx conferences the past 2 years. Dr. Kersh has published over 50 academic articles, and does frequent media commentary on U.S. politics, health policy, and the millennial generation. He has been a Mellon Fellow in the Humanities, a Luce Scholar, a Robert Wood Johnson Fellow, and is an elected Fellow of the National Academy of Public Administration. In 15 years of teaching at Yale, Syracuse, and NYU, he won four university-wide teaching awards. He is past president of the American Political Science Association's section on Health Politics & Policy, and serves on the editorial board of the *Journal of Health Politics, Policy, & Law*. Kersh received his PhD in political science from Yale in 1996, and has professional experience in the U.S. Congress, the British Parliament, and at think tanks in Tokyo and Washington, DC. In Winston-Salem, he serves on the boards of the United Way and the RiverRun Film Festival, and chairs the Mayor's Thought Force on Poverty.

Anthony R. Kovner, PhD, is professor emeritus of public and health management at New York University's Robert F. Wagner Graduate School of Public Service. He was director of Wagner's program in health policy and management for 20 years, the executive MPA for nurse leaders and the advanced management program for clinicians. Kovner was a senior program consultant to the Robert Wood Johnson program for two rural hospital programs and senior health consultant to the United Autoworkers Union. He was a full-time manager in several health care organizations for 12 years, including a large community health center, a nursing home, an academic faculty practice, and as CEO of a community hospital. Professor Kovner is the author or editor, with others, of 11 books, 48 peer-reviewed articles, and 33 published case studies. He was the fourth recipient, in 1999, of the Filerman Prize for Educational Leadership from the Association of University Programs in Health Administration.

Paul L. Kuehnert, DNP, NP, is associate vice president for the Robert Wood Johnson Foundation where he provides leadership and management direction for the Foundation's work related to leadership and transforming health and health care systems. As an executive leader for more than 25 years, Kuehnert has led both governmental and community-based organizations in order to help people lead healthier lives. In the late 1980s, he was a founder and later CEO of Community Response, Inc., one of the Chicago area's largest housing, nutrition, and social service providers for people living with HIV/AIDS. He moved to Maine in 1999 and served in the state health department, leading the development of a regional public health system and becoming deputy director of the department in 2005. From 2006 to 2012 when he joined the Robert Wood Johnson Foundation, Kuehnert was the county health officer and executive director for health in Kane County, Illinois, a metro-Chicago county of 515,000 people. There he led four departments—Public Health, Community Reinvestment, Animal Control, and Emergency Management—and worked with leaders from the private and public sectors to create the first county-level master plan in Illinois that integrated health, land use, and transportation. Dr. Kuehnert is a pediatric nurse practitioner and holds the Doctor of Nursing Practice in executive leadership as well as the Master of Science in public health nursing degrees from the University of Illinois at Chicago. He was named a Robert Wood Johnson Foundation Executive Nurse Fellow in 2004 and inducted into the American Academy of Nursing in 2015.

Amy Yarbrough Landry, PhD, is an associate professor in the Department of Health Services Administration at the University of Alabama at Birmingham. She is the MSHA Program Director and the Howard W. Houser Professor of Health Services Administration. Dr. Landry teaches Introduction to Health Systems and Comparative Health Systems to master's and doctoral students in her department. Dr. Landry's research interests pertain to the strategic management of health care organizations in a variety of contexts, including acute care hospitals, long-term care organizations, Medicaid managed care organizations, and physician organizations. Dr. Landry has also done research surrounding leadership in health care organizations. In particular, she is interested in executive selection, training, and development. Dr. Landry is a past board member of the Alabama Healthcare Executives Forum, the state chapter of the American College of Healthcare Executives (ACHE), and currently serves as the Chair of the Health Care Management Division of the Academy of Management.

Christy Harris Lemak, PhD, FACHE, is professor and chair of the Department of Health Services Administration at the University of Alabama at Birmingham. Dr. Lemak teaches and conducts scholarship in the areas of health care management and leadership with an emphasis on how leadership and organizational factors lead to high performance in health care. Her research includes studies of a complex pay-for-performance incentive program for physicians, and relationships among organizational culture, management practice, and surgical outcomes in a multihospital surgical collaborative. Dr. Lemak has extensively studied how Medicaid policy demonstrations affect hospitals, health plans, and relationships among provider organizations. She is currently examining new ways of measuring hospital and health system performance. She holds a PhD in health services organization and policy from the University of Michigan, MHA and MBA degrees from the University of Missouri-Columbia, and a BS in health planning and administration from the University of Illinois.

Laura C. Leviton, PhD, is senior adviser for evaluation at the Robert Wood Johnson Foundation. She has overseen evaluations in most of RWJF's areas of focus. Previously, Leviton was a professor of public health at the University of Alabama at Birmingham and on the faculty of the University of Pittsburgh School of Public Health. During this time, she collaborated on the earliest randomized experiment on effective ways to prevent HIV infection in gay and bisexual men. She is a leading writer on evaluation methods and practice, in particular for disease prevention. She was president of the American Evaluation Association in 2000. She is the co-author of three books—*Foundations of Program Evaluation* (1991), *Confronting Public Health Risks* (1997), and *Managing Applied Social Research* (2017)—and has served on several editorial boards for evaluation journals. For her work in HIV prevention and worksite health promotion, she received the 1993 award for Distinguished Contributions to Psychology in the Public Interest from the American Psychological Association. Dr. Leviton also served on three National Academy of Medicine committees and on the National Advisory Committee on HIV and STD Prevention of the Centers for Disease Control and Prevention. She received her PhD in social psychology from the University of Kansas and postdoctoral training in research methodology and evaluation at Northwestern University.

John Marchica, PhD, is the founder and CEO of Darwin Research Group and is a faculty associate in the W.P. Carey School of Business and the graduate College of Health Solutions at Arizona State University. John began his career at SRG as a health systems analyst, followed by a successful stretch in general management at Abbott Laboratories. He's a two-time health care entrepreneur, and his first company, FaxWatch, was listed twice on the *Inc. 500* list of fastest growing American companies. John is the author of *The Accountable Organization* and has advised health care executives on strategy and organizational change for more than a decade. John did his undergraduate work in economics at Knox College, has an MBA and master's degree in public policy from the University of Chicago, and completed his PhD coursework at The Dartmouth Institute. He serves as an active member of the American College of Healthcare Executives and is an advisor to the Global Council on Alzheimer's Disease.

James Morone, PhD, is the John Hazen White Professor of Political Science, Public Policy and Urban Studies at Brown University. He has been elected to the National Academy of Sciences, Engineering and Medicine as well as the National Academy of Social Insurance. Professor Morone received his BA from Middlebury College and his PhD from the University of Chicago. He has published eleven scholarly books and over 150 articles, reviews, and essays on American political history, health care policy, and social issues. Dr. Morone's first book, *The Democratic Wish,* was named a "notable book of 1991" by *The New York Times* and won the

Political Science Association's Kammerer Award for the best book on the United States. His *Hellfire Nation: The Politics of Sin in American History* was nominated for a Pulitzer Prize and named a top book of 2003 by numerous newspapers and magazines (including both *Christianity Today* and *Playboy* Magazine). His *The Heart of Power: Health and Politics in the Oval Office* (written with David Blumenthal, MD) was featured on the front page of *The New York Times Book Review*. Dr. Morone was distinguished Fulbright lecturer to Japan, has served on the editorial board of eight scholarly journals (chairing two of them), was editor of the *Journal of Health Politics, Policy and Law* and has testified before the U.S. Congress numerous times. He has been president of the New England Political Science Association, the Politics and History section of American Political Science Association, and chaired the faculty at Brown University. The senior class at Brown University has selected him five times as the winner of the Barrett Hazletine Citation for the professor who most inspired them.

C. Tracy Orleans, PhD, is the senior scientist for the Robert Wood Johnson Foundation and has led or co-led the foundation's public policy and health care system grantmaking in the areas of health behavior change, tobacco control, chronic disease management and prevention, physical activity promotion, and childhood obesity prevention during the past 18 years. During the past six years, she has focused mainly on discovering, evaluating, and applying effective policy and environmental strategies for reversing the rise in childhood obesity and reducing the disparities in its prevalence and health tolls. She is now working to develop metrics and research that will help to create a broad culture of health nationwide. Dr. Orleans has authored or coauthored more than 250 publications, served on numerous journal editorial boards, on national scientific panels and advisory groups (e.g., Institute of Medicine, U.S. Preventive Services Task Force, Community Preventive Services Task Force, National Commission on Prevention Priorities, National Collaborative on Childhood Obesity Research), and as the associate policy editor for the *American Journal of Preventive Medicine*. Dr. Orleans has received many awards for her national work in the fields of behavioral medicine, tobacco control, and childhood obesity prevention. Most recently, she was deeply honored, along with Drs. Jim Sallis and Mary Story, to receive the CDC's Weight of the Nation Pioneering Innovation Award for Applied Obesity Research in 2012.

David C. Radley, PhD, is a senior study director in Healthcare Delivery Research and Evaluation at Westat and Senior Scientist at the Commonwealth Fund. He is a health services researcher with experience in health policy evaluation, quality and performance measurement, and public reporting and visualization of health care delivery and social determinants of health-related data. His methodological expertise focuses on small-area analysis and the design, implementation, and interpretation of observational studies using large administrative and survey-based datasets. Dr. Radley previously worked as a senior scientist at the Institute for Healthcare Improvement and as an associate in Domestic

Health Policy at Abt Associates, Inc., where he oversaw projects related to the measurement of long-term care quality and the evaluation of various health IT initiatives. Dr. Radley has a Master of Public Health (MPH) degree from Yale University and a PhD in Health Policy from The Dartmouth Institute for Health Policy and Clinical Practice.

Lourdes J. Rodríguez, DrPh, serves as the director for the Center for Place-Based Initiatives at Dell Medical School at The University of Texas at Austin, which focuses on supporting and implementing health solutions proposed by and for residents of Austin and Central Texas communities. She holds an appointment as associate professor in the Department of Population Health. Dr. Rodríguez also serves in two University of Texas at Austin interdisciplinary grand challenges. The first, Planet Texas 2050, examines the impact on human health of rapid population growth and urbanization in the context of extreme weather events and climate change. The second, Whole Communities Whole Health, is redesigning the traditional cohort study design by starting with a strong foundation of community engagement and partnerships. Both projects are setting an ambitious 10-year research agenda. Her previous role was program officer for the New York State Health Foundation (NYSHealth) in the prevention area, where she disseminated evidence-based programs, supported promising prevention strategies, and leveraged additional resources for New York State. Before her current position, Dr. Rodríguez served as associate director of community partnerships for healthy neighborhoods at City Harvest, overseeing community engagement activities. From 2004 to 2012 she was on the faculty at the Columbia University Mailman School of Public Health. She coedited a book examining community mobilization for health and has authored numerous publications on violence prevention, mental health, and active living. Dr. Rodríguez received a BS in industrial biotechnology from the University of Puerto Rico, an MPH from the University of Connecticut, and a DrPH from Columbia University.

Victor G. Rodwin, PhD, MPH, professor of health policy and management at the Robert F. Wagner Graduate School of Public Service, New York University, conducts research and teaches courses on community health and medical care, comparative analysis of health care systems, and health system performance and reform. He has lectured widely on these topics in universities around the world, most recently at Sun Yat Sen University in Gouangzhou, Fudan University in Shanghai, Renmin University in Beijing, London School of Economics, London School of Hygiene and Tropical Medicine, and the Institut d'Etudes Politiques in Paris. Professor Rodwin was awarded the Fulbright-Tocqueville Distinguished Chair during the spring semester of 2010 while he was based at the University of Paris–Orsay. In 2000, he was the recipient of a three-year Robert Wood Johnson Foundation Health Policy Investigator Award on "Megacities and Health: New York, London, Paris, and Tokyo." His research on this theme led to the establishment of the World Cities Project (WCP)—a collaborative venture between Wagner/NYU and the International Longevity Center USA, which focuses on aging, population health, and the health care systems in New York, London, Paris, Tokyo, and Hong Kong, and among neighborhoods within these world cities.

Pamela G. Russo, MD, MPH, is a senior program officer at the Robert Wood Johnson Foundation (RWJF) in Princeton, New Jersey. She was recruited to RWJF to lead the Population Health: Science and Policy team in 2000. Her areas of focus include health impact assessments; bringing a health lens to decisions made in sectors not traditionally associated with health; community resilience; and innovations in funding that can sustain community health improvement. She is a member of the NASEM Population Health roundtable. Before RWJF, she was an associate professor of medicine, director of the Clinical Outcomes Section, and program co-director for the master's program and fellowship in clinical epidemiology and health services research at the Cornell University Medical Center in New York City. Dr. Russo earned her BS from Harvard College, with a major in the history and philosophy of science; her MPH in epidemiology from the University of California, Berkeley, School of Public Health; and her MD from the University of California, San Francisco. She completed a residency in general internal medicine at the hospital of the University of Pennsylvania and a combined clinical epidemiology and rheumatology fellowship at Cornell and the Hospital of Special Surgery.

Joanne Spetz, PhD, is a professor at the Philip R. Lee Institute for Health Policy Studies, the Department of Family and Community Medicine, and the School of Nursing at the University of California, San Francisco. She is also the associate director for research at Healthforce Center at UCSF and the director of the UCSF Health Workforce Research Center on Long-Term Care. Her fields of specialty are labor economics, public finance, and econometrics. She has led research on the health care workforce, the impact of nursing care, organization of the hospital industry, and medical marijuana policy. Dr. Spetz's teaching is in the areas of quantitative research methods, health care financial management, and health economics.

Matthew D. Trujillo, PhD, joined the Robert Wood Johnson Foundation in 2013 as a research associate with the Foundation's Research-Evaluation-Learning unit. Previously, Dr. Trujillo served an adjunct researcher with the RAND Corporation. He received a BS in Psychology from Arizona State University and a PhD in Psychology and Social Policy from the Woodrow Wilson School of Public and International Affairs at Princeton University. Specifically, his areas of expertise are prejudice, stereotyping, and discrimination. His dissertation examined the impact of microaggressions on ethnic identity and behavior. His work at the Foundation includes behavioral science and communications research on how to create healthy communities.

Monique J. Vasquez, MSSW and MPH candidate, is a graduate research assistant at the Department of Population Health, in the Dell Medical School at The

University of Texas at Austin (UT). She studies at the Steve Hicks School of Social Work at UT, and the School of Public Health through the University of Texas Health Science Center of Houston, Austin Regional Campus. She has completed several internships in her undergraduate studies as a peer advisor for higher education programs, young adult mentor, psychology research assistant, and case management intern with the International Rescue Committee. Her two graduate field placements in Austin focused on health care for uninsured and vulnerable populations through the non-profits Volunteer Healthcare Clinic and Migrant Clinicians Network. Monique is a Returned Peace Corps Volunteer and worked in Madagascar for two years in the health sector. She has experience in the mental health field as a former case manager and intake specialist for Medicaid clients. She previously graduated with a BS in both Psychology and Political Science at the University of Arizona in Tucson.

Elizabeth A. Ward, BS, BA, is a senior program assistant at the New York State Health Foundation (NYSHealth). Ms. Ward supports NYSHealth's Building Healthy Communities priority area, which leads neighborhood-level and policy interventions to increase residents' access to healthy, affordable food options, improve the built environment, and link communities with healthy lifestyle programming. She works closely with program staff to help design and develop grant opportunities and is responsible for assisting senior management and program staff with grants management, grantee communications, event coordination, programmatic research, and financial accounting. Ms. Ward also provides programmatic and administrative support to NYSHealth's veterans health program. Prior to joining NYSHealth, Ms. Ward worked as an executive assistant for a woman-owned New York City-based lobbying firm. She also worked as a paralegal for the Consumer Assistance Program at Health Law Advocates and as a development intern at Health Care for All in Boston. Ms. Ward earned a Bachelor of Science in Public Health, a Bachelor of Arts in Political Science, and a certificate in Public Policy and Administration from the University of Massachusetts at Amherst. She is currently pursuing her Master of Public Administration with a concentration in Urban Development and Sustainability at the CUNY Baruch Marxe School of Public and International Affairs.

Y. Claire Wang, MD, ScD, is associate professor of Health Policy and Management at Columbia Mailman School of Public Health and senior program advisor at the National Academy of Medicine. She is trained as a physician epidemiologist and a population health and decision scientist. She co-directs the Obesity Prevention Initiative, a cross-disciplinary team focusing on environmental and policy approaches to preventing obesity at the community level. She also co-directs the MPH certificate in Comparative Effectiveness and Outcomes Research. In 2015–2016, she was selected as a Robert Wood Johnson Foundation health policy fellow, serving in the U.S. Department of Health and Human Services. She is currently leading projects related to health IT interoperability and quality measurement with the National Academy of Medicine. She obtained her medical degree from National Taiwan University and her doctorate from Harvard School of Public Health.

Kathryn E. Wehr, MPH, senior program officer, joined the Robert Wood Johnson Foundation in 2010. Wehr works to increase the visibility and impact of solutions that advance health and that incorporate emerging research, practice, and policy tools to put evidence into action and create policy and system changes that enable all people to lead healthy, productive lives. As she puts it: "It takes all of us to improve the quality of people's lives, prevent illness, and make our communities vibrant, healthy places—no matter where people live, learn, work and play." To that end, Wehr's interests range from identifying innovations occurring across the country to developing new collaborations and solutions to improve the nation's health—especially those that nurture and strengthen early childhood development and health across the life course. Wehr received an MPH, Maternal and Child Health, from the University of North Carolina-Chapel Hill and is a Phi Beta Kappa graduate in Sociology from Illinois Wesleyan University.

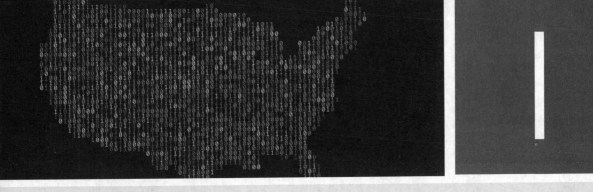

Health Policy

1

The Challenge of Health Care Delivery and Health Policy

Brian Elbel and James R. Knickman

LEARNING OBJECTIVES

▶ Understand the importance of health and health care to American life
▶ Describe defining characteristics of U.S. health care delivery
▶ Discuss major issues and concerns
▶ Identify key interest groups (stakeholders)
▶ Explain the importance of engaging a new generation of health leaders

KEY TERMS

▶ access to health care
▶ consumers
▶ customer friendly
▶ fee-for-service system
▶ health care delivery
▶ health maintenance
▶ health system
▶ Patient Protection and Affordable Care Act
▶ population health
▶ stakeholder
▶ value
▶ workforce

TOPICAL OUTLINE

▶ Why health is so important to Americans
▶ Defining characteristics of the U.S. health care delivery system
▶ Factors that shape the structure of the delivery system
▶ Seven key challenges facing the health system
▶ Stakeholders who shape and are affected by how the health system is organized and how it functions
▶ The organization of the book

INTRODUCTION

Our goal in editing this book is to provide a vibrant introduction to the U.S. health care system in a way that helps new students understand the wonders of health and health care. The book lays out the complexities of organizing a large sector of our economy to keep Americans healthy and to help people get better when they become ill. In addition, the book provides a framework to help professors engage students, with room for each professor to bring his or her perspective to the materials covered.

> Most of us are consumers of health care, and some are both consumers *and* providers, employers, or policy makers. This means *all* of us have a stake in improving the performance and delivery of U.S. health care.*

To introduce students to the many parts of the health system in the United States, we have engaged some of the leading thinkers and "doers" in the health sector to explain the parts of the system in which they are expert. Each author brings a different perspective, and it is not our aim to present one voice on this topic. Rather, we have asked each author to lay out the facts about a given topic and to offer ideas about what he or she thinks must happen to improve a specific aspect of the health system.

In many ways, the text lays out a serious "to do" list facing our health system and offers individuals beginning a health-related career a guide to the types of challenges that could engage them. The authors explain how the health system works, its challenge, and how individuals can contribute to the process of strengthening our system to ensure it works efficiently and effectively at the task of keeping all of us healthy.

In this first chapter, we explain the importance of the health system, provide an overview of how the system is organized, sketch out some of the challenges facing the overall system addressed in the book, and discuss the roles of five types of key stakeholders involved in the health enterprise. We also provide the logic behind the topics the book addresses and explain the book's organization.

---

*To hear the podcast, go to https://bcove.video/2PkbOe0 or access the ebook on Springer Publishing Connect™.

THE IMPORTANCE OF GOOD HEALTH TO AMERICAN LIFE

Our nation is built on the idea that society should ensure an opportunity for "life, liberty, and the pursuit of happiness." These words, of course, are from the second sentence of our Declaration of Independence. The aspiration of ensuring "life" is the core goal of the health system. It is obvious that nothing is possible for an individual without life, and most of us would agree that health is among the core needs to live a vibrant, viable life. Good health is essential to participate in the political and social system, to work to support ourselves and our families, and to pursue happiness and a good life.

Our nation has invested a tremendous amount to learn how to keep people healthy and how to restore health when disease, injury, or illness occurs. In the 19th century, researchers and public health experts from the United States and other countries began to understand the role of germs in communicating disease and the importance of basic public health practices, such as ensuring clean water and safe sanitation to maintain health. In the 20th century, the science and art of medicine exploded, creating amazing know-how to treat people who have diseases, injuries, and illnesses.

In response to the emerging know-how for delivering medical care, a large and complex health enterprise developed throughout the 20th century and continues to evolve. The pipeline of new ideas for better treating illnesses is quite full and promises to lead to ever-expanding methods to restore health when Americans have life-threatening medical problems. We are now faced with "personalized medicine" or the promise or hope that big data can solve many problems related to health or health systems.

We use the word *enterprise* deliberately because the health system is a blend of an altruistic-oriented set of providers and activities mixed with a huge industry that accounts for a sizable portion of all economic activity in our society. The **value** we put on health has led us to devote just under 20% of our economic resources to medical care and health promotion (see Chapter 10, Figure 10.1). Fully 11% of all jobs in America are in the health sector (Altarum, 2018). Each of us spends a sizable share of our income on the health care we need. We spend this money through taxes, which support a good share of the health enterprise; through foregone wages used by our employers to pay for health insurance; and by sizable out-of-pocket health care expenses for which each of us is responsible.

Thus, the pursuit of life, listed as a core principle in the Declaration of Independence, not only has resulted in a set of social and political norms about the importance of good health to everyone in America but also has spurred a huge industry that affects and is affected by society's economic activity and economic decisions. To understand the health system, we need to understand not only the art and practice of medicine and public health but also the economic, organizational, and management issues that must be addressed to keep the health system effective, efficient, and affordable in our overall economic life. How we go about organizing and managing the health system and changing it over time can hurt or help both our health status and our economic status.

DEFINING CHARACTERISTICS OF THE U.S. HEALTH SYSTEM

It is ironic that most health professionals think of themselves as working within the **health system** when in truth one of the first defining features of what we call a system is that health-related activities are not ordered or organized as a single enterprise. Rather, efforts to improve health and health care involve many types of actors and organizations working independently and with little coordination to make contributions to improving health status. In particular, our current approach to delivering medical care has evolved and keeps evolving in a haphazard way shaped more by economic incentives and opportunities than by a central or logical design. Equally importantly, this is not just about medical care, but social services and other systems in place that could have an even larger impact on health.

In recent years, we also have begun to recognize the clear difference between **health maintenance** and restoring health to a person who has a medical problem. The medical care system clearly takes charge of restoring health when people are ill. Often the medical care system takes charge of caring for people even if restoring health is impossible; the goal may be to limit the spread of a medical problem, to alleviate the symptoms of a medical problem, or to help a person cope with the pain and suffering and loss of function when major medical problems emerge. Doctors, nurses, technicians of various types, hospitals, nursing homes, rehabilitation centers, pharmaceutical companies, and medical device companies are among the actors who engage in efforts to care for people when they have medical problems.

The goal of maintaining health also involves many actors and activities. To some extent, medical providers help with this huge task by providing screening and prevention services that can keep people from becoming ill and help to identify illnesses very early when they might be easier to treat. However, good health among a population also requires a vibrant public health and social service system that works to help people avoid illness. Public health activities include preventing epidemics; making sure food, water, and sanitation are safe; monitoring environmental toxins; and developing community-based, public awareness, and education initiatives to help people eat healthy foods, exercise, and not engage in unhealthy behaviors such as smoking, drinking alcohol in excess, and using recreational drugs or abusing prescription drugs.

Increasingly, we also recognize that the health of populations is determined by social and economic factors. Adequate family incomes, high-quality educational opportunities, and being socially connected are all key factors that predict the health of a given person. Social issues such as discrimination, abuse, and social respect all are important determinants of health. To ensure attention to these issues and others like them requires involvement from many

> Adequate family incomes, high-quality educational opportunities, and being socially connected are all key factors that predict the health of a given person.

sectors of our society as well as political leadership to guide collective action to ensure our society encourages pro-health norms and practices. Some people term this a "health in all" approach to social policy. The relatively new concept of **population health** has also worked its way into the health system, with such systems increasingly taking into account the lives of patients outside the walls of their buildings.

We have organized this book so that it addresses both types of health issue challenges: (a) keeping the population healthy and (b) providing effective medical care when needed. Other key defining characteristics of the U.S. health care system guide the organization of this book:

- **The importance of organizations in delivering care.** These include hospitals, nursing homes, community health centers, physician practices, social services agencies, and public health departments.
- **The role of professionals in running our system.** These include physicians, nurses, managers, policy advocates, policy makers, researchers, technicians, and those directing technology and pharmaceutical businesses.
- **The emergence of new medical technology, smartphones, big data, and new pharmaceuticals.** New techniques in imaging, smartphone-based apps, big data, machine learning, pharmaceuticals, surgical procedures, DNA coding, and stem-cell technology are remarkable but often expensive ways of improving health care.
- **Tension between "the free market" and "governmental control."** This tension shapes America's culture but is sharply present, among the points of debate, in the health care sector. Relative to citizens of other countries, Americans have more diversity of opinion about whether health care, or certain health care services, are "goods" or "rights." How one feels about this issue often determines whether a person thinks the delivery of health care should be done by nonprofit or for-profit organizations and whether health care should be financed by taxes or private payments.
- **A dysfunctional payment system.** The traditional way we have paid health care providers rewards them for providing more and more billable services rather than rewarding them for being efficient and delivering effective care. This **fee-for-service system** has begun to change with more frequent use of payment approaches that reward valued services. But, we still have a long way to go to make it economically logical for providers to be efficient, to be customer or patient friendly, and to focus on the delivery of high-value services. Also, the payment approach is not transparent for individuals who use health care. For example, patients frequently have no idea what a service costs until after it is delivered. This is rarely true for other goods and services in the U.S. economy.

These defining characteristics make **health care delivery** a challenging part of U.S. politics and the economy. Addressing the challenges of delivering health care is worth the best effort and thinking of our readers, who are tomorrow's health care leaders.

> Addressing the challenges of delivering health care is worth the best effort and thinking of our readers, who are tomorrow's health care leaders.

MAJOR ISSUES AND CONCERNS

Our health system can be improved in many ways. The chapters that follow address a long list of specific concerns. Many of these issues flow, however, from seven overarching themes regarding challenges that each of us in the health sector can address:

- **Improving quality.** Reliable studies have indicated that between 44,000 and 98,000 Americans die each year because of medical errors. Other well-regarded studies show that people with mental health or substance use problems, asthma, or diabetes receive care known to be effective only about half the time. In addition, the health system could do much more to improve the experience of patients receiving care. The system is not always **customer friendly** and has not adopted many practices routinely used in other service sectors to improve the consumer experience. We have a good knowledge base about how to organize care so that high-quality services happen virtually all of the time. The challenge is spreading this knowledge into practice across the nation.

- **Improving access and coverage.** Millions of Americans still lack insurance coverage, and millions more have inadequate coverage for acute care. The federal health reform, the **Patient Protection and Affordable Care Act** (ACA; Obamacare), has dramatically reduced the number of people who lack insurance coverage, though gaps in coverage persist. Many states (though a decreasing number) have chosen not to adopt some of the expansions for low-income residents because of political opposition. Even when Americans have insurance coverage, **access to health care** is not always ensured. Many rural areas have shortages of doctors and other providers, and many doctors refuse to see patients with certain types of insurance (generally coverage for low-income residents, or Medicaid coverage) because of low payment rates.

- **Slowing the growth of health care expenditures.** Health care expenditures are simply the price of services multiplied by the volume (or number) of services. Total expenditures are growing much more rapidly than the rest of the economy because both prices and volume of services have increased relentlessly over the past 50 years. To keep health care affordable for middle-class and low-income residents—as well as for taxpayers and employers—we need to devise ways to moderate the ever-increasing share of our nation's economy devoted to the health sector. The challenge is to determine how to restructure delivery and payment so we can focus on high-value care as we get more efficient, with less waste. There has been progress in bringing costs of care down, especially due to the dynamics put in place by the great recession that started around 2008. Unfortunately, progress in reducing costs has helped businesses and government payers of care much more than it has helped individuals who have to buy health insurance in the private market place.

- **Encouraging healthy behavior.** Healthy behavior can help people avoid disease and injury or prevent disease or injury from getting worse. For millions of Americans, leading healthy lives is not of the highest priority relative to other more pressing factors in their lives. Changing health-related behavior is a difficult challenge, and one that health systems are increasingly taking on, but we need to identify effective prevention programs and ways to make our social and built environments more encouraging of healthy choices.

- **Improving the public health system.** The governmental public health infrastructure maintains population health and regulates aspects of the health care delivery system.

State and local health departments monitor the health of residents, provide a wide range of preventive services, and regulate health care providers and businesses, such as restaurants, that affect population health. The effectiveness and funding of state, municipal, and county health departments vary widely.

- **Improving the coordination, transparency, and accountability of medical care.** Problems of quality, cost, and access are caused by fragmentation and lack of coordination at the community level. This fragmentation exists both within and between health care organizations. It is affected by a lack of integrated and electronic record systems and by a lack of cooperative relationships among different types of providers who treat the same patient. For example, primary care physicians, hospitals, and specialty physicians often fail to work as teams or in coordinated ways. Consumers often are not given all of the information they deserve to make adequate medical choices. Providers often refuse to reveal the prices they will charge patients, second opinions are still not encouraged as frequently as they should be, and patients often do not get clear explanations of treatment options or the pros and cons of these options.

- **Addressing inequalities in access and outcomes.** In the United States, medical care and its associated outcomes depend on one's income level, race, and geographical location. In many cases, the care received by those with less income is subpar. Moreover, studies demonstrate that access and outcomes vary by race, even for Blacks, Latinos, and Whites who have the same incomes and education levels. Marked differences also exist in access, quality, and outcomes across different regions of our country. Best practices do not spread easily or quickly. Addressing these inequalities is a major challenge facing the health sector.

KEY STAKEHOLDERS INFLUENCING THE HEALTH SYSTEM

A complicated enterprise like the health system includes many types of stakeholders. A **stakeholder** group is a set of people who have a strong interest in how something in our society is done. In addition, stakeholders generally have some power in shaping what happens. Finally, different stakeholders may have very different goals and views about what should be done and how.

To understand the health system, one needs a good scorecard of the interests and roles of distinct stakeholder groups. Each contributor to this book gives attention to roles of stakeholders. The stakeholders that keep appearing as the story of the health system unfolds include five key groups: (a) **consumers**, (b) providers and other professionals engaged in the health system, (c) employers, (d) insurers, and (e) public policy makers.

Individuals

Individual consumers (or patients) should be at the center of the health system. After all, it is their needs and wants that are the

> A stakeholder group is a set of people who have a strong interest in how something in our society is done.

reason for this giant enterprise. In some ways, however, individuals sometimes seem like bystanders in health care decisions. Often, physicians and other providers assert that they know best and fail to have a patient co-manage a medical problem or be a full partner in selecting a choice of action. Or, perhaps worse, an insurer decides what is best or "allowed" given a specific health condition.

Individuals are also bystanders in issues about payments. Providers sometimes think their "customer" is an insurance company because the insurer pays much of the bill. In addition, the same provider (unknown to many individuals) may charge astonishingly different prices to different groups and individuals. The usual norm in our economy, unlike in health care, is that the person receiving goods or a service is the customer, and the customer has a right to know what the charge will be before purchasing the good or service.

Even so, individuals are influential stakeholders in many ways. For example, when there is widespread dissatisfaction among them, change happens. Insurers changed the rules of early managed care payment systems in the 1990s due to consumer complaints. Similarly, a major federal program offering a new form of catastrophic insurance to elders was repealed after sharp dissatisfaction among seniors.

Most experts argue that individuals need to be at the center of health care choices. Additionally, individuals need to understand the crucial role their behavioral choices play in determining their health status. Choosing to eat healthy foods, stay physically active, drink alcohol moderately, and abstain from tobacco products are among the most important choices they make to protect their health.

What do individuals want as key stakeholders? Most importantly, they want good access to health care for themselves and their families. Polls indicate that individuals value good-quality care and affordable care. They would also like to be treated well by providers and have a good experience when they need care.

Providers and Other Professionals Engaged in Making the Health System Operate

Many professionals work to advance medical knowledge, medical practice, and the business of health care. The vast majority of this **workforce** is motivated principally by the social goal of keeping people healthy. Medical providers, caregivers, pharmaceutical and medical device companies, and researchers have created an impressive set of interventions that can help people who are sick.

In recent years, however, many members of the broad health workforce have faced great financial pressure to prevent the costs of health care from increasing as quickly as in the past. Payment systems keep lowering the fees paid for goods and services, and consumers and payers have been demanding better quality, better outcomes, more value, and better patient experiences. In addition, the organization of services has begun to evolve quickly.

More and more physicians and other providers are working in large practices compared with the small ones that used to be the norm. Hospitals are merging with other types of medical providers, and the approach insurers use to pay for services is changing rapidly. A greater number of professionals, inside and outside the health system, are also increasingly engaged in working to improve health.

> Understanding the views and needs of the health workforce and the organizations dedicated to improving health is crucial to understanding how the system works and how to improve the system.

Understanding the views and needs of the health workforce and the organizations dedicated to improving health is crucial to understanding how the system works and how to improve the system. The following chapters suggest that providers and professionals engaged in the health enterprise would value simpler rules that govern how care is provided and fair opportunities to earn incomes that reflect their expertise and their large investments in training.

Employers

Employers are stakeholders because most businesses offer employees private health insurance as a key element of their compensation package. In this sense, the cost of health insurance is a cost of doing business for employers and can greatly affect the profitability of a business. For example, employee health care costs add approximately $1,500 to the cost of producing every automobile manufactured in the United States.

In their role as stakeholders, employers want to see a slowdown in their health care cost responsibility as compared with the last 50 years. In addition, employers want healthy employees who are productive and do not have to take time off from work due to illness. These desires lead some employers to advocate for high-quality health care and for wellness and prevention programs that help employees stay healthy.

Insurers

Insurance companies act as the intermediary among payers (often employers), providers (who need a system for getting paid), and consumers (who need a system to determine the kinds of health care covered by the employer's insurance plan).

In some cases, insurers take some financial risk: If the payments they make to providers exceed the premiums set for employers, the insurer loses money. Increasingly, however, the insurer leaves the employer to bear the risk and plays the role of a pure intermediary, setting rules to determine when a health service is eligible for reimbursement and other rules to determine what payment is made. Of course, an insurer must negotiate these rules with employers and providers.

As stakeholders, insurers always face pressure. Employers, consumers, and providers often have tense relationships with insurers, who in many ways play the role of referees in health care. Payers often feel that the costs of running the insurance process are too expensive.

Some approaches to payment currently exist that could compete with traditional insurance companies. Some health systems are starting their own insurance companies, and it is possible that capitated payment systems (payment of a premium for a person/family for the year regardless of use of covered benefits) could bypass traditional insurance systems and go directly from payers to providers. Insurers want to protect their role in the health sector. They also seek to expand their role by offering analytical services that can support higher-quality and more efficient delivery approaches.

Public Policy Makers

The final type of stakeholder we consider is policy makers; both appointed public officials and elected politicians are included in this category. However, policy makers do not act as a single stakeholder group. Instead, various components of this group set agendas, which often conflict with one another.

Elected officials differ strikingly in their views about how the health system should work and about the role government should play in health care. At times, differences in views reflect different ideologies. Sometimes, however, different views emerge about how best to manage the extensive responsibilities that have fallen to government over the past 80 years.

Consensus does exist on some policy issues, however, within this stakeholder group. Most elected officials and civil servants working on health issues would like to see slower inflation rates in the health sector. In addition, there is consensus that the U.S. health system should use state-of-the-art medical care and prevention interventions. Finally, there is a common sense that quality and the patient experience should be important concerns of health providers.

ORGANIZATION OF THIS BOOK

The book is organized into four parts:

Part I: Health Policy—has chapters on the current state of health care delivery, charts depicting key statistics, a discussion of the important role of policy, and a comparative analysis of health care delivery in other countries.

Part II: Keeping Americans Healthy—has four chapters on population health, public health, behavioral health, and the health of vulnerable populations.

Part III: Future of Health Care Delivery and Health Policy in the United States—has six chapters on organization of care, workforce, financing, cost and value, quality of care, health care management and governance, and information technology.

Part IV: Futures—summarizes key ideas addressed in the book, with a look to the future about how change in the health system might play out.

CONCLUSION

The editors remain optimistic that pragmatism, flexibility, consensus building, and attention to objective, high-quality evidence can bring about positive change. We remain stimulated by the challenges we face as we work hard at the local, state, and national levels to create and sustain a viable and effective health care system.

Certainly, we have observed that best practices are now used to improve health care and health across a wide range of settings in the United States and worldwide. How do we speed up the process of getting more for the money we spend, and how do we engage every type of stakeholder to bring about more effective services by insisting on best practices in everything we do? This book gives the reader the motivation and skills to get engaged.

The future U.S. health care delivery system will see improvements if committed and informed Americans choose to enter the field and engage effectively. Future leaders who are knowledgeable about the health sector and who know how to implement effective change are needed. The system also needs to improve quality, get more value for cost, improve patient participation in self-care, and encourage provider transparency and accountability.

▶ CASE EXERCISE—HEALTH CARE DELIVERY PLAN

You are an aide to the governor of State X. A billionaire has said he will give the governor $3 billion if he comes up with a satisfactory plan to improve health and medical care for the state. Assume the state currently spends $300 billion on health care annually. The goal is ensuring quality of health care, improving the patient experience, improving the overall health of the state's population, and containing the increase in health care costs. Develop the criteria for assessing the success of the plan. Where will the major shifts in resources occur? Give a rationale for your recommendations.

As you consider this case, you might address the following questions:

1. How might the billionaire evaluate whether the governor's plan is satisfactory?
2. After the money is given to fund the plan, what must happen to improve health care delivery performance substantially in State X?

DISCUSSION QUESTIONS

1. What is the real and perceived performance of the U.S. health care system? How do views differ among different groups of patients, providers, payers, and politicians?
2. Why do we spend so much money on health care?
3. Why isn't the population healthier?
4. How is the ACA part of the problem or part of the solution to improving health care delivery in the United States?
5. What are your priorities to improve the value of health care Americans get for the money we spend? What is your rationale for these priorities?

REFERENCE

Altarum. (2018). Health care jobs engine propels share of total jobs to all-time high. Retrieved from https://altarum.org/news/health-care-jobs-engine-propels-share-total-jobs-all-time-high

2

Organization of Care

Amy Yarbrough Landry and Cathleen O. Erwin

LEARNING OBJECTIVES

▶ Describe the current care delivery system
▶ Define and distinguish between types of health care services along the continuum of care
▶ Identify and discuss types of organizations in the U.S. health care delivery system
▶ Increase awareness of new mechanisms for health system performance improvements
▶ Understand and discuss future trends in the health delivery system
▶ Describe innovative approaches to improving care delivery

KEY TERMS

▶ academic health center
▶ accountable care organizations (ACOs)
▶ accreditation
▶ ambulatory care
▶ average length of stay (ALOS)
▶ centers of care
▶ certification
▶ chronic care
▶ community health improvement
▶ continuing care retirement community
▶ continuity of care
▶ continuum of care

- ▶ corporate practice of medicine (CPOM)
- ▶ emergency care
- ▶ end-of-life care
- ▶ health homes
- ▶ horizontal integration
- ▶ hospice care
- ▶ inpatient
- ▶ instrumental activities of daily living (IADLs)
- ▶ long-term care
- ▶ multispecialty group practice (MSGP)
- ▶ outpatient
- ▶ palliative care
- ▶ patient-centered medical home (PCMH)
- ▶ population health
- ▶ prehospital care
- ▶ primary care
- ▶ private practice
- ▶ privileges
- ▶ public health agencies
- ▶ quaternary care
- ▶ rehabilitation clinics
- ▶ same-day surgery
- ▶ single specialty group practice
- ▶ solo practice
- ▶ specialty care
- ▶ special hospitals
- ▶ subacute care
- ▶ tertiary care
- ▶ urgent care centers
- ▶ vertical integration

TOPICAL OUTLINE

- ▶ The current organization of the health care delivery system
- ▶ Types of health care delivery organizations
- ▶ Health system performance
- ▶ The future of the health care delivery system
- ▶ Examples of best practices in the organization of medical care

INTRODUCTION

In the United States, health care is delivered through a complex and multifaceted system of private and public institutions that operate in cooperation with, but largely independent of, each other. Unlike many other countries, the United States has no central governmental agency to control the delivery of health care, although delivery is heavily influenced through health care legislation and the government's role as a major purchaser of health care services through Medicare, Medicaid, and other public

> The organization of the nation's complex and multifaceted health care system can evolve as patients' needs and government regulations and policies change.*

programs. The **continuum of care** in the United States encompasses care from the cradle to the grave and includes services focused on both the prevention and the treatment of medical conditions and diseases as well as end-of-life care.

The individuals and organizations that provide care in the United States are faced with increasing pressure and scrutiny from the government, private insurance organizations, and the public to provide the highest quality of care while controlling costs and increasing access to underserved populations. Consequently, health care services and organizational structures are continuously being adapted to meet the demands and mandates of health care policy and to survive and thrive in this dynamic health care environment.

This chapter describes the current health care delivery system in the United States, including services, organizations, health system performance, and new innovations in care delivery.

DESCRIPTION OF THE CURRENT CARE DELIVERY SYSTEM

The World Health Organization (WHO) defines *health* as a "state of complete physical, mental and social 'wellbeing' and not merely the absence of disease or infirmity" (WHO, 2017). By definition, the health system includes all organizations, institutions, and resources that have a primary purpose of promoting, restoring, and/or maintaining health (WHO, 2015). From a broad, comprehensive perspective it includes care delivered through traditional clinical and public health settings as well as contributions to health from a variety of community organizations that have a stake in or can affect the health of individuals and communities.

The following sections provide a general discussion of the types of clinical health care services available in the United States, the types of organizations through which these services are delivered, and how these and other organizations are involved in the fields of community health, community benefit, and population health.

Health Care Services

Health care services are provided for the purpose of contributing to improved health or to the diagnosis, treatment, or rehabilitation of sick people. Health care

---

*To hear the podcast, go to https://bcove.video/2E1WuAY or access the ebook on Springer Publishing Connect™.

Health care services are provided for the purpose of contributing to improved health or to the diagnosis, treatment, or rehabilitation of sick people.

services include prevention, cure, rehabilitation, and palliation efforts oriented to either individuals or populations.

Prevention

Prevention of disease and maintenance of general good health are the focus of health promotion and preventive services. Health status is affected by a number of factors, including health policy, individual behavior, social determinants, physical determinants, biology and genetics, and availability of health services. Services associated with prevention may be focused on the health of an individual or the health of a population. Although prevention services have always been available in the United States, an even greater emphasis is placed on prevention because of its prominence in the Patient Protection and Affordable Care Act of 2010 (ACA) as an essential component of health insurance benefits. Most health plans must cover a set of preventive services at no cost to the beneficiary. Additionally, a variety of new reimbursement mechanisms used by both private and governmental payers incentivize provider organizations to keep patient populations healthy and out of the hospital.

The prevention field often distinguishes interventions delivered by a health care provider (clinical prevention services) from those delivered by non–health care providers (community-based prevention initiatives). According to the Institute of Medicine (IOM, 2012), a holistic view of community-based prevention incorporates cultural, social, and environmental changes; also, community-based prevention is often more difficult to fund and staff than clinical interventions. Certain preventive services may be offered through a clinical–community relationship that might entail a primary care provider making a connection with a community-based organization to provide specific services (such as a community-based weight-loss program) or collaboration between clinical and community-based organizations to network, coordinate, or cooperate on preventive services delivery. Additionally, the field sometimes distinguishes between prevention initiatives that focus on individuals one at a time and initiatives that are more population-based, working with larger groups of people (e.g., efforts to increase the availability of healthy food in low-income neighborhoods).

PUBLIC HEALTH, COMMUNITY HEALTH, AND POPULATION HEALTH It's important to distinguish between the fields of public health, community health, and **population health**, which are sometimes used interchangeably yet differ somewhat in definition and scope. Traditionally, public health has been viewed as a function of federal, state, and local public health departments to address health concerns affecting the public at large, such as preventing epidemics, containing environmental hazards, and promoting healthy living (IOM, 2003).

A more expansive view of public health is the concept of **community health improvement** or community benefit, which focuses on collaboration among a wide array of organizations (e.g., public health departments, health care delivery organizations, social service agencies, government entities) to address issues impacting the health of a particular community. The interest in how health care and public health activities could be coordinated to improve the health of communities was accelerated in the mid-1990s, fueled by organizations such as the Robert Wood Johnson Foundation, Institute of Medicine, and U.S. Department of Health and Human Services and organized hospital groups such as the Catholic Hospitals of America and Voluntary Hospitals of America (VHA), among others. The Association for Community Health Improvement is an affiliate organization of the American Hospital Association (AHA) and serves as a national association for community health, community benefit, and population health professionals. This is one avenue through which hospitals and health systems receive educational resources, tools, networking opportunities, and professional development to assist in achieving organizational community health goals.

Although many health care organizations actively engaged in community health needs assessment and activities prior to the passage of the ACA, the ACA mandates that all nonprofit hospitals complete a community health needs assessment (CHNA) process every 3 years. CHNAs are a tool that have long been used by hospitals, public health departments, and other social service agencies (e.g., United Way) to identify and prioritize significant health needs in the community. Community health also encompasses a broad perspective on the various components or factors that affect the health of a community, such as employment, crime, education, housing, transportation, food, and medical care.

More recently, the concept of *population health* has become an important topic and focus for health care delivery organizations and payers. It has been defined as "the health outcomes of a group of individuals, including the distribution of such outcomes within the group" (Kindig & Stoddart, 2003). In general, population health focuses on health status indicators for a defined group of people, and the goal of population health management is to improve the health of the population and reduce inequities or disparities between population groups. Ways that organizations approach population health management will be described later in this chapter.

Clinical prevention services are often categorized as primary, secondary, or tertiary, based on the stages of the disease they target.

PRIMARY PREVENTION SERVICES Primary prevention services are focused on preventing or reducing the probability of the occurrence of a disease in the future. Services are provided through public and private institutions and are often focused on educating the public about the risks associated with individual behaviors that can negatively affect their short- and long-term health.

Examples of primary prevention include immunizations for prevention of childhood diseases, smoking cessation programs to reduce the risk of lung cancer and heart disease, weight loss programs, prenatal and well-baby care, programs to increase workplace safety, and the promotion of hand washing to reduce the spread of influenza or other diseases. The services are provided through a wide variety of institutions, such as public health departments, physician offices, hospitals, social service agencies, places of employment, houses of worship, and broadcast media, among others.

SECONDARY PREVENTION SERVICES These services are focused on the early detection and treatment of disease in order to cure or control its effects. The goal is to minimize the effects of the disease on the individual. Secondary services are largely focused on routine examinations and tests such as blood pressure screenings, Pap smears, routine colonoscopies, examination of suspicious moles, and mammograms. Early detection and treatment often increases the probability of a successful outcome.

TERTIARY PREVENTION SERVICES These services are targeted at individuals who already have symptoms of a disease in order to prevent damage from the disease, to slow down its progression, to prevent complications from occurring as a result of the disease, and ultimately to restore good health to the person with the disease.

Tertiary prevention includes services such as providing diabetic patients with education and counseling on wound care. It also includes institutional practices such as infection control in a hospital facility to prevent illness or injury caused in the process of providing health care.

Acute Care

Acute care is short-term, intense medical care providing diagnosis and treatment of communicable or noncommunicable diseases, illness, or injury. The definition of acute care varies across the scholarly literature and textbooks. Acute care is sometimes defined as *primary, specialty, tertiary*, or *quaternary* in nature, centered around the care delivered by physicians and other providers in clinical settings (such as physician offices and hospitals). Acute care services may be provided on an **outpatient** basis (i.e., not requiring an overnight hospital or health care facility stay) or on an **inpatient** basis (i.e., requiring an overnight stay).

A more comprehensive definition of acute care includes not only these services but also the emergency services provided in the community given the time-sensitive nature of the need for diagnosis and treatment. One proposed definition of acute care includes the components of the health system where acute care is delivered to treat unexpected, urgent, and emergent episodes of illness and injury that could lead to disability or death without rapid intervention (Hirshon et al., 2013). Based on this definition, acute care encompasses a range of functions including emergency care, trauma care, prehospital emergency care, acute care surgery, critical care, urgent care, and short-term inpatient stabilization (Figure 2.1). The following sections outline the types of acute care based on the framework illustrated in Figure 2.1, although not all of the domains are discussed because of obvious overlaps. The primary, specialty, tertiary, and quaternary care definitions are incorporated into the framework to show where these levels of care best fit within the acute care model and to note relationships to other forms of care.

EMERGENCY AND URGENT CARE Emergency care is designed to provide immediate care for sudden, serious illness or injury, although it is sometimes utilized for nonemergent care by individuals who are uninsured or underinsured. A medical emergency is defined by what is known as the prudent layperson standard:

[A] condition with acute symptoms of sufficient severity (including severe pain) such that a prudent layperson, who possesses average knowledge of health and medicine, could reasonably expect the absence of immediate medical attention to result in (i) placing the health of the individual (or unborn child) in serious jeopardy, (ii) serious impairment of bodily functions, or (iii) serious dysfunction of any bodily organ or part. (Social Security Act § 1867)

Emergent types of care (such as trauma) can be classified by the triage level, that is, by the emergency severity index (ESI). The ESI is a five-level triage algorithm that clinically stratifies patients into groups based on immediacy of the need to be seen, which includes the following levels:

1. Immediate (less than 1 minute)
2. Emergent (1–14 minutes)
3. Urgent (15–60 minutes)
4. Semiurgent (61–120 minutes)
5. Nonurgent (121 minutes–24 hours)

In 2015, .7% of ED visits were classified as immediate, 7.4% as emergent, and 29.8 as urgent; the remaining 61.2% were either semiurgent, nonurgent, not triaged, or unknown (Centers for Disease Control and Prevention [CDC], 2017).

The Emergency Medical Treatment & Labor Act of 1986 (EMTALA) requires that all patients who present themselves for treatment at an ED must be screened and evaluated, provided the necessary stabilizing treatment, and admitted to the hospital when necessary—regardless of ability to pay.

Urgent care is used for an illness, injury, or condition that is serious enough for a reasonable person to seek care right away but not so severe as to require ED care. It is considered **ambulatory care**, which means that the person in need of care can walk (or ambulate) into the facility. However, a patient in need of "ambulatory" care may need some assistance entering the facility, depending on the nature of the illness or injury (e.g., severe ankle sprain). Services are provided by physicians and advanced practice providers (such as nurse practitioners or physician assistants) typically on a walk-in basis without a previously scheduled appointment because of the immediacy of the need. Urgent care services may be provided through a traditional physician practice or an urgent care center.

PREHOSPITAL CARE **Prehospital care** includes medical services provided in the community, such as stabilization by emergency services before or during transportation to a health care facility. It also includes evaluation and treatment provided through local, community-based providers, as in a private physician practice setting.

Primary care. **Primary care** is the first and most general source for routine treatment of illness and disease. Primary care providers may be physicians, physician assistants, or nurse practitioners who have trained in family medicine, internal medicine, pediatric medicine, gerontology, or other primary care "specialties," such as obstetrics and gynecology. In the managed care environment,

FIGURE 2.1   DOMAINS IN ACUTE CARE

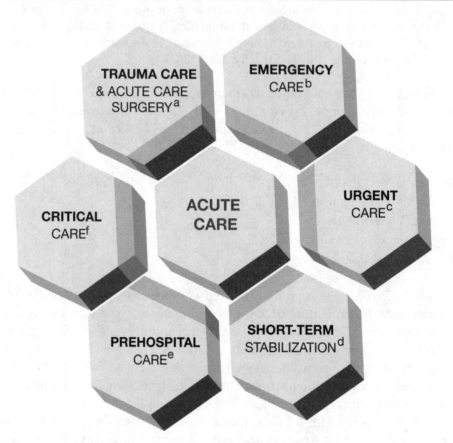

[a]Treatment of individuals with acute surgical needs, such as life-threatening injuries, acute appendicitis, or strangulated hernias.

[b]Treatment of individuals with acute life- or limb-threatening medical and potentially surgical needs, such as acute myocardial infarctions or acute cerebrovascular accidents, or evaluation of patients with abdominal pain.

[c]Ambulatory care in a facility delivering medical care outside a hospital emergency department, usually on an unscheduled, walk-in basis (e.g., evaluation of an injured ankle or fever in a child).

[d]Treatment of individuals with acute needs before delivery of definitive treatment (e.g., administering intravenous fluids to a critically injured patient before transfer to an operating room).

[e]Care provided in the community until the patient arrives at a formal health care facility capable of giving definitive care (e.g., delivery of care by ambulance personnel or evaluation of acute health problems by local health care providers).

[f]Specialized care of patients whose conditions are life-threatening and who require comprehensive care and constant monitoring, usually in intensive care units (e.g., patients with severe respiratory problems requiring endotracheal intubation and patients with seizures caused by cerebral malaria).

Source: Hirshon, J. M., Risko, N., Calvello, E. J. B., de Ramirez, S. S., Narayan, M., Theodosis, C., & O'Neill, J. (2013). Health systems and services: The role of acute care. *Bulletin of the World Health Organization, 91,* 386–388. doi:10.2471/BLT.12.112664. Used with permission.

primary care delivery plays an important role in the coordination of care to help control costs and ensure that the appropriate level of care is sought for the health concern. Primary care providers are involved in delivering both acute care and preventive care.

Specialty care. **Specialty care** refers to care delivered through providers who are trained as specialists or subspecialists in the field of medicine. This type of care sometimes requires a referral from a primary care physician. Specialists focus on a particular body system or on a specific disease or condition; they have the knowledge and expertise to handle medical conditions beyond the realm of primary care. For example, cardiologists diagnose and treat conditions involving the heart, endocrinologists focus on hormone systems and may specialize in a disease such as diabetes, and neurologists are trained to diagnose and treat disorders associated with the nervous system—brain, spinal cord, and so on. Similarly to primary care, specialty care may be utilized to address both acute and preventive care needs.

Chronic care. **Chronic care** is the continual treatment and monitoring of conditions that can be controlled but not cured; it includes both physical and behavioral conditions. Examples of chronic conditions include diabetes, hypertension, and depression. As the life expectancy of the population has increased, so have the incidence and prevalence of chronic conditions. It is estimated that more than one-fourth of all Americans and two out of three older Americans have at least two chronic conditions, and approximately 66% of the nation's health costs are attributable to the treatment of people living with multiple chronic conditions (Agency for Healthcare Research and Quality, 2013).

The management and treatment of chronic conditions may be delivered by primary and/or specialty care providers. By definition, chronic care is not considered acute care; however, chronic conditions can cause or exacerbate acute episodes of illness. Chronic care also fits within the category of preventive services, which include services that focus on the early detection and management of chronic conditions.

TERTIARY CARE **Tertiary care** typically involves hospitalization for specialty care that requires highly specialized equipment and expertise and involves more complex therapeutic interventions, such as coronary bypass surgery, neurosurgery, advanced neonatal intensive care, or treatments for severe burns or injuries. Some tertiary care services may be provided on an outpatient basis, such as same-day surgeries. Patients are admitted to a tertiary facility through a *practitioner order* from a qualified provider who has been granted admitting privileges by the facility.

QUATERNARY CARE **Quaternary care**, an extension of tertiary care, entails providing the most complex medical and surgical care for highly specialized and unusual cases. It may involve experimental procedures, experimental medications, or very uncommon surgeries or procedures. Examples of quaternary care are advanced trauma care and organ transplantation. Quaternary care is not offered by every hospital or medical center; it is more likely to be found in academic medical centers.

SUBACUTE INPATIENT CARE **Subacute care** is a level of inpatient care needed by a patient immediately after or instead of hospitalization for an acute illness, injury, or exacerbation of a disease process. This level of care centers on providing one or more active medical conditions or administering one or more technically complex treatments. It requires more intensive skilled nursing care than is provided to the majority of patients in a skilled nursing facility (i.e., nursing home).

The term "subacute care" has been applied to a broad range of medical and rehabilitative services and settings that provide care to patients after an acute care episode. It combines rehabilitation and convalescent services for patients who typically need 10 to 100 days of treatment and is provided in settings other than in acute care hospital beds. Subacute care is delivered in facilities licensed to provide the appropriate level of care, which includes special units established by acute care hospitals and skilled nursing facilities.

Rehabilitative Care

Rehabilitative health care services are aimed at restoring a person to his or her original state of health (or as close as possible). Rehabilitation services help a person keep, regain, or improve skills and functioning for daily living that have been lost or impaired because of illness or injury. Services include physical therapy, occupational therapy, speech–language pathology, and psychiatric rehabilitation. Rehabilitative services are offered in a variety of inpatient and outpatient settings.

Long-Term Care

Long-term care encompasses a range of services and support provided to meet personal care needs on a long-term basis, most of which is not medical care. It encompasses an array of services provided in a variety of settings for people who have lost some independence because of a medical condition, injury, or chronic illness. Long-term care is often used to provide assistance with *activities of daily living (ADLs)*, such as bathing, dressing, using the toilet, transferring to or from a bed or chair, and eating, among others. Other common services and support assist with **instrumental activities of daily living (IADLs)**, which are everyday tasks, such as housework, taking medication, preparing meals, shopping, and responding to emergency alerts, among others.

The duration and level of long-term care needed by individuals vary and often change over time. Long-term care services may be provided in an individual's home or in a community setting or institution.

End-of-Life Care

End-of-life care is provided in the final hours or days of an individual's life. This type of care includes physical, mental, and emotional comfort as well as social support for people who are living with and dying of terminal illness or a condition that is advanced, progressive, and incurable. End-of-life care requires a range of decisions. These decisions may include preparing advance directives to make end-of-life wishes clear to family and providers as well as determining the types of treatment and care that will be utilized.

Palliative care is the treatment for discomfort, symptoms, and stress of serious illness, providing relief from pain, fatigue, nausea, shortness of breath, loss of appetite, or problems with sleep. Palliative care can be received at any stage of an illness but is always included in hospice care.

When the focus shifts from cure to care, a patient moves to hospice care. **Hospice care** is end-of-life care utilized when a patient is expected to live 6 months or less. It is provided by a team of health care professionals and volunteers in the home, a hospice center, a hospital, or a skilled nursing facility. Hospice programs also provide services to support a patient's family. The interdisciplinary hospice team usually consists of the patient's personal physician; hospice physician or medical director; nurses; hospice aides; social workers; bereavement counselors; clergy or other spiritual counselors; trained volunteers; and speech, physical, and occupational therapists, if needed.

Health Care Delivery Organizations

This section discusses the wide range of organizations that exist to deliver health care services, including hospitals, health systems, physician offices, specialty hospitals, long-term care facilities, rehabilitation hospitals, home health agencies, and other health-related organizations.

Hospitals

By definition, a hospital (other than psychiatric) is an institution primarily engaged in providing, by or under the supervision of physicians, to *inpatients*, diagnostic and therapeutic services for medical diagnosis, treatment, and care of injured, disabled, or sick persons; or rehabilitation services for injured, disabled, or sick persons. *Outpatient* services are optional but have been growing in importance over time as more and more medical interventions can be done in an outpatient setting and as the field sees growing importance to integrating primary care, specialty care, and inpatient care for reasons of both quality and efficiency.

According to the AHA (2018), the United States has approximately 5,534 registered hospitals, which include all community, federal, psychiatric, and long-term care hospitals and hospital units located in institutions (such as prison hospitals, college infirmaries, and so on). Hospitals can be categorized in a number of ways, such as by purpose, size, ownership, location (urban or rural), teaching status, or system affiliation. Most hospitals in the United States provide general medical and surgical services on a short-term basis. The four primary categories for hospitals according to the AHA are (a) *community*, (b) *special*, (c) *rehabilitative* and *chronic disease*, and (d) *psychiatric*.

Hospitals are subject to federal and state regulations. A hospital must be *licensed* to operate; licensing is handled at the state level by the agency or entity designated with such authority for the state. Licensure focuses on physical plant requirements, sanitation, personnel, and equipment. To receive reimbursement for services provided to Medicare and Medicaid patients, hospitals must receive **certification** from the federal government. Hospitals may choose to pursue **accreditation** by The Joint Commission, an independent, nonprofit organization that accredits hospitals and other types of health care institutions. This voluntary participation in accreditation is a symbol of quality that indicates the organization has met certain performance standards. The Centers for Medicare & Medicaid Services (CMS) recognize accreditation as suitable proof that a hospital has met the minimum requirements to receive certification.

Patients are referred to the hospital for services on the authority of a member of the medical staff (i.e., a physician) who has been granted admitting **privileges** in accordance with state law and criteria for standards of medical care established by the facility. Hospitals provide both *inpatient* (requiring an overnight stay) and *outpatient* services (not requiring an overnight stay). Outpatient services are sometimes referred to as *ambulatory care,* which means the patient is able to walk (ambulate) into the facility to receive diagnostic or therapeutic treatment. However, in actuality not all patients who receive outpatient services can ambulate (e.g., patients brought to the ED by ambulance).

COMMUNITY HOSPITALS By AHA definition, community hospitals are all nonfederal, short-term *general,* and other *special* hospitals accessible by the general public. General hospitals provide patient services, diagnostic and therapeutic, for a variety of medical conditions; the **average length of stay (ALOS)** is less than 25 days. Hospitals also provide diagnostic x-ray services, clinical laboratory services, and operating room services with facilities and staff for a variety of procedures. Services are provided on both an *inpatient* and an *outpatient* basis. Traditionally, hospitals primarily have delivered care on an inpatient basis, but over the past three decades more services have been moved to an outpatient, or *ambulatory,* basis to contain costs. In addition to cost containment, medical practices have advanced enabling many procedures that previously required an overnight stay to become less invasive and therefore require a shorter recovery period that can be achieved at a patient's home without nursing care.

Special hospitals provide diagnostic and treatment services for patients who have specified medical conditions, both surgical and nonsurgical. These hospitals must provide the services deemed appropriate for the specified medical conditions for which services are provided.

Community hospitals are grouped by ownership in three categories:

- Voluntary, not-for-profit (nonprofit)
- Investor-owned (for-profit, proprietary)
- Public (state or local government owned and managed)

Some community hospitals operate as free-standing single hospital entities, whereas others are part of a health system. A system is defined as either a multihospital or diversified single hospital system. Community hospitals may also be classified as participating in a network, which is defined as a group of hospitals, physicians, other providers, insurers, and/or community agencies that work together to coordinate and deliver a broad spectrum of services to the community (AHA, 2018).

Hospitals may also be classified by teaching status—teaching hospitals are affiliated with medical schools and provide clinical education, residencies, and internships for medical and dental students. These teaching hospitals (along with other hospitals not affiliated with a medical school) also provide clinical education and training for nursing and allied health professions students. Teaching hospitals are typically voluntary, not-for-profit or public, government-sponsored hospitals. Some teaching hospitals operate as part of an **academic health center**, which comprises an allopathic or osteopathic medical school, one or more health professions schools (e.g., allied health, dentistry, nursing, pharmacy, public health, veterinary medicine), and one or more owned or affiliated teaching hospitals or health systems. Academic health centers are heavily involved in clinical research and high-level tertiary and quaternary care, in addition to providing advanced training and education for clinicians in primary and specialty care.

REHABILITATION HOSPITALS Rehabilitation hospitals specialize in providing therapeutic interventions to help patients regain functional ability to the highest possible level after an injury or illness that has caused some loss of ability. By Medicare definition, 75% of a rehabilitation hospital's patients must require intensive (at least 3 hours per day) rehabilitative services to treat conditions related to stroke, spinal cord injury, major trauma, brain injury, or other debilitating disease or injury. Rehabilitative services provided within these facilities include physical therapy, occupational therapy, and speech-language therapy. Other services may also be provided to assist patients with psychological, vocational, or social needs related to their condition.

PSYCHIATRIC HOSPITALS The primary function of a psychiatric hospital is to provide diagnostic and treatment services for patients who have a psychiatric-related illness. Some facilities specialize in short-term or outpatient therapy, whereas others may specialize in temporary or permanent care of residents who require routine assistance, treatment, or a specialized and controlled environment as a result of a psychological disorder. General hospitals may also operate psychiatric units within their organizations.

Psychiatric hospitals are required to provide clinical laboratory and diagnostic x-ray services in addition to psychiatric, psychological, and social work services. Psychiatric hospitals have written agreements with general hospitals for the transfer of patients in need of medical or surgical services not available at the psychiatric institution (AHA, 2018).

OTHER HOSPITALS The federal government operates approximately 209 hospitals that are not accessible to the general public. Included among these hospitals are those operated by the Veterans Administration (VA) for the nation's military veterans, the Department of Defense (DOD) for active duty military personnel, and the Indian Health Service (IHS) for American Indians and Alaska Natives.

Physician Organizations

In the United States, physicians have traditionally been self-employed, working in private medical practices that they own either solely or in partnership with other physicians. Hospitals establish relationships with physicians by granting them admitting privileges to provide inpatient and outpatient procedures and services to their patients that cannot be delivered within the physician practice setting. In recent years, however, there has been a trend toward the employment of physicians by hospitals and other health care organizations and toward larger practice sizes. This trend has been attributed to a number of reasons, including stagnant reimbursement rates, a desire for better work-life balance for physicians, and efforts by hospitals to increase market share. The results of a physician practice benchmark survey in 2016 conducted by the AMA indicate that only 47.1% of physicians have an ownership stake in their practices, and an equal amount (47.1%) are employees of either a medical practice or hospital organization. This marks the first year that the majority of physicians are not practice owners, with a 6% decrease observed from a prior study conducted in 2012. Additional trends indicate that having an ownership stake is less common among women physicians than men and less common among younger physicians than older physicians (Kane, 2017).

As mentioned, physicians may be employed by others (e.g., hospitals, government, medical schools) or be self-employed (i.e., in **private practice**). A variety of physician practice settings are utilized in the United States, which include **solo practice**, **single specialty group practice**, **multispecialty group practice** **(MSGP)**, corporate medical practice, and **urgent care centers**, among others.

SOLO PRACTICES A physician practice operated by one physician is known as a solo practice. Approximately 20% of physician practicing in the United States are in solo practices, compared with 40.5% in 1983 (AMA, 2013). According to the AMA (2013), a majority of physicians in solo practices own their practice.

SINGLE SPECIALTY GROUP PRACTICES The most common type of physician practice is the single specialty group practice: a practice with two or more physicians who have the same medical specialty, such as internal medicine or cardiology. Forty-two percent of the physicians in the United States are in a single specialty group practice (Kane, 2017).

MULTISPECIALTY GROUP PRACTICES A multispecialty group practice consists of two or more physicians who practice different medical specialties. Approximately 25% of physicians in the United States are in a multispecialty group practice (Kane, 2017).

CORPORATE MEDICAL PRACTICES Corporate medical practices are physician practices owned by business corporations or entities. This is commonly known as the **corporate practice of medicine (CPOM)**. CPOM is prohibited in some states: The types of prohibitions vary by state and may be found in various laws, regulations, or court rulings. A typical exception allows hospitals and health maintenance organizations (HMOs) to employ physicians because these businesses were established for the purpose of providing treatment to patients and are licensed entities. Most states allow physicians to provide services through a professional service corporation (P.C.), a business entity formed for the purpose of providing professional services, such as medical services. Some states have CPOM laws but do not enforce them. Such laws were established in an earlier era when concern about the commercialization of medicine led to great efforts to ensure that medicine would be practiced only by licensed professionals.

URGENT CARE CENTERS Urgent care centers offer walk-in, extended-hour access to individuals with acute illness and injuries that are not bona fide emergencies. In addition to services found in the typical physician's office, urgent care centers usually can treat minor fractures and provide intravenous fluids as well as perform on-site x-ray and laboratory test processing. These centers are typically staffed by physicians and other providers and operate 7 days a week, including holidays, from 8 or 9 a.m. until 7 or 9 p.m. This is a growth area in the health care delivery system, with more than 9,000 centers operating nationwide and approximately 300 new centers opening each year.

COMMUNITY HEALTH CENTERS Community health centers (CHCs) provide health care services, focusing on primary and preventive care, to medically underserved and indigent populations. Approximately 27 million people are served by CHCs in 10,400 communities in the United States (National Association of Community Health Centers, n.d.). To receive care at a CHC, an individual must be a resident of the state in which the center is located, be uninsured, and be poor as defined by federal poverty guidelines. CHCs contract with the state or local health department to provide services to eligible individuals; they also help to provide linkages to social services and government-sponsored health insurance programs, such as Medicaid and the Children's Health Insurance Program (CHIP). CHCs may be organized as part of a public health department or another health service organization, or as a nonprofit organization.

Ambulatory Surgery Centers

Ambulatory surgery centers (ASCs) are facilities that provide surgical services for procedures that are done on an outpatient basis. This is sometimes referred to as same-day surgery. ASCs are not physician offices, although physicians have taken the lead in their development.

The first ASC was established in 1970 by two physicians. Today, more than 5,400 ASCs are in operation across the United States. Physicians have some ownership in approximately 90% of the licensed ASCs in the United States. Community hospitals have also partnered with physicians to open and operate ASCs, and a small percentage of ASCs are entirely hospital owned.

Patients treated at an ASC have already been diagnosed by a physician and have elected to have an outpatient surgical procedure. All ASCs must have at least one dedicated operating room and the appropriate equipment to perform surgery safely and provide quality patient care. The most prevalent specialties served by ASCs are ophthalmology, orthopedics, gastrointestinal, pain management, plastic surgery, and urology (Ambulatory Surgical Center Association, 2018).

Long-Term Care Organizations

Long-term care organizations operate facilities for individuals who are not able to manage independently in the community. The services provided in these facilities vary depending on the level of assistance needed; services may range from custodial care and chronic care management to short-term rehabilitative services. Long-term care facilities (LTCFs) may be owned by government entities, nonprofit organizations (including churches), or investor-owned corporations. LTCFs may be independent facilities that are either freestanding or operated within a **continuing care retirement community**. LTCFs may be part of a multifacility organization (that is, a chain) or may be hospital-owned as either an attached or a freestanding facility.

INDEPENDENT LIVING FACILITIES Independent living facilities are multiunit housing developments that may provide support services such as meals, transportation, housekeeping, and social activities. These facilities are typically utilized by active senior adults who do not require assistance with ADLs.

Independent living facilities are sometimes operated as part of a *continuing care retirement community*, which provides a full range of LTCFs and other services—an assisted living facility and a skilled nursing facility. This arrangement enables seniors to make a transition into a residence that meets their physical needs as they begin to require more medical assistance. Independent living facilities that do not provide many services beyond a residence are sometimes referred to as senior apartments.

ASSISTED LIVING FACILITIES Assisted living facilities are available for individuals who are basically able to care for themselves but may need some assistance with some daily activities. Assisted living facilities are residential facilities that provide services that may include meals, laundry, housekeeping, medication reminders, and assistance with ADLs and IADLs.

Most states require licensure for assisted living facilities, and the exact definition of what constitutes an assisted living facility varies among states. Approximately 90% of assisted living services in the United States are paid through private funds, although a few states allow payment for assisted living through Medicaid waivers.

SKILLED NURSING FACILITIES A skilled nursing facility (or nursing home) is licensed by the state in which it operates to provide 24-hour nursing care, room and board, and activities for convalescent residents and residents with chronic or long-term illnesses or conditions. Special populations served by skilled nursing facilities include physically or mentally challenged children and adults, and children and adults with debilitating diseases and/or conditions. Regular medical supervision and rehabilitation services must be available. The facilities are staffed by health care professionals including a physician as medical director, registered nurses (RNs), licensed practical nurses (LPNs), and trained nursing assistants. Skilled nursing facilities are reimbursed through a variety of mechanisms, including private funds, long-term care insurance, Medicare (for short-term rehabilitation or subacute care), and Medicaid. Medicaid is the source of payment for 6 out of 10 residents in skilled nursing facilities.

Rehabilitation Organizations

Rehabilitative services are provided in a variety of inpatient and outpatient settings, including inpatient rehabilitation hospitals, rehabilitation units in acute care hospitals, skilled nursing facilities, outpatient rehabilitation centers and units, and other medical rehabilitation providers.

INPATIENT REHABILITATION FACILITIES An inpatient rehabilitation facility is either a freestanding inpatient rehabilitation hospital or a unit of an acute care hospital. Intensive acute rehabilitation services are provided and generally include at least 3 hours of therapy per day for 5 to 7 days each week. Therapy may include physical, occupational, speech, or recreation therapy.

Patients who cannot tolerate intensive therapy in an acute rehabilitation setting may be transferred to a transitional care, *long-term care,* or *subacute* care facility, where less intensive rehabilitation services are provided along with other medical services (e.g., 24-hour skilled nursing care) needed for convalescence and recovery.

OUTPATIENT REHABILITATION PROVIDERS Rehabilitation services may be provided on an outpatient basis—that is, the patient lives at home and visits the facility for therapy. Therapy plans are developed on an individual basis and typically include 2 to 3 days of treatment per week. Nursing services are usually not included in the outpatient setting. **Centers of care** are facilities that provide outpatient rehabilitative services for patients with a particular specific illness, such as multiple sclerosis, Parkinson's disease, or stroke.

Three types of providers may qualify for reimbursement for outpatient rehabilitation services by Medicare:

- Rehabilitation agencies are organizations that provide integrated, multidisciplinary programs designed to upgrade the physical functions of handicapped and disabled individuals through a specialized team of rehabilitation personnel.
- **Rehabilitation clinics** are facilities established primarily to provide outpatient rehabilitative services by physicians. To meet the definition of a clinic, medical services must be provided a group of three of more physicians practicing rehabilitation medicine together, and a physician must be present in the facility at all times during the hours of operation to perform medical services.
- **Public health agencies** are official agencies established by state or local government that provide environmental health services, preventive medical services, and, sometimes, therapeutic services.

Integrated Delivery Systems

An integrated delivery system (IDS) is a collaborative network of providers who work together in a coordinated fashion to provide a continuum of care to a particular patient population or community. Within an IDS, providers work together through information sharing, shared responsibility, and collaborative resource utilization (Enthoven, 2016). Many believe integrated delivery systems can help to address some of the problems associated with the fragmented delivery system in the United States and move toward the goals of improving the quality and accessibility of care while containing or reducing costs.

Integrated delivery systems have existed since the early 1900s, but interest in the IDS concept began to spread in the 1990s when hospitals and physician practices consolidated through mergers and acquisitions in the face of changing reimbursement methodologies from public and private insurers. Interest in IDSs has surged in recent years during the national health reform debate as experts have suggested that the IDS approach to health care delivery can improve quality and reduce costs. Research has shown that IDSs have a positive effect on quality, but there is little evidence of an effect on costs or health care utilization (Hwang, Chang, LaClair, & Paz, 2013).

Two types of integration—horizontal and vertical—are used to create an IDS. **Horizontal integration** involves linking organizations that provide the same level of care, such as a multispecialty group practice. **Vertical integration** involves linking organizations that provide different levels of care, for example, preventive, primary, secondary, tertiary, and long-term care. One of the goals of an IDS is to provide **continuity of care** for the patient, which includes continuity of information (e.g., shared medical records), continuity across primary and secondary care (e.g., discharge planning from specialist to generalist care), and provider continuity (e.g., seeing the same provider each time).

Emergency Medical Services

An emergency medical service (EMS) provides acute care for medical emergencies that take place outside the hospital setting. EMS is utilized within a community to treat those in need of urgent medical care or to stabilize and transport patients with illness or injuries who are unable to transport themselves to the appropriate medical facility. It is a system of coordinated response and emergency medical care involving multiple people and agencies.

EMS is regulated by federal and state governments and may be provided by paid professionals or, in some communities, by volunteers. The organization of EMS varies from community to community, based on state regulation, population density, and topography, and may be provided via public institutions, private institutions, or a public–private configuration. Prehospital EMS can be based in a fire department, a hospital, an independent government agency (such as a public health agency), or a nonprofit corporation (such as a rescue squad); EMS may also be provided by commercial for-profit companies. The essential components of an EMS system are the same regardless of the provider.

Home Health Care Organizations

Home health agencies and organizations provide medical services in a patient's home. Services are typically provided for elderly or disabled patients, or for patients who are unable to visit a hospital or physician's office because of weakness after surgery or other reasons. Care provided in the home may be acute, long-term, or end-of-life. Home health primarily involves the provision of skilled nursing services and therapeutic services (e.g., physical, occupational, and/or speech and hearing). A home health agency may be a public, nonprofit, or proprietary agency and may be a subdivision of a larger organization. The agency must be licensed by the state in which it operates or receive approval that it has met all standards and requirements to operate. These agencies are also subject to certification requirements by CMS and may also seek accreditation from an independent accrediting organization. Home health agencies and organizations must have policies established by a governing body that must include at least one physician and one RN, and the services it provides must be overseen by a physician or a registered professional nurse.

Hospice and Palliative Care Organizations

Palliative care services are available for anyone with a serious illness as well as for patients who are terminally ill. Palliative care may be provided in a hospital, outpatient clinic, long-term care facility, or hospice facility. It is delivered by a team of specialists, including physicians, nurses, and social workers, and may include other professionals, such as massage therapists, pharmacists, and nutritionists. Each facility where palliative care is provided typically has its own palliative care team; these professionals work in partnership with a patient's primary physician and others involved in treating the individual.

Hospice care is provided to terminally ill patients either in their homes (*hospice residential care*) or in a health care facility (*hospice inpatient care*) owned and operated by a hospice organization or health system. According to the National Hospice and Palliative Care Organization (2018), hospice care programs were first established in 1974 and have grown in number to more than 4,199 Medicare certified programs, including both primary locations and satellite offices, as of 2015. The majority of hospice programs are offered by freestanding, independent agencies (72.2%), and the remainder are part of a hospital system (14.2%), home health agency (12.9%), or nursing home (0.6%). Hospice programs range in size from small organizations serving fewer than 50 patients on an annual basis to large, corporate chains operating programs on a national basis and caring for thousands of patients each year. In 2015, 32% of hospice programs registered with Medicare were nonprofit organizations, 63% were for-profit organizations, and about 5% were government owned and operated.

Pharmacies

Medication is an integral part of health care delivery, and pharmacists play a significant role in ensuring the safe and effective use of medication to achieve desired health outcomes. The role of the pharmacist has traditionally been to dispense medication; that role is now expanding into the direct care of patients as the use of medication has grown and new technologies are employed in the medication dispensing and utilization processes.

Licensed pharmacies include retail pharmacies in the community setting and hospital or other institutional pharmacies. Community pharmacies include chain pharmacy organizations (e.g., CVS, Walgreens); pharmacies located within other large retail organizations (e.g., Walmart, Kroger); and independent, locally owned and operated pharmacies. The community pharmacy provides the public with access to medication, including administering flu shots, and serves as a source of advice on health issues. Approximately 6 out of 10 licensed pharmacists work in the community setting. Institutional pharmacies control drug distribution within a health care facility and help to ensure each patient receives the appropriate drug and dosage. Institutional pharmacies are involved in highly specialized areas, including nuclear medicine, intravenous therapy, and drug and poison information. A hospital or health system may also operate a retail pharmacy within its facilities in addition to its clinical pharmacy operation.

Pharmaceutical Companies and Medical Device Manufacturers

Another integral part of the health care delivery system are the pharmaceutical companies and medical device manufacturers that develop and supply medications, medical supplies, durable medical equipment, and medical devices to health care organizations and sometimes directly to the public. Not only do these organizations supply materials needed for the direct care of patients, but they also play an important role in helping ensure safe and effective care.

Medical device manufacturers provide essential products for modern medical care, including devices that range from CT scanners and surgical robotic devices to blood pressure cuffs and thermometers. These products also constitute a significant portion of the national health expenditure. The CMS estimates retail spending on durable medical equipment in the amount of $51 billion and spending for other nondurable medical products at approximately $62.2 billion in 2016. The biopharmaceutical industry comprises the pharmaceutical and biotechnology industries. Biopharmaceutical companies develop, manufacture, market, and distribute drugs and vaccines used to prevent and treat diseases. It is made up of four sectors: pharmaceutical and medicine manufacturers, pharmacy wholesalers, research and development services, and management of companies and enterprises. Biopharmaceutical companies spend up to $135 billion annually on research and development, and it is estimated that it takes up to 15 years to develop a medicine or vaccine. The biopharmaceutical industry accounts for nearly 20% of all research and development investment in the United States, where new drugs must be approved by the Food and Drug Administration (FDA) as safe and effective.

The industry is sometimes referred to as "Big Pharma" because of its size, its influence over health care legislation, and its effect on the cost of health care delivery. Thirty-six of the largest pharmaceutical companies make up the membership of the industry's professional association, the Pharmaceutical Research and Manufacturers of America (PhRMA), and invest more money in lobbying than any other industry in the United States.

Other Delivery Organizations

TELEMEDICINE Telemedicine uses electronic communications to exchange medical information between sites to improve a patient's clinical health status. Telemedicine services may include primary care and specialist referral services, remote patient monitoring, consumer medical and health information, and medical education. Hospitals, specialty clinics, home health agencies, and physicians' offices all use telemedicine. The services may be offered within a single health care organization or between health care organizations.

According to the American Telemedicine Organization (2018), more than half of U.S. hospitals are participating in some form of telemedicine, and more than 200 telemedicine networks with 3,500 service sites exist in the United States. Emerging models of telemedicine delivery include offering specialty consultation services through membership associations that match people in need of services with providers, and independent businesses that are organized to provide telemedicine consultation services but are not health care providers. These independent businesses recruit appropriately licensed specialists to provide telemedicine services and then market these services and handle contract negotiations and all legal and technical aspects of delivery.

Retail Clinics

Retail clinics are medical clinics located in pharmacies, grocery stores, and "big box" stores such as Target. These clinics provide routine care for acute conditions (e.g., bronchitis) as well as preventive care. Retail clinics began emerging in 2000, and more than 2,000 clinics were operating in the United States by 2016. Retail clinics are often open extended hours and on weekends, offering a convenient alternative for routine care, particularly when conventional physician offices are closed. A study by the Rand Corporation indicated that young adults (ages 18–44) account for 43% of patient visits, although the utilization of retail clinics by seniors is increasing (Rand Health, 2016). In 2016, three-quarters of the retail clinics in the United States were operated by two companies—CVS and Walgreens (Rand Health, 2016). Retail clinics are also operated by hospital chains and physician groups, accounting for about 11% of the market. Although some critics of retail clinics voiced concern about the quality of care provided, research suggests that these facilities provide equivalent quality of care to care offered in other provider settings for a select group of conditions. Most commonly, patients seek care at retail clinics for acute conditions including respiratory infections and sore throats. However, these clinics are viewed as promising settings for vaccinations and chronic care management.

Health System Performance

Although the United States spends more money per capita on health care than any other nation in the world, we are lagging behind other countries on a variety of quality indicators, including average life expectancy and infant mortality rates. The Institute of Medicine (IOM) estimates that more Americans are killed every year by medical errors than in automobile accidents. As a response to these staggering statistics, the IOM released *Crossing the Quality Chasm* (2001), a landmark report that issued a mandate for improvement in U.S. health system performance. Additionally, a portion of the ACA is dedicated to improving quality and health system performance through funding research, aligning financial incentives with performance outcomes, and identifying a national quality strategy. Although marginal improvements in quality and performance have been observed in the past decade, we still have a long way to go to achieve a high-performing health system.

Organizations such IOM, the Institute for Healthcare Improvement (IHI), and the National Committee for Quality Assurance (NCQA) are leading the health system improvement movement through initiatives including patient centeredness, the Triple Aim, and the **patient-centered medical home (PCMH)**. The CMS is financially incentivizing the "meaningful use" of electronic health records (EHRs) by health care providers to promote quality improvement in health care. Quality improvement efforts of this type promote collaboration among health care providers, payers, the government, and other stakeholders with the goal of achieving real health system change. In the next section of this chapter, we provide an overview of some of the quality improvement initiatives that demonstrate the most promise in improving U.S. health system performance.

> The idea behind the Triple Aim is that to improve the delivery of health care in the United States, organizations must simultaneously pursue three dimensions: improve the patient experience of care, improve the health of populations, and reduce the per-capita cost of health care.

The Triple Aim

The IHI is a not-for-profit organization that is dedicated to improving health and health care worldwide. The IHI (2018) promotes a learning initiative and a framework called the Triple Aim for health care organizations and communities. The idea behind the Triple Aim is that to improve the delivery of health care in the United States, organizations must simultaneously pursue three dimensions: (a) improve the patient experience of care, (b) improve the health of populations, and (c) reduce the per-capita cost of health care.

Achieving this triple aim is difficult because one organization is rarely accountable for all three dimensions. However, the IHI has identified five system components necessary for fulfillment of the Triple Aim:

- *Focus on individuals and families*: Care should be customized at an individual level utilizing families and caregivers as partners.
- *Redesign primary care services/structures*: A team of professionals must be established that can deliver the majority of necessary care.

- *Population health management*: Partnerships within the community are necessary to promote prevention and wellness.
- *Cost control platform*: Cooperative relationships with provider groups must be in place to control costs.
- *System integration and execution*: Services across the continuum of care must be coordinated.

Although the Triple Aim initiative is ambitious, a few health systems have taken on the challenge and have succeeded. A strong focus on primary care, coupled with community alignment, is necessary to achieve positive patient experiences and improvement in population health. Additionally, active physician participation is crucial to reduce costs. A model of care utilizing a multidisciplinary approach is one way to approach the Triple Aim. Signature Healthcare achieved success with this approach by initiating a Complex Care Clinic focused on high-risk Medicare Managed Care patients

Signature Healthcare, located in eastern Massachusetts, provides services to approximately 10,000 residents over the age of 65. Their most vulnerable patient population includes elderly with multiple chronic illnesses, social challenges, and functional limitations. Signature decided to develop a process focused on providing quality care for this population, and they used the principles of the Triple Aim for guidance.

1. Signature created a Complex Care Clinic led by nurse practitioners to facilitate the management of chronic diseases among this patient population. Appointments were lengthened from 15 minutes to 40 minutes per visit to accommodate patient needs. Nurse practitioners, in consultation with physician partners and a care coordination team, took over care management for these patients.
2. Signature engaged community stakeholders in patient care. For example, many elderly patients needed assistance with transportation, finances, and meals. Signature engaged local organizations, including the Alzheimer's Association and the Visiting Nurse Association, as partners in care. Additionally, they worked with the local public transportation system to facilitate subsidized transport for these patients.
3. Signature updated its infrastructure to best serve this patient population. Internal roles were reassessed, guidelines specific to geriatric conditions were put into place, and screening protocols to help identify seniors at risk for falls were implemented and integrated into the health record.

Signature's initiative aimed at managing elderly patients with complex conditions was successful on a variety of fronts. Patients participating in the Complex Care Clinic had decreased ED utilization and decreased hospital admissions. Billing and coding practices improved as a result of the coordinated approach to providing care. Finally, patient feedback on the new approach to care was extremely positive, and approximately 98% of patients rated their care as "very good" (IHI, 2015).

Patient Centeredness

The IOM identified patient centeredness as one of six domains that define quality care. Patient-centered care is "care that is respectful of and responsive to individual patient preferences, needs, and values and ensures that patient values guide all clinical decisions" (IOM, 2001). Six dimensions to patient-centered care have been identified (Gerteis, Edgman-Levitan, & Daley, 1993):

- Respect for patients' values, preferences, and expressed needs
- Coordination and integration of care
- Information, communication, and education
- Physical comfort
- Emotional support
- Involvement of family and friends

Providing patient-centered care means giving patients the information they need to participate actively in decision making about their care with the goal of obtaining the most desirable outcome. If a patient is incapacitated or unable to participate in decision making regarding his or her care, then a family member or caregiver should be engaged. When a health care intervention cannot provide a cure, it should aim to alleviate the patient's suffering. The likelihood that an outcome desired by a patient can be achieved is increased by actively involving patients and family members in decision making regarding the provision of care.

Although we are making progress in this direction, research suggests that certain patient-centered practices are still rare. Movements toward the PCMH and patient-centered research are continuing to shift the momentum in the right direction; however, there is still a long way to go. The achievement of a truly patient-centered health system will require the participation of patients, family members, physicians, nurses, and other health care providers involved in the provision of care.

Population Health Management

In terms of the organization of care, there is a growing interest among the payer community (insurance companies, Medicare, etc.) for providers to engage in population health management of definable patient populations for which they provide coverage. Provider organizations are engaging in a variety of population health management activities that involve managing a patient's care across provider settings. First, effectively managing the network of providers that patients see can help ensure they are receiving the most efficient and effective care for their conditions. Helping patients navigate physician and specialty care visits can facilitate information sharing among providers and led to better care outcomes. Providers are also making efforts to manage patient transitions of care. A transition in care occurs when a patient moves from one health care delivery setting to another. For example, a patient might be discharged from an acute care hospital and require home health services to facilitate recovery. A hospital can manage this transition of care by proactively planning for the discharge with the patient, family, and home health service.

Provider organizations are also beginning to invest in providing care within the home for seriously ill patients. Hospitals are trying new ways to embed resources within the homes of high-risk patients to ensure they remain compliant with medication protocols and remain healthy. Outreach may involve phone calls, telemedicine services, or simply deploying a practitioner to the patient's home. Finally, provider organizations understand that chronic diseases are the primary drivers of death and disability in the United States. Using data analytics can help organizations identify chronically ill patients so that their conditions can be carefully managed (Optum, 2014).

THE FUTURE OF THE DELIVERY SYSTEM

Recent years have seen the introduction of several innovative new models of care that have potential to realign incentives and improve overall health system performance in terms of cost, quality, and access. The ACA encouraged the adoption of these new models, and a variety of new organizational forms have emerged from the private sector. Renewed interest in physician employment models also demonstrates potential for increased integration and more closely aligned clinical and financial incentives between physicians and other providers.

Innovative Models of Care Delivery

Patient-Centered Medical Homes

The *PCMH* model of primary care emphasizes communication and care coordination. Patient centeredness is an important goal of PCMHs. Physician practices must meet certain standards to be designated as PCMHs. The NCQA released revised standards for PCMHs in 2017 focused around six concepts which represent the overall themes for PCMH (see Table 2.1). Evidence suggests that the PCMH is effective at improving health care quality and reducing costs.

> Evidence suggests that the PCMH is effective at improving health care quality and reducing costs.

Group Health Cooperative (GHC) in Seattle, Washington, provides an example of a successful PCMH model. GHC is a nonprofit health system that consists of physician groups, medical facilities, and health plans that serve Washington and northern Idaho. In 2006, the system decided to pilot test a PCMH practice. GHC's pilot practice expanded staffing and emphasized the use of care teams. The ratio of patients to primary care providers was reduced for the pilot practice, and their enhanced staffing model included physicians, medical assistants, LPNs, physician assistants/nurse practitioners, RNs, and pharmacists. The idea behind this increased staffing was to facilitate

TABLE 2.1 STANDARDS FOR PATIENT-CENTERED MEDICAL HOMES

CONCEPT AREAS	CONTENT
Team-Based Care and Practice Organization	Helps structure a practice's leadership, care team responsibilities, and how the practice partners with patients, families, and caregivers
Knowing and Managing Your Patients	Sets standards for data collection, medication reconciliation, evidence-based clinical decision support, and other activities
Patient-Centered Access and Continuity	Guides practices to provide patients with convenient access to clinical advice and helps ensure continuity of care
Care Management and Support	Helps clinicians set up care management protocols to identify patients who need more closely managed care
Care Coordination and Care Transitions	Ensures that primary and specialty care clinicians are effectively sharing information and managing patient referrals to minimize cost, confusion, and inappropriate care
Performance Measurement and Quality Improvement	Improvement helps practices develop ways to measure performance, set goals, and develop activities that will improve performance

Source: Adapted from National Committee for Quality Assurance. (2018). *Structure of concepts, criteria, and competencies.* Washington, DC: Author.

patient relationships and to allow for comprehensive coordinated care. Additionally, patient encounters with clinical staff increased from approximately 20 minutes to 30 minutes in duration, and time was set aside each day for teams to create coordinated care plans (Reid et al., 2010). The pilot clinic was so successful that HGC spread implementation of the PCMH model across 25 additional clinics. The clinics that implemented PCMH practices experienced better health outcomes, increased access to care, and improved physician and staff satisfaction (Reid, 2015).

Health Homes

Health homes were created by the ACA to give states an option for providing patient-centered, medical home–type services to Medicaid beneficiaries suffering from severe or multiple chronic conditions. The purpose of health homes is to create a system of care that facilitates and coordinates access to primary care, acute care, behavioral care, and long-term community-based services. Medicaid beneficiaries with (a) at least two chronic conditions, (b) one chronic condition and high risk for another, or (c) a serious mental health condition are eligible for health home services.

Promoting care for the whole person, care that is individually tailored to each patient and family, is a goal of health homes.

Health home services are offered by designated providers, teams of health professionals that link to a designated provider, or a health team. Physicians, group practices, community health centers, home health agencies, or any other provider deemed appropriate by the state is considered a designated provider. Health teams consist of a physician and other health care professionals such as nurses, social workers, and other appropriate professionals. Health homes provide care management, care coordination, health promotion, transitional care from inpatient to other settings, individual and family support, follow-up care, and referral to community social support services. Additionally, health homes use health information technology (IT) to coordinate such services. Health homes must provide quality-driven, cost-effective, culturally appropriate care. Promoting care for the whole person, care that is individually tailored to each patient and family, is a goal of health homes.

Accountable Care Organizations

Accountable care organizations (ACOs) are groups of providers that share responsibility and financial accountability for providing high-quality, coordinated care to Medicare patients. The goal of ACOs is to ensure that patients get the right care at the right time in the most efficient way. ACOs are organized around primary care providers, and the high level of care coordination provided by ACOs is particularly important for the chronically ill. If ACOs are successful at meeting quality and cost savings targets, these organizations qualify for financial incentives or shared savings from the Medicare program.

The ACA facilitated the creation of ACOs for the Medicare program. Some ACO models allow for sharing of financial risk and reward for a defined population of patients, while other ACOs allow for shared savings based on financial and quality targets Family Foundation. In 2018, more than 550 Medicare ACOs represented approximately 12 million Medicare beneficiaries. Additionally, provider groups are creating "ACO-like" organizations that strive to facilitate comprehensive care coordination for patient populations beyond Medicare beneficiaries.

Medicare ACOs have demonstrated moderate success in reducing costs and improving quality for patient populations. In 2016, all ACO types generated significant net savings and demonstrated lower spending on Medicare services. In terms of quality, all ACO models had equivalent or better quality than traditional Medicare providers (Kaiser Family Foundation, 2018). Although early indicators of success are limited, ACOs remain a promising model for improving care coordination and lowering the cost of care for particular populations of patients.

Beth Israel Deaconess Care Organization (BIDCO) achieved success as one of the early Medicare "Pioneer" ACOs. It is currently participating with the Medicare program as a "Next Generation" ACO, a program designed for organizations with experience coordinating care for Medicare beneficiaries. BIDCO includes more than 2,500 physicians, a variety of community hospitals, and a network of providers allowing it to function as an IDS. They support providers with a robust population health program that facilitates regular provider meeting and information sharing among network participants. BIDCO attributes its success as an ACO to several factors:

1. First, BIDCO created an IT infrastructure that allows information sharing among providers. This gives providers the information needed to make evidence-based care decisions.
2. Second, BIDCO worked with a variety of stakeholders from within and outside the health care industry to redesign processes and find a fresh approach to providing care.
3. Third, BIDCO increased transparency surrounding quality indicators and this approach resulted in collaboration and competition among providers. This ultimately led to improved outcomes.
4. Fourth, BIDCO began to look at data in different ways that factored in the role that social determinants of health can play in predicting someone's utilization of services.
5. Finally, BIDCO created an incentive model to motivate physicians to increase individual and system level performance. (Hulbert, 2017)

BIDCO is currently aligned with more than 30,000 Medicare beneficiaries. The organization was able to achieve significant cost savings and perform well on quality indicators as a Pioneer ACO. After its first year of participation as a "Next Generation" ACO, BIDCO again demonstrated cost savings and produced high-quality outcomes (CMS, 2018).

Community-Based Solutions

Social needs of individuals play an important role in contributing to health. These needs include issues such as housing conditions, access to healthy food, crime in the community, and poverty. In the current health care environment, the emphasis on population health and prevention has facilitated the interests of provider organizations in addressing social issues to keep community members healthy and out of hospitals. Keeping patients healthy is not only the right thing to do, it is also financially beneficial under new payment methodologies that incentivize health. Although the linkage between social factors and health has long been recognized, more collaboration between community resources and provider organizations to provide social services has emerged in recent years.

One example of such a collaborative is the *Staten Island Performing Provider System (PPS)*. In 2015, Staten Island University Hospital and Richmond Hill Hospital received funding through the state of New York to form the Staten Island PPS. The PPS engaged community-based organizations that provide social services for citizens such as homeless shelters, food banks, community health centers, and physicians serving large numbers of uninsured and Medicaid patients. The provider organizations and social services organizations are working collaboratively on a variety of projects aimed at improving the health status of the community and reducing avoidable hospital admissions. Projects include efforts to better coordinate care and social services for people with serious conditions, improve health literacy, and implement substance abuse initiatives for at-risk youth (Sparer, Muennig, & Brown, 2016). Although the PPS is still in its early stages, this type of collaboration shows promise in improving the health of communities.

Provider organizations are also developing community-based programs aimed at reducing avoidable hospital readmissions. According to CMS, almost one of every five Medicare patients is likely to be readmitted to the hospital within 30 days of discharge. These readmissions may occur because of inadequate care management resulting from a bumpy transition in care from one setting to another. Unnecessary readmissions are extremely costly to the Medicare system, and acute care hospitals face financial penalties if their readmission rates are too high. Most importantly, inappropriate readmissions are bad for patient care. In an effort to better coordinate transitions of care, health care providers have found success in reducing readmission rates by seeking community-based solutions.

The *Care Transition Choices (CTC)* program presented by the Partners in Care Foundation is one example of a successful community-based program aimed at improving transitions of care for high-risk patients. The *CTC* started as a pilot program established through CMS under the Community Care Transition Program. The program has been so successful that private health plans and physician groups have adopted the program and kept it in operation. The *CTC* program works by assigning care transition coaches to work with high-risk patients on cultivating health self-management skills, review appropriate medication use, and recognize warning signs of a worsening condition. Coaches visit patients in the hospital and in their homes. In addition to clinical monitoring, coaches link patients with community resources, including meal delivery and wheelchair-accessible transportation. The program has been successful in significantly reducing hospital readmissions among Medicare patients and reducing costs (Partners in Care Foundation, 2018).

Clinical Integration

Physician–Hospital Alignment

The alignment of physician and hospital goals and incentives is a critical success factor in the era of health reform. Traditionally, both types of provider have been reimbursed based on volume or productivity. However, reimbursement mechanisms are becoming more focused on quality and efficiency. Identifying ways to align the incentives of physicians and hospitals is vitally important to maximize the clinical quality of care while minimizing costs.

> Identifying ways to align the incentives of physicians and hospitals is vitally important to maximize the clinical quality of care while minimizing costs.

Different economic levels and approaches to physician–hospital alignment involve a variety of organizational arrangements. Loosely aligned physician-hospital arrangements involve a traditional independent practice model, in which physicians are still "volunteer" members of a hospital's medical staff and alignment is sought through contractual arrangements to secure medical directors and physician administrators. In this traditional alignment model, economic integration is not achieved. Closer alignment might be achieved through more strategic approaches, such as joint ventures or co-management agreements between physicians and hospitals with some level of shared economic interests. The ultimate level of physician–hospital alignment is achieved through employment relationships with full economic integration. With this level of alignment, physicians are truly employees and are required to comply with hospital policies and share goals (Sowers, Newman, & Langdon, 2013).

A well-regarded example of an integrated health system is Scripps Health (www.scripps.org), which includes acute care hospitals, outpatient centers, and home health and hospice services in the San Diego, California, area. Scripps employs more than 15,000 workers, and approximately 3,000 affiliated physicians provide care at Scripps facilities. Scripps Health is a success story in the area of physician–hospital alignment. In 1999, Scripps was losing millions of dollars a year and physician and employee confidence was at an all-time low. A new CEO created an organizational turnaround by aligning physician and hospital interests more closely through a co-management approach. Although California law makes direct physician employment difficult, closer alignment was achieved through an integrated foundation model that emphasizes transparency and open communication between physician and administrative leadership. The CEO was able to regain physician trust and leverage close alignment with physicians to achieve financial and quality improvements. Since the turnaround, Scripps Health has been well positioned for growth, and the system has received numerous awards and accolades, including becoming one of *Fortune* magazine's "100 Best Companies to Work For" (Scripps Health San Diego, n.d.). In 2017, Scripps announced the implementation of a new dyad leadership model that pairs hospital administrators with physician leaders to further align mutual interests.

Physician Employment Models

More complex reimbursement systems are emerging from health reform and the quality movement. Physician payment is moving from a primarily fee-for-service or volume-based methodology to a model more dependent on quality and clinical outcomes. As a result of this shift, many physicians are no longer interested in private practice models. Instead, they are seeking affiliation and employment opportunities with health systems and hospitals. Physician employment models free up clinician time so they can focus on providing patient care rather than the business of running a practice. Employment can be advantageous for hospitals and health systems by increasing their level of alignment with physician providers. Physician employment models often tie compensation to quality and productivity metrics.

The Mayo Clinic (www.mayoclinic.org) is one successful model of physician employment. Physicians work together with other clinic staff to care for patients, and their work is centered on the philosophy that "the needs of the patient come first" (Mayo Clinic, n.d.). The culture of Mayo is unique, rooted in the values of its founders: teamwork, collegiality, professionalism, mutual respect, and commitment to progress for the organization and individuals. Care is provided by integrated teams of physicians, health care professionals, and scientists. The Mayo culture emphasizes team success over individual success. Although physician employees are provided with a vast array of resources and support, they are compensated with a salary. This salary structure eliminates any incentives to perform tests or procedures for financial gain. Treatment is purely focused on what is best for the patient (Mayo Clinic, n.d.).

BEST PRACTICES
Innovative Approaches to Improving Care Delivery

So far in this chapter, we have described several organizations that use innovative approaches to deliver high-quality health care. Health care delivery organizations must continue to innovate if they hope to deliver high-quality care while controlling costs. This section highlights two organizations that have strong reputations as long-term innovators.

Intermountain Healthcare—Salt Lake City, Utah

Intermountain Healthcare (www.intermountainhealthcare.org) fosters a culture of innovation. Intermountain is a nonprofit health care system comprising 22 hospitals, more than 185 physician clinics, and an affiliated insurance company. The system has more than 33,000 employees who serve patients in Utah and southeastern Idaho. The mission of Intermountain Healthcare is "helping people live the healthiest lives possible" (Intermountain Healthcare, n.d.). In addition to pursuing the typical health care delivery activities of an integrated health system, Intermountain has several programs that nurture a learning environment and culture of innovation.

Intermountain has several initiatives centered around using technology and innovation to provide high-quality care at a sustainable cost. Intermountain Innovations is an effort to develop new revenue streams by commercializing proven clinical and technological innovations. The Intermountain Simulation Center capitalizes on technology to provide training for clinicians and employees that will help promote safety and reduce medical errors among its health team. Intermountain hosts the Homer Warner Center, a research facility dedicated to the discovery and implementation of technology through medical informatics.

Of particular prominence is the Intermountain Transformation Lab. The purpose of this lab is to bring innovation and technology to the patient's bedside at a rapid pace. In addition to working with external technology partners, Intermountain's Healthcare Transformation Lab also provides opportunities for Intermountain employees to develop ideas into new technology. The lab provides a place for clinicians to work with technology experts in developing innovative ideas that will improve the delivery of health care. Examples of projects targeted by the lab include designing the patient room of the future, creating a hand-washing sensor for providers, 3D printing of medical devices for clinical purposes, and creating a "Life Detector" to notify caregivers of changes in vital signs of patients.

Intermountain hopes to affect change in the delivery of health care through providing educational opportunities and conducting research throughout the system. Its culture of innovation capitalizes on the knowledge of caregivers and employees to improve quality and reduce costs (Intermountain Healthcare, n.d.).

The Cleveland Clinic—Cleveland, Ohio

The Cleveland Clinic (www.clevelandclinic.org) is a multispecialty academic medical center with a focus on clinical care and research. It houses more than 1,400 hospital beds at its main campus and works with more than 3,000 physicians and scientists. The Cleveland Clinic's mission is "to provide better care of the sick, investigation into their problems, and further education of those who serve" (Cleveland Clinic, 2018). Quality and innovation are among its core values, and the clinic is consistently named in *U.S. News and World Report's* "America's Best Hospitals" survey.

Cleveland Clinic is innovating care delivery by negotiating directly with self-insured employers as part of its Program for Advanced Medical Care (PAMC). The idea behind PAMC programs is to allow employers to provide their employees with access to world-class health care at a reasonable price. Bundled payment programs and transparency in quality outcomes make the Cleveland Clinic a natural choice for large employers interested in securing greater value in their health care purchases. PAMC's first agreement of this kind began with Lowe's Companies in 2010 to provide heart care for its more than 200,000 employees. The clinic recently expanded its cardiac program by contracting with Walmart and is now focusing on marketing packages of orthopedic procedures to large employers. Promoting this form of "domestic medical tourism" may change the way care is delivered, or at least promote transparency among health care providers in terms of quality and pricing (Cleveland Clinic, 2018).

CONCLUSION

The U.S. health care delivery system can look forward to many changes on the horizon. Uncertainty surrounding the ACA continues to push providers to continually improve quality and manage costs. Innovative new forms of delivering health care will continue to emerge to meet the demands of both patients and purchasers of health care. Health care delivery organizations that fail to evolve and learn will face a difficult road. Those organizations that focus on innovation and knowledge creation will be well positioned for the future.

► CASE EXERCISE—INNOVATIVE IDEAS

You have just been promoted to work as the assistant to the CEO of a large, partially integrated health care delivery system. Your first assignment is to identify several innovative ways to improve health system quality, control costs, and maximize access to care for citizens in your community. Opportunities exist to improve physician-hospital alignment and to provide more integrated care across health system entities. Draft a memo to your CEO that answers the following questions:

1. What are five innovative ideas your health system could implement to meet improvement goals around cost, quality, and access?

2. What innovation or innovative idea is the most critical to ensure the health system achieves its goals?

3. What innovation will be the most difficult to achieve? Why?

4. Why will the implementation of these innovative ideas improve health system performance?

DISCUSSION QUESTIONS

1. The U.S. health system is shifting its focus to wellness and prevention. Give an example of the three forms of prevention. How should emphasis on prevention alter the delivery of health services in a particular community?

2. The baby boomer generation, which represents a significant portion of the U.S. population, is reaching an age when its utilization of health services will most likely increase. Additionally, life expectancy continues to improve with advancements in medicine and community health. Discuss how this aging of such a large segment of the population will affect specific health care delivery services and organizations.

3. Most health care in the United States is delivered in traditional settings such as hospitals, physician organizations, and long-term care organizations. However, access to new delivery settings is becoming more readily available, and demand for care delivery through telemedicine and retail clinics is increasing. Give an example of an application for telemedicine. Discuss how the utilization of telemedicine might affect cost, quality, and access to care in the U.S. health care system.

4. Although the United States spends more money per capita on health care than any other country in the world, its performance has much room for improvement. How can ideas such as the Triple Aim initiative or patient centeredness help to improve performance in the U.S. health system?

5. Discuss why coordinated care delivery approaches, such as PCMHs or ACOs, might improve care for patients. Discuss barriers and opportunities for implementation of such coordinated care delivery approaches.

REFERENCES

Agency for Healthcare Research and Quality. (2013). Retrieved from https://www.ahrq.gov

Ambulatory Surgical Center Association. (2018). What is an ASC? Retrieved from https://www.ascassociation.org/AdvancingSurgicalCare/aboutascs/industryoverview

American Hospital Association. (2018). Fast facts on U.S. hospitals, 2018. Retrieved from https://www.aha.org/statistics/fast-facts-us-hospitals

Centers for Disease Control and Prevention. (2017). *National hospital ambulatory medical care survey: 2015 emergency department summary tables.* Retrieved from https://www.cdc.gov/nchs/data/nhamcs/web_tables/2015_ed_web_tables.pdf

Centers for Medicare & Medicaid Services. (2018). Next Generation ACO Model. Retrieved from https://innovation.cms.gov/initiatives/Next-Generation-ACO-Model

Cleveland Clinic. (2018). Facts & figures. Retrieved from http://my.clevelandclinic.org/about-cleveland-clinic/overview/who-we-are/facts-figures.aspx

Enthoven, A. C. (2016). What is an integrated health care financing and delivery system (IDS)? and what must would-be IDS accomplish to become competitive with them? *Health Economics & Outcome Research, 2*(2), 1–9. doi:10.4172/2471-268X.1000115

Gerteis, M., Edgman-Levitan, S., & Daley, J. (1993). *Through the patient's eyes: Understanding and promoting patient-centered care.* San Francisco, CA: Jossey-Bass.

Hirshon, J. M., Risko, N., Calvello, E. J. B., de Ramirez, S. S., Narayan, M., Theodosis, C., & O'Neill, J. (2013). Health systems and services: The role of acute care. *Bulletin of the World Health Organization, 91,* 386–388. doi:10.2471/BLT.12.112664

Hulbert, J. (2017, October 30). Five ACO success tips from Beth Israel Deaconess Care Organization CEO. *Managed Healthcare Executive.* Retrieved from http://www.managedhealthcareexecutive.com/hospitals-providers/five-aco-success-tips-beth-israel-deaconess-care-organization-ceo

Hwang, W., Chang, J., LaClair, M., & Paz, H. (2013). Effects of integrated delivery systems on cost and quality. *American Journal of Managed Care, 19*(5), e175–e184. Retrieved from https://www.ajmc.com/journals/issue/2013/2013-1-vol19-n5/effects-of-integrated-delivery-system-on-cost-and-quality

Institute for Healthcare Improvement. (2015). *Signature Healthcare: A Triple Aim improvement story.* Cambridge, MA: Author. Retrieved from http://www.ihi.org/resources/Pages/Publications/SignatureHealthcareTripleAim.aspx

Institute for Healthcare Improvement. (2018). *The IHI triple aim initiative.* Retrieved from http://www.ihi.org/Engage/Initiatives/TripleAim/Pages/default.aspx

Institute of Medicine. (2001). *Crossing the quality chasm: A new health system for the 21st century.* Washington, DC: National Academies Press.

Institute of Medicine. (2003). *The future of the public's health in the 21st century.* Washington, DC: National Academies Press.

Institute of Medicine. (2012). *An integrated framework for assessing the value of community-based prevention.* Washington, DC: National Academies Press.

Intermountain Healthcare. (n.d.). Transforming healthcare. Retrieved from https://intermountainhealthcare.org/about/transforming-healthcare

Kaiser Family Foundation. (2018). Medicare delivery system reform: The evidencellink: 8 FAQs: Medicare ACO models. Retrieved from https://www.kff.org/faqs-medicare-accountable-care-organization-aco-models

Kane, C. K. (2017). *Policy research perspectives: Updated data on physician practice arrangements: Physician ownership drops below 50 percent.* Chicago, IL: American Medical Association. Retrieved from https://www.ama-assn.org/sites/default/files/media-browser/public/health-policy/PRP-2016-physician-benchmark-survey.pdf

Kindig, D., & Stoddart, G. (2003). What is population health? *American Journal of Public Health, 93*(3), 380–383. doi:10.2105/AJPH.93.3.380

Mayo Clinic. (n.d.). Culture. Retrieved from https://jobs.mayoclinic.org/culture

National Association of Community Health Centers. (n.d.). About our health centers. Retrieved from http://www.nachc.org/about-our-health-centers

National Committee for Quality Assurance. (2018). *NCQA PCMH recognition: concepts (PCMH) 2017*. Washington, DC: Author. Retrieved from https://www.ncqa.org/programs/health-care-providers-practices/patient-centered-medical-home-pcmh/pcmh-concepts/

National Hospice and Palliative Care Organization. (2018). Retrieved from http://www.nhcpco.org

Optum. (2014). *The four steps of population health management*. Retrieved from https://cdn-aem.optum.com/content/dam/optum3/optum/en/resources/white-papers/Four_steps_population_health_management.pdf

Partners in Care Foundation. (2018). Avoid re-hospitalization of high-risk patients and cut costs with Care Transition Choices. Retrieved from https://www.picf.org/community-care-transition-program-cctp

Rand Health. (2016). *The evolving role of retail clinics*. Retrieved from https://www.rand.org/pubs/research_briefs/RB9491-2.html

Reid, R. (2015). *Transforming primary care: Evaluating the spread of group health's medical home*. Retrieved from https://www.ahrq.gov/sites/default/files/wysiwyg/professionals/systems/primary-care/tpc/tpc-profile-reid.pdf

Reid, R., Coleman, K., Johnson, E., Fishman, P., Hsu, C., Soman, M.,... Larson, E. (2010). The group health medical home at year two: Cost savings, higher patient satisfaction, and less burnout for providers. *Health Affairs, 29*(5), 835–843. doi:10.1377/hlthaff.2010.0158

Scripps Health San Diego. (n.d.). About us: Chris Van Gorder. Retrieved from http://www.scripps.org/about-us__executive-team__chris-van-gorder

Social Security Act, 42 U.S.C. § 1867(e)(1)(A).

Sowers, K., Newman, P., & Langdon, J. (2013). Evolution of physician-hospital alignment models: A case study of comanagement. *Clinical Orthopaedics and Related Research, 471*(6), 1818–1823. doi:[10.1007/s11999-013-2911-0]

Sparer, M., Muennig, P., & Brown L. (2016). (Re)*defining the healthcare delivery system: The role of social services*. Newark, DE: KPMG Government Institute. Retrieved from https://assets.kpmg.com/content/dam/kpmg/pdf/2016/07/9-salud-re-defining-the-healthcare-delivery-system-the-role-of-social-services.pdf

World Health Organization. (2015). Health systems strengthening glossary. Retrieved from http://www.who.int/healthsystems/hss_glossary/en/index5.html

World Health Organization. (2017). Constitution of WHO: Principles. Retrieved from http://www.who.int/about/mission/en

3

The Politics of Health Care in the United States

Rogan Kersh and James Morone

LEARNING OBJECTIVES

▸ Understand the health care infrastructure

▸ Explain the effect of spending on the health care infrastructure

▸ Describe the politics of Medicare and Medicaid

▸ Discuss the impact of politics on the health care delivery system

▸ Explore how personal health decisions become public

KEY TERMS

▸ access

▸ administrative efficiency

▸ innovation

▸ patient outcomes

▸ policy issue

TOPICAL OUTLINE

▸ Costs for health care infrastructure

▸ Many dollars are spent on health care but to what effect?

▸ The politics of Medicare and Medicaid

▸ The role of politics in equitable health care services

▸ Personal health decisions become public: obesity

INTRODUCTION

It is the best of health care systems; it is the worst of health care systems—at least among rich nations. Health care in the United States is a point of cultural pride ("finest in the world!"). It is the nation's largest economic sector, at $3.5 trillion in annual costs and approaching 20% of U.S. GDP (gross domestic product). It is a moral issue, given low-income Americans' terrible health care outcomes, dragging the national average below other rich countries on most measures of population health, including maternal mortality and life expectancy at birth. It is a **policy issue** because every one of these dimensions (quality, costs, injustice) feed into heated congressional, White House, and state/local legislative discussions. And health care is, of course, a deeply personal matter: It is about the human condition, about wellness and suffering, sickness and death.

> Despite the United States' enormous spending on health care—the highest in the world—patient outcomes lag behind those of comparable countries.*

The modern American health care system was forged by political choices. The United States experienced furious debates about whether to cover all citizens through a government program (in the 1940s), even as most other wealthy democracies were organizing such programs. It deployed tax policy to foster a private, employer-sponsored health insurance coverage industry (1950s). It filled the gaps in coverage for some of America's poor and almost all people over 65 with two programs, Medicare and Medicaid, legislated in 1965 (and now swallowing a quarter of the federal budget and, on average, a fifth of state budgets). Every presidential administration in the past 80 years—Democratic and Republican, liberal and conservative—has proposed major changes in health policy. Both the Barack Obama and the Donald Trump administrations zoomed in on health care in their first months. In short, the battle over the shape of American health care is constant (Blumenthal & Morone, 2008; Henry Kaiser Foundation, 2016).

This chapter takes up three main dimensions of the U.S. health care system, emphasizing throughout the central role of politics and policymaking. We begin with the basics—America's national health infrastructure and how medical services are financed. Next we zero in on health insurance, which inspires especially heated policy debates (more technical reviews of issues related to financing and health insurance are presented in Chapters 10 and 11). A third primary theme is health disparities among Americans: Geography, a proxy for wealth and poverty, is a major determinant of health outcomes (this topic is covered in more detail in Chapter 8). After describing the political context for health care, we take up a specific issue—obesity—and detail how political maneuvering shapes health matters that many Americans still consider personal, not a matter of government regulation. As both history and contemporary practice show, many ostensibly private matters in the health domain have

---

*To hear the podcast, go to https://bcove.video/2zHJ1v7 or access the ebook on Springer Publishing Connect™.

been the subject of public regulation—even in the famously individualistic, anti-government United States.

At the core of health politics and policy is the question of whether individuals have a right to health care or whether it should be treated as any other market good, like clothes or food or cars. Most wealthy democratic countries view health care as a foundational human right and provide at least a basic level of health services to all residents; some, like Canada, aim for a universal right to equal care (Chapter 4 focuses in more detail on a comparative global health perspective). Uniquely among advanced democracies, the United States views health care not as a right but a patchwork: an entitlement for most people over 65, a perquisite of employment in some companies and sectors, and a service to be purchased either as insurance or at point of service for millions of others. The United States is among a handful of countries not to have ratified a UN treaty declaring health care a fundamental human right (UN official text, 2018).

> At the core of health politics and policy is the question of whether individuals have a right to health care or whether it should be treated as any other market good, like clothes or food or cars.

Our idiosyncratic health system has always been shaped by political debates—drawing in policymakers as well as large employers, private insurance companies, and professional medical decision makers. This chapter examines whether the result of all that politicking is better health outcomes for most Americans. Our main aim in this chapter is to clarify the roles of policymaking and politics in the U.S. health system. Our discussions of financing, insurance, and obesity as a behavioral health issue and comparative health care are meant to complement other chapters in the book and to provide context for the exploration of the dynamics of politics and policymaking in the world of the U.S. health system. Our aim is to communicate how politics and policy impact the health system and how political scientists approach the topic of health care.

HEALTH CARE INFRASTRUCTURE AND SPENDING: MANY DOLLARS, TO WHAT EFFECT?

The U.S. system of delivering and financing health care is the most complicated among advanced countries. Some nations, like Great Britain, manage health care through the government; others, like Switzerland, rely on the private market (with government subsidizing care for the least well-off). Still others—Singapore, for example—mix government-run care for low-income residents with a private system (Gusmano & Rodwin, this volume). The United States includes elements of all three. Complicating matters further, treating patients and paying for those treatments are managed by different collections of institutions. The one-word summary: fragmentation.

Providing Health Care

Let's start with government-provided care. American military veterans receive health care from more than 1,200 hospitals and clinics managed by the Veterans Health Administration (VHA). More than 305,000 VHA health professionals and support staff tend to some 9 million veterans each year, making this the largest health system in the United States. Veterans' complaints in recent years about long waits for care and elaborate eligibility rules have resulted in diminished approval ratings for the VHA, even as it spends nearly $200 billion annually (VA Health Care, 2017). Along with this federal management of veterans' care, state and local governments also run public clinics and hospitals, which help serve those who can't otherwise afford care. Moreover, members of the armed forces and their families receive care through services organized by each branch of the federal military. Overall, about a quarter of U.S. health care delivery is through these various government-run entities.

The remaining three-quarters of hospitals and clinics are run by private companies, which are deeply enmeshed in the U.S. health care system. Of those clinics and hospitals that are private, about 70% are nonprofit—managed by universities, religious institutions, charities, or nonprofit networks. The remainder are for-profit, often organized into large systems: the Hospital Corporation of America, for example, based in Nashville, Tennessee, manages more than 175 hospitals in the United States and the United Kingdom, with annual revenues of more than $3 billion.

What about prescription drugs and other pharmaceuticals? The U.S. drug industry is almost entirely private—an economic behemoth with global reach, approaching $500 billion in annual sales. By comparison, in most other advanced democratic countries, the government purchases and distributes prescription drugs.

> The U.S. drug industry is almost entirely private—an economic behemoth with global reach, approaching $500 billion in annual sales. By comparison, in most other advanced democratic countries, the government purchases and distributes prescription drugs.

What difference does it make that so much of the U.S. health infrastructure is outside government supervision? A lot: In most advanced countries, a central government body (like the United Kingdom's National Health Service, or China's Ministry of Public Health) provides strategic planning; determines where additional doctors, nurses, and other health professionals are needed (and whether there are sufficient hospitals and clinics to house them); and pays most of the cost of care. In the United States, privately managed care facilities are free to open or close where and when they wish. America has no national health planning; individual states and large cities monitor their health systems, regulate providers, and collect reams of health data—but do not wield direct influence on the provision of care. The result is a hodgepodge of some often-superb facilities, especially in higher-income neighborhoods, and many places (especially inner cities and rural areas) devoid of first-rate medical institutions or professionals.

Although the U.S. system lags behind almost every wealthy nation in health outcomes—more on that later—America does lead the world in health **innovation**: developing new treatments, medical instruments, and drugs for the bewildering array of diseases and health conditions that beset us. More than 60% of health research and development (R&D) funding is carried out by private industry; another quarter is funded by the government, often as grants to university researchers, many of whom

> Although the U.S. system lags behind almost every wealthy nation in health outcomes, America does lead the world in health innovation: developing new treatments, medical instruments, and drugs for the bewildering array of diseases and health conditions that beset us.

work closely with private companies to license their discoveries for sale. Nearly 150 U.S. universities also manage large health care systems, organized around teaching hospitals where the next generation of medical professionals are trained.

In sum, if you get sick in the United States, are not in the military or a military veteran, and need to see a doctor, chances are high that she will be privately employed—though likely in a nonprofit hospital or clinic. If you are under 65, unemployed, and uninsured, you may seek care at an emergency room or a low/no-cost public clinic. Should you receive a prescription, you'll probably go to a private pharmacy like CVS or Walgreens and buy (with help from insurance, which we talk about below) drugs or other palliative services. Those pharmaceuticals (or insulin treatments, special bandages, etc.) were likely produced by private companies, though the R&D may well have involved government-funded research in university or public laboratories at places like the Centers for Disease Control and Prevention (CDC), a government agency.

Perplexed yet? Health care provision in the United States is a tangled mixture of national, state, and local government; private companies, both for-profit and nonprofit; universities and nonprofit health-advocacy organizations; and medical professionals spread across all these groups. This multi-layered complexity—sitting atop an equally complicated financing arrangement, discussed in detail in the following—is part of the reason that Americans far outstrip the rest of the world in health care spending. Let's take a look at where that annual $3.5 trillion goes.

Health Care Spending

Figure 3.1 provides a summary of how American health care dollars are spent.

Note that this arrangement—nearly a third of total funds spent on hospital care, for example—is not ordained by law or medical best practices but

FIGURE 3.1   DISTRIBUTION OF U.S. HEALTH CARE SPENDING: 2018

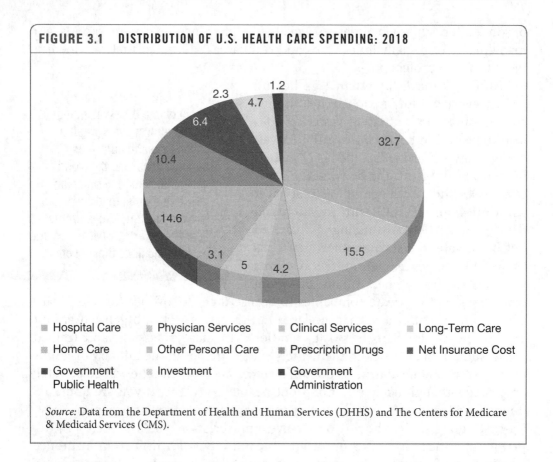

Source: Data from the Department of Health and Human Services (DHHS) and The Centers for Medicare & Medicaid Services (CMS).

reflects a mix of tradition, strategic decisions, investor choices, and political compromises. Many other countries spend a higher percentage of their health dollars on government administration (1.2% in the United States) because their systems are subject to central control. Most others also spend a far lower proportion of their health dollars on prescription drugs (approaching 11% in the United States)—mainly because their national government purchases drugs in bulk quantities and manages their distribution. As we will see below, U.S. political debates on funding prescription drugs tend to rule out such centralized government purchases.

The United States is also distinctive in terms of *how much* it spends on health care: by a considerable margin, the world's most per capita. Figure 3.2 lists the top health-spending countries per person.

With the United States considerably ahead of other wealthy nations—spending twice as much as the average peer country—questions arise about what lies ahead. "Bending the health cost curve" downward has been a priority for health policymakers for decades; President Richard Nixon warned darkly that "we face ... a breakdown in our medical system," caused by rising costs, back in 1969 (Nixon, 1969). Fifty years later, costs continue to rise.

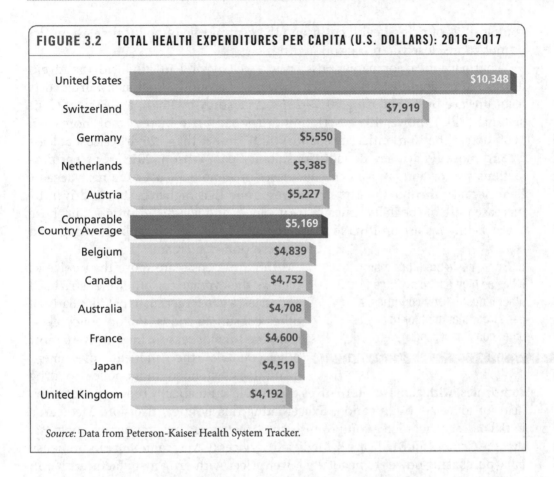

FIGURE 3.2   TOTAL HEALTH EXPENDITURES PER CAPITA (U.S. DOLLARS): 2016–2017

United States	$10,348
Switzerland	$7,919
Germany	$5,550
Netherlands	$5,385
Austria	$5,227
Comparable Country Average	$5,169
Belgium	$4,839
Canada	$4,752
Australia	$4,708
France	$4,600
Japan	$4,519
United Kingdom	$4,192

Source: Data from Peterson-Kaiser Health System Tracker.

Bending the Cost Curve? Health Spending in Coming Years

Given the convoluted U.S. infrastructure, the job of providing high-quality health services is demanding—and becomes more difficult as costs soar. After a drop in annual increases after the Affordable Care Act (ACA)'s passage, costs have begun again to rise steadily, with prescription drug increases leading the way. Other drivers of the current boost in U.S. health expenses include higher costs for out-of-pocket care, rising Medicare expenses as a swelling number of baby boomers age into the program, and ACA premium hikes—the latter a consequence of executive branch regulatory actions designed to weaken the ACA.

> Given the convoluted U.S. infrastructure, the job of providing high-quality health services is demanding—and becomes more difficult as costs soar.

In a sentence, why do Americans pay so much for health care? Because U.S. providers charge more for the same service. Without a single regulator negotiating prices, costs are simply passed along (Cuckler et al., 2018). To understand the complexities of rising health costs, and the central role of political decisions, let us look more closely at prescription drugs.

Pharmaceutical companies raised prices well beyond inflation with the advent of the Trump administration: After growing by around 2% annually, drug costs leapt upward by 4.4% during 2017–2018. As a study by Pharmacy Benefit Consultants (PBC) shows, 40 prescription drugs had price increases of more than 100% across the 15 months since January 2017; more than 225 drugs cost at least a third more (Pharmacy Benefit Consultants' comparison, 2018). Current projections are for annual drug cost increases of some 6.5% over the next decade. Pharmaceutical company representatives argue that higher costs are driven by increased use of specialty drugs to treat cancer and genetic disorders, but those skyrocketing fastest on PBC's list include drugs for bee stings, bedwetting, and prescription skin cream.

> U.S. drug costs are more than twice as high as the average for other industrialized countries, a gap larger than that for nearly all other consumer goods.

U.S. drug costs are more than twice as high as the average for other industrialized countries, a gap larger than that for nearly all other consumer goods. Public policy decisions are a major reason. In contrast to most other countries, the American government guarantees extended monopolies to drug companies, with generic alternatives that would dramatically reduce prices often held up for years by litigation. Exacerbating this political decision, Medicare's initial passage included a compromise, since reaffirmed many times by Congress, that the Centers for Medicare & Medicaid Services (CMS) cannot use its immense bulk-purchasing power to negotiate lower prices with drug manufacturers. CMS payment plans are also required by Congress to cover nearly *all* drugs, rather than concentrating on the most frequently prescribed (and/or cheaper) medications (Kesselheim, Avorn, & Sarpatwari, 2016). Companies routinely claim that the high costs of research and development, along with long delays in Food and Drug Administration (FDA) approval of new drugs, keep their costs high. But academic analyses find at best mixed evidence of association between R&D expenses and drug prices (Jaroslawski, Auquier, & Toumi, 2017; Kesselheim, Avorn, & Sarpatwari, 2016), and the FDA's swifter drug approval processes in recent years has not resulted in a commensurate price reduction for new pharmaceuticals.

A final reason for unusually high prescription drug prices is the fragmentation of the industry. Drug companies utilize distributors for their products, who add a hefty premium to the price of every drug. How much do they add? Drug companies are not permitted to list their prices before the distributor markup. It is a fragmented system is rife with opportunities for "investment." Budget-minded policymakers, restricted at every turn from addressing these well-protected political decisions, can agree only that innovative policy moves are an essential part of the solution to sharply rising prescription drug prices (Alexander et al., 2017; Frank & Zeckhauser, 2018).

For a blend of reasons, then—manifestly including politics—U.S. health spending is the world's highest. What do we get for all those dollars expended?

Across the first two-thirds of the 20th century, America was among world leaders in terms of health outcomes, ranking near the top in areas like infant mortality and life expectancy. In recent decades, almost every wealthy nation has surpassed the United States on primary measures of mortality and morbidity. As we will explore, these are *average* measures; they mask enormous differences between rich and poor.

Patient Outcomes and Beyond: Evaluating American Health Care

Assessing health care systems is a complex science (Gusmano & Rodwin, this volume). A hospital that rates highly on curing patients may actually turn away the sickest cases. Nuanced assessment measures are therefore required. Along with **patient outcomes**, analysts now evaluate health care systems in four additional areas: **access** (is health care availability timely and affordable?), care process (including such vital aspects as patient safety, preventive care, coordinating care across different health providers, and health professionals' engagement with patients), **administrative efficiency** (measuring whether the immense bureaucracy required to operate health systems work smoothly and swiftly), and equity (do all who seek care receive similar treatment?). Chapter 12 reviews the topic of quality improvement in more detail.

Since health care systems exist to enhance people's health and well-being, *patient outcomes* top the list of evaluative criteria. Here the United States performs poorly, compared to peer nations. On an Institute of Medicine comprehensive study of 17 high-income countries, Americans scored at or near the worst on nearly all of nine measures, including frequency of homicides, incidence of heart and lung disease, infant mortality, obesity, disability rates, frequency of car accidents, and sexually transmitted infections among teens (Woolf & Aron, 2013). Together, these features drive down life expectancy. According to latest Organisation for Economic Co-operation and Development (OECD) estimates, Americans born in recent years can expect to live to age 78.8 on average—a full 5.1 years less than in Japan, and not in the world's top 30 countries—ranking below Chile, Slovenia, and Cuba (Kochanek, Murphy, Xu, & Arias, 2017; OECD, 2017).

On the other above-listed dimensions, from system efficiency through equity, the United States is also a relatively low performer. Figure 3.3 summarizes an analysis of all five evaluative dimensions by the Commonwealth Fund, a global health policy research organization (Schneider et al., 2017). As you can see, the United States scores highest—fifth overall—on care process, thanks to preventive measures like mammography screening and provider–patient engagement, ranging from wellness counseling on healthy behaviors to end-of-life discussions with health providers. Otherwise, American health systems perform poorly. The United States ranks next to last in administrative efficiency and finishes at the bottom in the other three areas. Add up the results and America finishes last overall among wealthier countries.

The American combination of high health spending per capita—31% higher than Switzerland, the second most expensive—and lagging patient outcomes is

FIGURE 3.3   EVALUATING HEALTH SYSTEMS: COMPARING 11 WEALTHY COUNTRIES

	OVERALL RANKING	Care Process +	Access +	Administrative Efficiency +	Equity +	Health Care Outcomes +
AUS	2	2	4	1	7	1
CAN	9	6	10	6	9	9
FRA	10	9	9	11	10	5
GER	8	8	2	6	6	8
NETH	3	4	1	9	2	6
NZ	4	3	7	2	8	7
	4	10	5	4	5	3
NOR	6	11	6	5	3	2
SWE	6	7	8	8	4	4
UK	1	1	3	3	1	10
US	11	5	11	10	11	11

Source: Retrieved from Commonwealth Fund.

a source of concern for U.S. health providers and policymakers alike (Papanicolas, Woskie, & Jha, 2018). Figure 3.4 combines these two comparative features—higher costs and poorer results—in a compelling juxtaposition. Among the world's 25 largest economies, the United States outstrips all others on expense (farthest right, along *x* axis) and lags most on life expectancy (farthest down on *y* axis).

Part of the reason U.S. health care is so expensive—and partly why outcomes are poor compared to other advanced countries—involves how it is financed. When it comes to who *pays* for insurance and delivering health care services, here again complexity rules. And also again, political debates and deals are central to America's convoluted architecture of health financing.

WHO PAYS? THE POLITICS OF MEDICARE, MEDICAID, AND MUCH MORE

Some 18% of the U.S. GDP (all goods and services a nation produces) is devoted to health services, a percentage that continues to rise—and that is higher than peer nations, which typically spend around 10% of GDP on health care. Financing those huge health costs involves a jumbled mixture of national, state, and local government; private insurance companies; individual payers; and private charities. Figure 3.5 illustrates the mix of payment sources for U.S. health care.

Look carefully at the figure and you're probably in for a surprise. The largest source of health insurance in the United States is the government: Medicare (a federal government program), Medicaid (joint federal and state), and other

FIGURE 3.4   LIFE EXPECTANCY VS. HEALTH EXPENDITURE: 25 COUNTRIES, 35 YEARS

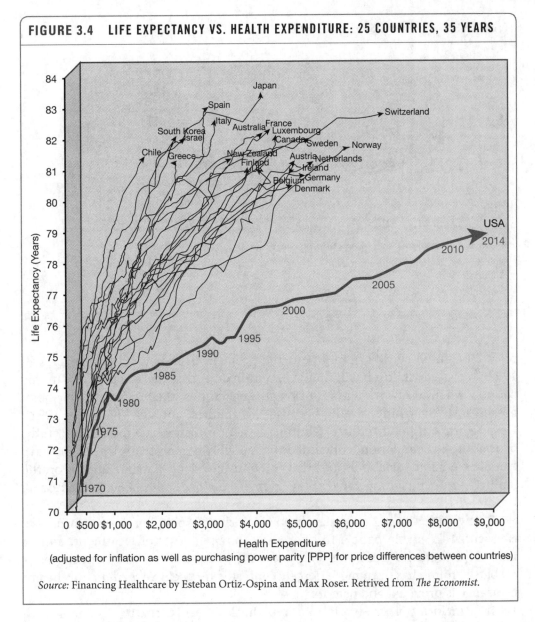

Source: Financing Healthcare by Esteban Ortiz-Ospina and Max Roser. Retrived from *The Economist*.

programs amount to 41% of insurance coverage. Together, these giant entitlement programs (only Social Security is larger) account for approximately $1.18 trillion in government spending, a figure that by 2026 is expected to top $2 trillion. Private plans account for 34% of health care insurance (see Figure 3.5). The next biggest slice: "out of pocket." People pay at the point of service, either to cover cost sharing (which can run to thousands of dollars) or because they have no insurance.

Ironically, because they have no negotiating leverage, uninsured individuals face higher prices than the insurance companies

> Ironically, because they have no negotiating leverage, uninsured individuals face higher prices than the insurance companies pay.

FIGURE 3.5 PAYMENT SOURCES FOR U.S. HEALTH CARE

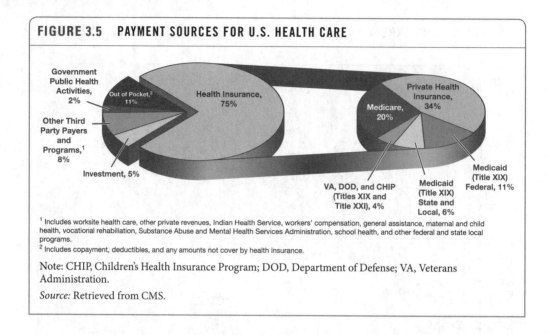

[1] Includes worksite health care, other private revenues, Indian Health Service, workers' compensation, general assistance, maternal and child health, vocational rehabiliation, Substance Abuse and Mental Health Services Administration, school health, and other federal and state local programs.

[2] Includes copayment, deductibles, and any amounts not cover by health insurance.

Note: CHIP, Children's Health Insurance Program; DOD, Department of Defense; VA, Veterans Administration.

Source: Retrieved from CMS.

pay. Bill Clinton starkly pointed out the problem of individual payers back in 1993: "our grandchildren will find it ... unthinkable that there was a time in this country when hardworking families lost their homes, their savings, their businesses, lost everything, simply because the children got sick" (Clinton, 1993). Despite years of policy efforts, Clinton's lament remains true today. One study, by the Kaiser Foundation, concluded that roughly a quarter of Americans have trouble paying medical bills and that the bills have had "a major impact on the family"—often including bankruptcy (Hamel, Norton, Pollitz, Levitt, Claxton, & Brodie, 2018).

Along with soaking up a significant majority of spending, health insurance is essential to enable people to afford the spiraling costs of treatment, among many other benefits (Sommers, Gawande, & Baicker, 2017). No American political battleground has been more fiercely contested in recent years than how health insurance is provided and paid for.

In a majority of the world's nations, health care is free to residents, with insurance provided mainly by the national government. Fall ill in any of 160 countries—from Costa Rica to Zambia, Pakistan to Denmark—and you can seek care secure in the knowledge that government-paid insurance will cover the cost of your treatment. In a smaller group of countries, the private market is a main source of insurance. In Switzerland, for example, the government mandates that everyone have health coverage but does not provide it: Instead, Swiss purchase individual plans from more than 100 private companies. (Government subsidies are provided to people in lower income brackets, on a sliding-scale basis.)

The U.S. system is a patchwork, the result of political compromises on Capitol Hill, state legislatures, city councils, employers, health care institutions, health care professionals, the White House, and more. How did we get to this tangled and fragmented nonsystem? We turn now to a closer look at the peculiar political history of health insurance in America.

Health Insurance Reform: A Brief Political History

President Harry S. Truman (1945–1953) ran for reelection in 1948 touting his national health insurance plan; it was his top domestic priority. However, Congress—dominated by conservative Southern Democrats—buried the issue. The powerful chair of the Senate Finance Committee declined even holding hearings on the proposal. If the United States operated as a parliamentary democracy, like Germany or Canada, the president would have been able (indeed, expected) to pass the program he promised in the campaign. National health insurance fell short—thanks to the American government of checks and balances (Blumenthal & Morone, 2008).

Republican President Dwight D. Eisenhower (1953–1961) was eager to build a private insurance alternative to Truman's plan. His administration made permanent a tax deduction to encourage employers to offer health insurance to workers—and the private health insurance system took off. Note that it was financed by a conscious policy decision: what political economists call a tax expenditure, one that cost the federal government $253 billion in 2018.

With John F. Kennedy's win in 1961, Democrats resurrected the Truman plan, reduced its scope to cover only those over 65, and renamed it Medicare. Their hope was that it would prove so popular that the rest of the population would demand coverage, too. In a legislative coup, planned by President Lyndon Johnson (1963–1969) and the chair of the Ways and Means Committee, Wilbur Mills (D-AK), Congress passed not just Medicare but two counterproposals introduced by the Republicans and the American Medical Association. The final legislation included a federal program that paid hospital and physician costs for people over 65 (Medicare) and a federal state program, administered on the state level, that paid for some categories of poor people, mainly families with dependent children (Medicaid). Even with these limits, opponents denounced the Johnson/Mills program as "socialized medicine." Only 10 House Republicans voted for it, though most changed to "aye" votes after failing to bury the bill (Berkowitz, 2005; Blumenthal & Morone, 2008).

These two programs eventually came to cost a quarter of the entire U.S. federal budget. Periodic expansions of Medicare and Medicaid still left millions of Americans without insurance, at the mercy of a frayed health care safety net. By the early 1990s, nearly 20% of Americans under 65 (the cutoff age after which Medicare provides insurance), or just under 40 million people, had no health insurance. President Bill Clinton, after signing in 1993 a massive bill designed to bring the federal budget back into balance, turned to health care reform. A multiplicity of health care changes were blended into one of the most ambitious legislative efforts since World War II, with extension of insurance at the measure's heart. Opponents, again trumpeting the dangers of government-mismanaged health care, were able to defeat the effort, thanks in part to widely watched television advertisements starring an innocuous American couple, Harry and Louise, worrying aloud about the devastating effects of "letting government choose: We lose."

The Clinton administration assisted opponents by taking a year to design and submit its plan. As Lyndon Johnson well understood, such massive proposed changes very rarely can navigate the American system of multiple vetoes beyond a year after a presidential election. A more focused expansion of insurance for around 660,000 low-income children, known as the Children's Health Insurance Program (CHIP), won bipartisan support and passed in the wake of the Clinton health-reform collapse. Today an expanded CHIP serves nearly 9 million children annually.

Barack Obama submitted his health insurance expansion within 2 months of taking office and, after a year of blistering politics in Congress and in congressional town hall meetings dominated by the rising Tea Party, managed to win passage by February 2009. The legislation finally squeaked through without a single Republican vote. In marked contrast to past reforms (Social Security in 1935, Medicare/Medicaid in 1965), Republicans did not shift their final votes to "aye," but kept right on resisting (Hoffman, 2003).

> To date, "Obamacare" has extended coverage to some 20 million people, around two fifths of those uninsured before the ACA was enacted.

To date, "Obamacare" has extended coverage to some 20 million people, around two fifths of those uninsured before the ACA was enacted. It involves two major programs. First, it subsidized private insurance and required people to purchase it. Second, it put aside the state-by-state Medicaid patchwork and expanded the program to cover everyone under 138% of poverty (today, about $32,000 for a family of four). Notably, the first is the kind of program once sponsored by Republicans; the latter expands a classic big-government program legislated during the Johnson years.

Implacable Republican opposition continued. A Republican-led Congress staged more than 100 votes between 2011 and 2018 to repeal the law and twice advanced repeal to the U.S. Supreme Court, where it failed both times by a 5–4 margin. Donald Trump, whose 2016 presidential campaign was built in part around a promise to eliminate the ACA, dismantled portions of the law through executive orders and ordered sweeping cutbacks in federal advertisements during periodic enrollment periods.

One target of Republican ire is the ACA's individual mandate, which requires most people to have insurance. In order to finance care for sick people, healthy ones must pay into the system—and they, in turn, receive affordable health services should they fall ill. To ensure compliance with the mandate, a financial penalty is charged to those who fail to sign up for insurance (which is heavily subsidized for the poorest Americans). President Trump issued an executive order in 2017 ending that penalty; months afterward in summer 2018, his Justice Department issued a ruling that the mandate itself was unconstitutional (Beech & Lambert, 2018), despite congressional passage and two affirmative decisions in the Supreme Court. In contrast, the Medicaid expansion continues to spread, as we discuss below.

Peering in 2018 into the murky future, the nonpartisan Congressional Budget Office predicted a return to rising numbers of uninsured people, given continued peeling away of the mandate and other aspects of the ACA. What may fairly be viewed as a moral tragedy—that millions of people in the world's wealthiest country are unable to pay for health services—will continue for the forseeable future.

THE POLITICS OF PROVIDING EQUITABLE HEALTH SERVICES

Fifty-eight countries around the globe, including nearly all U.S. peer countries (wealthy democracies), provide universal care—every resident is guaranteed access to the health care system by their government. Of the world's 201 nations, 160 provide free health care: no cost to the patient. This does not mean that people in different income classes are all treated equally—it is possible in some of these 160 countries to buy private insurance, which can ensure superior care. But a minimum level of professional care is generally guaranteed to all. The United States is among the small handful of countries (most of them lower income, like Liberia, Iraq, and Haiti) that do not provide free care and do not seek to cover all residents. One result is significant health disparities in the United States: The quality of health coverage and care varies widely, depending on where you live and how much wealth you have.

> Fifty-eight countries around the globe, including nearly all U.S. peer countries (wealthy democracies), provide universal care—every resident is guaranteed access to the health care system by their government.

Take a look, for example, at Raleigh, North Carolina. Babies born in the 27617 zip code, generally home to wealthier households, have an average life expectancy of **88 years**. Mere miles away, in the 27610 zip code on Raleigh's southeast side, babies born today have a life expectancy of **76 years**: a shocking 12-year gap. That's the difference between Japan (number 1 in life expectancy) and Kyrgyzstan (number 106), or between Germany (ranked 24) and Iraq (121) (World Health Organization, 2016).

Health outcomes are worse in almost every respect: Residents of the 27610 zip code have higher rates of obesity, diabetes, and asthma and return to hospitals within a month of discharge far more often than their neighbors in the 27617 zip code. They miss work for illness far more frequently. And a much higher proportion are uninsured, so when poorer residents seek care at a first-rate medical facility like WakeMed Hospital—if available to them at all—it could break their bank account (VCU Center on Society & Health, 2018). Figure 3.6, produced by Virginia Commonwealth University's Center on Health & Society and the Robert Wood Johnson Foundation, graphically illustrates this Raleigh disparity in life expectancy.

FIGURE 3.6   DIFFERING LIFE EXPECTANCIES BY ZIP CODE: RALEIGH-DURHAM, NORTH CAROLINA

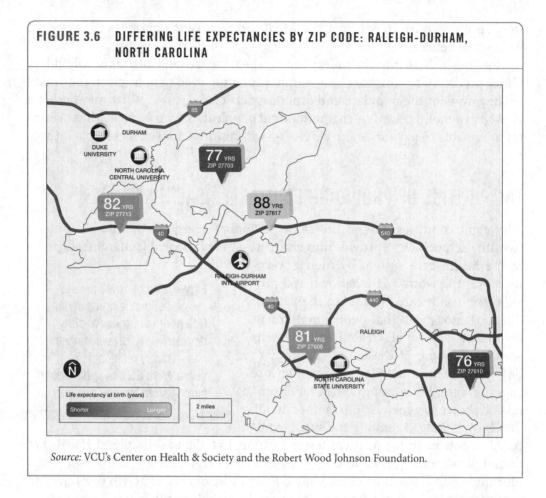

Source: VCU's Center on Health & Society and the Robert Wood Johnson Foundation.

Similarly disturbing divergences are evident across the country: from California, where two freeway exits separate neighborhoods with 9 years' difference in life expectancy, to New York City, where six subway stops also separate a 9-year gap. This stark illustration demonstrates what public health researchers have long known: Health disparities are endemic in the United States (Egen, Beatty, Blackley, Brown, & Wykoff, 2017). Health outcomes across most groupings of Americans rise steadily as education improves, income grows, housing is safer, access to good care exists, and public transportation services are readily available. Once again, all these topics are indelibly colored by political choices—in America's federalist system, decisions are variously made at the national, state, and local level, not infrequently with disagreements and tensions across office holders on each level.

Contributing to political complexity around care for America's less well-off, many rural residents of "red states"—those overwhelmingly voting Republican—both exhibit relatively poor health outcomes and staunchly oppose government efforts to improve their health. Versions of the sign "Keep your government hands off my Medicare!" regularly appeared at Tea Party rallies in the wake of the ACA's passage (Skinner, 2012)—the irony was noted publicly by President Obama, among many others (CNN, 2009).

With little national government efforts at present to address health disparities, some states and cities are taking action themselves. Virginia in June 2018 became the 33rd state (including the District of Columbia) to expand Medicaid to a wider set of needy residents, a policy passed as part of the ACA but left up to individual states. Although conservative governors tended to oppose this extension even though more than 90% of funds came from the national government, the benefits continue to spread (Sommers & Epstein, 2017). Figure 3.7 demonstrates, as of June 2018, which states have opted into this Medicaid expansion—and which have not. All 18 of the latter had Republican governors and/or large GOP majorities in their state legislature at the time of this writing.

HOW PERSONAL HEALTH DECISIONS BECOME PUBLIC: THE CASE OF OBESITY

The preceding discussions demonstrate that policy decisions, emerging from political fights and compromises, are essential to shaping the distinctive U.S. health care system. Certainly health providers, market forces, and patients are also vital contributors—but none of these act absent of political context. And

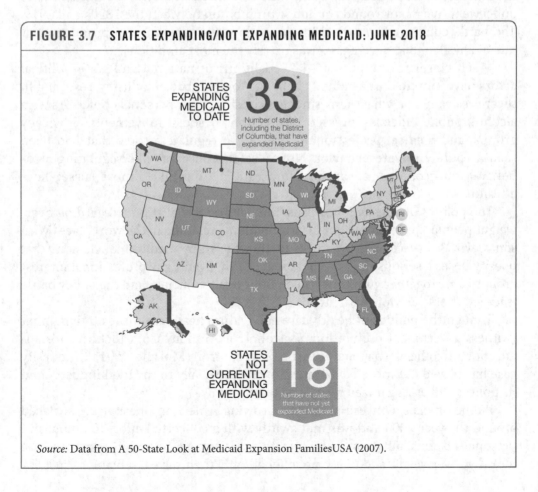

FIGURE 3.7   STATES EXPANDING/NOT EXPANDING MEDICAID: JUNE 2018

Source: Data from A 50-State Look at Medicaid Expansion FamiliesUSA (2007).

that context itself is the subject of a pitched battle among conflicting American ideals. On one hand, the U.S. policy is often described as among the world's most favorable to individual freedom—prizing personal liberty foremost. On the other, repeatedly across our national history government actors have charged freely into private arenas, regulating in the name of public health and safety personal matters like Americans' drinking habits, sexual practices, or tobacco use (Kersh & Morone, 2002a; Kersh & Morone, 2002b). Understanding this push–pull between liberty and government regulation in the name of improved public health is at the heart of health politics in the United States (Chapter 7 focuses on how health and behavior influence health status in further detail).

Alcohol provides one example of private behavior turned subject of public health regulatory regimes, helping to illustrate present-day trends. Alcoholic beverages were long more commonly consumed by Americans than water, given the dangers inherent in untreated water across the United States' first century. (The "revolutionary" first widespread disinfection regimen for water was not introduced until 1881 (McGuire, 2006).) When John Chapman, known as Johnny Appleseed, planted all those apple trees in the 1840s, their fruit was more often used to make fermented or "hard" cider than for eating (Kerrigan, 2012). Despite the ubiquity of cider, beer, rum, and wine on American tables, the United States underwent five major rounds of liquor prohibition between the 1820s and 1919. The battle culminating in the 18th Amendment—outlawing the production or sale of any alcoholic beverages—was merely the most ambitious.

Much closer to the present day, coalitions of national and state political actors have mounted a sustained challenge to the tobacco industry, resulting in severe restraints on what many smokers consider their personal choice. As with alcohol, public officials—pressed into action by social movements, advocacy groups, and medical professionals—moved to regulate a topic that had been seen as purely private behavior. Note also that in areas like regulating alcohol and tobacco, other advanced democratic nations take a more laissez-faire attitude.

The politics of obesity follow this familiar arc: Social stigma regarding overweight people tips into outright discrimination, including in the workplace (Watson, Levit, & Lavack, 2018)—and is further fueled by medical conclusions that obesity poses a serious threat to personal health. Eventually professional interest groups come together with concerned public health officials, and the policy battle is joined (Kersh & Morone, 2010).

Though the politics of health care can feature headlong rushes to judgment (witness government prohibition of alcohol, or Anthony Comstock's Victorian-era efforts to officially ban literature on birth control) (Morone, 2004), the obesity case has played out more deliberately, owing especially to the food industry and its political allies' organized resistance to change.

Public officials' concern about the growing American obesity rate surfaced around the year 2000 and was met swiftly with a concerted effort to emphasize personal responsibility, not "nanny state" government actors, in response. The idea that overweight and obese people had only themselves to blame—"just say no, and push back from the table," in the words of a widely reprinted editorial—tapped a deep individualistic strain in U.S. politics and, especially at the national level, stifled policymaking designed to address nutrition and diet. No significant policy addressing obesity passed Congress between 2000 and 2010, though dozens of bills were introduced; indeed, the only related measure that won approval in either chamber was the "Personal Responsibility in Food Consumption Act of 2005," which protected the food industry against lawsuits. It passed the U.S. House but failed in the Senate (Kersh, 2015; Kersh & Elbel, 2015).

National policy debates also play out in state and local arenas, and here more substantive achievements have been registered. Prominent policies considered and, in some locations, enacted include taxes on sugar-sweetened beverages and junk foods (Pomeranz, Wilde, Huang, Micha, & Mozaffarian, 2018); calorie labels on chain and fast-food restaurant menus (Kiszko, Martinez, Abrams, & Elbel, 2014); government encouragement for "reformulation" of popular snack foods to reduce sugar, salt, and/or fat content (Buttriss, 2013); and regulating the availability and nutritional quality of "competitive foods" served in schools (Datar & Nicosia, 2017).

National policy action on obesity since 2010 has focused on calorie menu labeling, passed as part of the ACA. New York, Philadelphia, Washington's King County, and the State of California were among jurisdictions that implemented a calorie-labeling rule. Even with ample precedent, it took nearly 8 years (and much lobbying on both sides) before the administrative rulemaking process finally yielded a formal labeling rule in May 2018. Meanwhile, U.S. obesity rates have risen inexorably, topping 37% of adults in 2018. Thirty years ago, most U.S. states reported adult obesity rates of 10% or lower, with none higher than 15%. The health consequences of obesity are well chronicled (Meldrum, Morris, & Gambone, 2017), but—much as with the U.S. health system as a whole—the American policymaking system, susceptible at every turn to veto points, interest group influence, and deliberately slowed action, has added layers of complexity rather than opening a path to better health outcomes or reduced expense.

CONCLUSION: BETTER NATIONAL HEALTH AHEAD?

We invited readers at the opening of this chapter to imagine whether the result of extensive politicization of U.S. health systems has led to enhanced patient care or greater efficiency. Comparisons to other countries, as well as a look toward the future—as we write, media alarms are being sounded about Medicare's impending bankruptcy, a few years hence (Edney, 2018)—would suggest that a rosy view is hard to apply. Much as with American society more generally, absent a strong movement for meaningful change, the likely road ahead involves a mixture of dazzling health care innovations, greater disparities in access to care, knee-buckling expenses, and immense investment of time and energy by political as well as health professionals—with little concrete improvement to show for it.

▶ CASE EXERCISE—INSURANCE PLANS

As you sit down to choose your insurance plan for the upcoming year, you have to answer two questions: (a) what is your BMI (body mass index)? and (b) how many cigarettes do you smoke a day? The second question is easy for you because you are not a smoker and never have been. But the first one—well, you are overweight. You need to decide how to answer the question. If you answer truthfully, your insurance rates go up. If you lie, your rates stay the same, but you run the risk of being caught and paying a fine.

1. How would you decide which choice to make? What factors would you consider?

2. Is it fair and equitable to be charged more for insurance if you are overweight or a smoker? What about those who drink or are hypochondriacs—shouldn't they be grouped, too?

DISCUSSION QUESTIONS

1. How is the U.S. health care system financed? How is that different from China and Great Britain?
2. If the government is not paying to support health care, what is it paying for?
3. What is the role of politics in Medicare and Medicaid?
4. How can average citizens use his or her influence on politicians to provide equitable health services?
5. Why are personal health decisions becoming public?

REFERENCES

Alexander, G. C., et al., (2017). Reducing branded prescription drug prices: A review of policy options. *Pharmacotherapy, 37*(11), 1469–1478.

Beech, E. & Lambert, L. (2018). U.S. Justice Department says Obamacare individual mandate unconstitutional. *Reuters.*

Berkowitz, E. (2005). Medicare and Medicaid: The past as prologue. *Health Care Financing Review, 27*(2), 11–23.

Blumenthal, D., & Morone, J. (2008). *The heart of power: Health and politics in the oval office: 1935–2008.* Berkeley, CA: Univ. of California Press.

Buttriss, J. (2013). Food reformulation: The challenges to the food industry. *Proceedings of the Nutrition Society, 72*(1), 61–69.

Clinton, W. J. (1993). *Address to a joint session of Congress on health reform.* Washington, DC: Office of Government Printing.

CNN. (2009). Obama pokes fun at "Don't Touch My Medicare!" People. Retrieved from https://www.youtube.com/watch?v=pJp-roulVsA

Cuckler, G. A., et al. (2018). *National health expenditure projections, 2017–2026: Despite uncertainty, fundamentals primarily drive spending growth. Health Affairs, 37*(3).

Datar, A., & Nicosia, N. (2017). The effect of state competitive food and beverage regulations on childhood overweight and obesity. *Journal of Adolescent Health, 60*(5), 520–527.

Edney, A. (2018). Medicare fund to fall short in 2026, sooner than last forecast. *Bloomberg News*. Retrieved from https://bloom.bg/2sSCzgt

Egen, O., Beatty, K., Blackley, D. J., Brown, K., & Wykoff, R. (2017). Health and social conditions of the poorest versus wealthiest counties in the United States. *American Journal of Public Health*, 107(1), 130–135.

Frank, R. G., & Zeckhauser, R. J. (2018). Excess prices for drugs in Medicare: Diagnosis and prescription. (HKS Working paper no. RWP18-005).

Government Accountability Office (2017). *VA health care: Opportunities exist for improving implementation and oversight of enrollment processes for veterans*. Washington, DC: GAO.

Gusmano, M., & Rodwin, V. G. (this volume). Comparative health systems.

Hamel, L., Norton, M., Pollitz, K., Levitt, L., Claxton, G., & Brodie, M. (2016). The burden of medical debt: Results from the Kaiser Family Foundation/New York Times medical bills survey. Retrieved from. https://kaiserf .am/2zooVau

Henry Kaiser Foundation. (2016). State health facts: Distribution of state general fund expenditures. Retrieved from https://kaiserf .am/2NOuKC2

Hoffman, B. (2003). Health care reform and social movements in the United States. *American Journal of Public Health*, 93(1), 75–85.

Jaroslawski, S., Auquier, P., & Toumi, M. (2017). No correlation between the prices of oncology orphan drugs in the US and their patient population sizes. *Journal of Cancer Policy* 14, 1–4.

Kerrigan, W. (2012). *Johnny Appleseed & the American orchard: A cultural history*. Baltimore, MD: The Johns Hopkins University Press.

Kersh, R. (2015). Of nannies and nudges: Current US food politics. *Public Health, 129*.

Kersh, R., & Elbel, B. (2015). Public policy & obesity: Overview and update. *Wake Forest Journal of Law & Policy*, 5(1), 105–123.

Kersh, R., & Morone, J. (2002a). How the personal becomes political: Prohibitions, public health, and obesity. *Studies in American Political Development*, 16(2), 162–175.

Kersh, R., & Morone, J. (2002b). The politics of obesity: Seven steps to government action. *Health Affairs*, 21(6), 142–153.

Kersh, R., & Morone, J. (2010). Obesity politics & policy. In J. Cawley, ed., *Oxford Handbook of the Social Science of Obesity*. New York: Oxford University Press.

Kesselheim, A. S., Avorn, J. & Sarpatwari, A. (2016). The high cost of prescription drugs in the United States: Origins and prospects for reform. *Journal of the American Medical Association 316*(8), 858–871.

Kiszko, K. M., Martinez, O. D., Abrams, C., & Elbel, B. (2014). The influence of calorie labeling on food orders and consumption: A review of the literature. *Journal of Community Health*, 39(6), 1248–1269.

Kochanek, K. D., Murphy, S. L., Xu, J., & Arias, E. (2017). *Mortality in the United States, 2016*. NCHS Data Brief No. 293.

McGuire, M. J. (2006). Eight revolutions in the history of US drinking water disinfection. *American Water Works Association Journal*, 98(3), 123–149.

Meldrum, D. R., Morris, M. A., & Gambone, J. C. (2017). Obesity pandemic: Causes, consequences, and solutions—but do we have the will? *Fertility & Sterility*, 107(4),833–839.

Morone, J. (2004). *Hellfire nation: The politics of sin in American history*. New Haven, CT: Yale University Press.

Nixon, R. (1969). Remarks at a briefing on the nation's health system.

OECD. (2017). OECD indicators: Health at a glance. Retrieved from https://bit.ly/1iCMVty.

Papanicolas, I., Woskie, L. R., & Jha, A. K. (2018). Health care spending in the United States and other high-income countries. *Journal of the American Medical Association*, 319(10), 1024–1039.

Pharmacy Benefit Consultants' comparison. (2018). Retrieved from https://bit.ly/2xR9OXi

Pomeranz, J. L., Wilde, P., Huang, Y., Micha, R., & Mozaffarian, D. (2018). Legal and administrative feasibility of a federal junk food and sugar-sweetened beverage tax to improve diet. *American Journal of Public Health, 108*(2), 203–209.

Schneider, E. C., et al. (2017). *Mirror, Mirror 2017: International comparison reflects flaws and opportunities for better American health care.* New York: Commonwealth Fund.

Skinner, D. (2012). Keep your government hands off my Medicare!: An analysis of media effects on Tea Party health care politics. *New Political Science, 34*(4).

Sommers, B. D., & Epstein, A. M. (2017). Red-state Medicaid expansions—Achilles' heel of ACA repeal? *New England Journal of Medicine, 376*(6), 1–3.

Sommers, B. D., Gawande, A. A., & Baicker, K. (2017). Health insurance coverage and health— What the recent evidence tells us. *New England Journal of Medicine, 377,* 586–593.

UN official text. (2018) Retrieved from https://bit.ly/J1E1V3

VCU Center on Society & Health. (2018). Mapping life expectancy. Retrieved from https://bit.ly/2FsfyWb

Watson, L., Levit, T., & Lavack, A. (2018). Obesity and stigmatization at work. In S. Thomson and G. Grandy, eds., *Stigmas, work and organizations.* New York: Palgrave Macmillan.

Woolf, S. H., & Aron, L. eds., (2013). *U.S. Health in International Perspective: Shorter Lives, Poorer Health.* Washington, DC: National Academies Press.

World Health Organization. (2016). Life expectancy increased by five years since 2000, but health inequalities persist.

Comparative Health Systems

Michael K. Gusmano and Victor G. Rodwin

LEARNING OBJECTIVES

▶ Understand the difference between national health insurance (NHI) and national health service (NHS) systems

▶ Highlight key features and issues in the health systems of Britain, France, Canada, and China

▶ View the U.S. health system from an international perspective

KEY TERMS

▶ national health insurance (NHI)

▶ national health service (NHS)

TOPICAL OUTLINE

▶ Looking abroad to promote self-examination at home

▶ Health system models

▶ NHS and NHI systems compared with the United States

▶ The health systems in England, Canada, France, and China

▶ Provider payment

▶ Coordination of care

▶ Workforce and information technology (IT)

▶ Health system performance

▶ Lessons

INTRODUCTION

Public opinion polls regularly find that medical professionals and the public are dissatisfied with the system and believe major change is necessary.

Price, volume, and technology diffusion are the most important factors driving health care costs, not an aging population.*

Windows can sometimes be mirrors. A look at health systems abroad can enable us to develop a better understanding of our health system in the United States. An international perspective reveals that the United States has the most expensive health care system in the world. Unlike other wealthy countries, however, the United States fails to provide universal health insurance coverage. Moreover, in contrast to most other wealthy nations, our population faces flagrant inequities in access to primary and specialty care. Health care costs are often a source of financial strain, even bankruptcy, for people with serious illness (Hacker, 2006), and Americans suffer from high rates of mortality that could have been avoided with timely and appropriate access to a range of effective health care services (Nolte & McKee, 2012). There is also evidence that the U.S. health care system squanders resources and fails to address many of its population's health care needs. Not surprisingly, public opinion polls regularly find that medical professionals and the public are dissatisfied with the system and believe major change is necessary (Blendon, Benson, & Hero, 2014; Hargreaves et al., 2015).

Looking Abroad to Promote Self-Examination at Home

International comparisons of health care system performance remind us that there are workable alternatives to our current system. Examining other systems provides "the gift of perspective" and helps us to understand our own system "by reference to what it is like or unlike" (Marmor, Freeman, & Okma, 2005). As Rudolf Klein (1997, p. 1270) explains:

> Policy learning ... is as much a process of self-examination—of reflecting on the characteristics of one's own country and health care system—as of looking at the experience of others ... the experience of other countries is largely valuable insofar as it prompts a process of critical introspection by enlarging our sense of what is possible and adding to our repertoire of possible policy tools. For policy learning is not about the *transfer* of ideas or techniques ... but about their adaptation to local circumstances. (emphasis in original)

This chapter attempts to provide a better understanding of the U.S. health care system by comparing it to health systems in wealthy countries, which share many characteristics in common, and by contrasting it to China, a more striking contrast. Our focus on wealthy nations draws on the experience of member nations of the Organisation for Economic Co-operation and Development (OECD), an organization based in Paris that studies economic trends, policies,

*To hear the podcast, go to https://bcove.video/2Pe60Tv or access the ebook on Springer Publishing Connect™.

and health data of its members. We pay special attention to England,[1] which operates a **national health service (NHS)**, and to Canada and France, which have **national health insurance (NHI)** systems. Our focus on China is an example of so-called BRIC nations (Brazil, Russia, India, and China) with large populations that have benefited from rapid economic growth over the past two decades and now are demanding access to state-of-the-art medical care.

Although England's NHS is one of the most public systems in the world, it also allows opportunities for private hospitals, private practice, and private insurance for those who prefer such options. Canada is frequently compared with the United States because of its physical proximity and similar political culture; until the mid-1960s, Canada's health care financing and delivery systems were nearly identical to those in the United States (Marmor et al., 2005). France's health system also shares many features with the U.S. health system. Like the United States, France relies on a multipayer system for financing care and offers a mix of public and private providers for delivering health care services. French citizens also enjoy freedom of choice among providers—to an even greater extent than Americans. The French experience (Rodwin, 2006) suggests that it is possible to achieve universal coverage without adopting a single-payer NHI system, such as Canada's, or an NHS, as in England. China has proclaimed a commitment to universal health care coverage and, given its size and progress over the past decade, represents an important case study. Despite its rapidly growing economy, China's national investments in public health and medical care are still far smaller than those of OECD nations, and out-of-pocket payments represent roughly one-third of all health care expenditures. We conclude the chapter with some lessons of comparative experience for U.S. policy makers.

HEALTH SYSTEM MODELS

NHS systems, such as those in the United Kingdom, Sweden, Norway, Finland, Denmark, Portugal, Spain, Italy, and Greece, may be traced back to Lord Beveridge, who wrote the blueprint for the English NHS immediately after World War II. Although such systems are characterized by a dominant share of financing derived from general revenue taxes, this does not preclude other forms of financing. For example, the relative size of private financing and provision is much higher in Italy and Spain than in Sweden or Denmark. In England, 76% of NHS funding comes from general taxation, 18% from a payroll tax, and the remainder from private payments (Thomson, Osborn, Squires, & Reed, 2012, p. 33). Historically, NHI systems have had a more open-ended reimbursement system for health care providers, but this distinction is blurring as NHI systems are increasingly under pressure to operate within budget limits.

NHI systems may be traced back to Chancellor Otto von Bismarck, who established the first NHI program for salaried industrial workers in Germany in 1883. With the exception of Canada, whose dominant share of financing is from general

---

[1] We focus on England, the largest constituent country within the United Kingdom, because there are important differences among the NHS in Scotland, Wales, and Northern Ireland.

tax revenues, these systems are characterized by payroll tax-based financing. In addition to income taxes, about a quarter of Canada's federal spending on health care comes from corporations. The provinces also supplement income and corporate taxes with additional sources of funding such as sales, tobacco, and alcohol taxes. As with NHS systems, NHI systems are characterized by significant variation in their financing and organizational arrangements. For example, the share of French public health care expenditures financed from an income tax on all earnings, including dividends and interest from capital, increased to 16% in 2016 (Rodwin, 2018).

Whether one's image of a health system is private and market-based, as in the United States and Switzerland; public and government-managed, as in the United Kingdom and Scandinavian nations; or at some intermediary point along such a continuum, as in France and Canada, it is possible to make some useful distinctions with respect to the public versus private provision of health care and methods of financing health services. Table 4.1 classifies health systems along these dimensions.

Provision of Health Services

The arrangements for providing health care in Table 4.1 distinguish whether health services are delivered by the public, private not-for-profit, or private for-profit sector. Within these categories, many distinctions may be added. For example, some publicly capitalized organizations (row A) are national (e.g., the Veterans Health Administration [VHA] in the United States), others are subnational (state mental hospitals), and many are local (municipal hospitals). Likewise, the not-for-profit category may include a variety of quasi-public organizations, such as hospital trusts in Britain (row B). The for-profit form of provision (row C) includes private for-profit hospitals and a distinctive subcategory in the United States – hospitals and managed care organizations (MCOs) that sell ownership shares to investors on publicly traded stock markets. Indeed, the growth of large investor-owned MCOs distinguishes the United States from most other OECD nations.

TABLE 4.1 HEALTH SYSTEM PROVISION AND FINANCING

DELIVERY APPROACH	FINANCING			
	Government Income Taxes and General Revenue 1	Social Security/NHI Payroll Taxes 2	Private Insurance 3	Out-of-Pocket Payments 4
Government Owned and Operated A				
Private Nonprofit/ Quasi-Government B				
Private For-Profit C				

Financing

The four methods of raising revenues to pay for health services correspond to columns 1 through 4:

- 1: General revenue financing through the fiscal tax system, including personal income taxes
- 2: Compulsory payroll tax financing through the Social Security system
- 3: Voluntary premiums assessed by private health insurance companies and often paid by either employees or individuals
- 4: Individual out-of-pocket payments made at the time a patient receives a service

Although all countries rely on blends of these four sources of revenue to finance health care services, most developed countries have adopted one of two distinct health system models for actually getting care delivered to patients. NHS systems generally rely on the government to organize the delivery of services directly and either employ providers directly or as private contract employees. In NHI systems, governments organize social insurance programs that reimburse health care providers for services rather than paying for health care directly through the government's budget. NHI systems generally rely mostly on payroll taxes to fund their health services. NHS systems, however, rely on general revenue taxation such as income taxes and a broad range of other taxes to fund the delivery system. Using income taxes and general revenues allows for greater redistribution of resources from the wealthy to the poor. Payroll types are generally not highly redistributive.

In contrast to England, Canada, and France, China and the United States rely, to varying degrees, on subnational and local governments to finance health care. In Canada, provinces and territories administer universal health insurance programs, and the federal government provides block grants that account for approximately 20% of health care expenditures. To qualify for the federal funds, provincial and territorial health insurance systems must meet five criteria specified by the Canada Health Act of 1984. They must be (a) administered on a nonprofit basis by a public authority; (b) comprehensive in the sense that they must cover most health services provided by hospitals, medical practitioners, and dentists; (c) universal in that all legal Canadian residents are covered; (d) portable so that coverage for all residents in each province or territory is transferable to all other parts of Canada; and (e) accessible, although "reasonable access" is not defined in the law.

In 2009, China adopted a reform that provided health insurance for all of its population. Between 2000 and 2013, the share of government total health expenditure doubled from 15.5% to 30.1% (Qian, 2015). Although China now provides some minimal health insurance to the majority of its population, coverage remains extremely limited, and as we noted earlier, roughly one-third of all spending on health care still comes from out-of-pocket payments (Table 4.1, column 4). In terms of public funding for health care, China relies—to an even greater extent than Canada—on subnational government revenues to finance the country's three NHI funds.

Below the national government, China has provincial, regional, and local governments. By the mid-1990s, these subnational government authorities financed 80% to 90% of total government spending on social services, including health care (Hipgrave et al., 2012). The adoption of health reform has increased central government contributions to health care, but local government taxes and out-of-pocket payments from individual patients still represent the two largest sources of revenue. This approach has exacerbated the large economic disparities between the wealthier coastal provinces and the poorer rural provinces in western China. The national government has attempted to address the country's rural-urban disparities, but with limited success.

NHS AND NHI SYSTEMS COMPARED WITH THE UNITED STATES

Table 4.1 enables one to highlight key features of NHS and NHI systems and to adopt an international perspective on the U.S. health care system. The most striking difference between the United States and NHS or NHI systems is that the United States—even after passage of the Patient Protection and Affordable Care Act of 2010 (ACA)—includes large elements of financing based on actuarial principles whereby private insurance premiums (column 3) are set with respect to estimated risk. In contrast, in NHS and NHI systems, most health care financing is based on ability to pay (columns 1 and 2). Ability-to-pay criteria lead to wealthier, younger, and healthier individuals paying disproportionately to finance the care of poorer, older, and sicker individuals. Aside from this important distinction, the rows and columns of Table 4.1 suggest that most health care systems have elements of many boxes ranging from socialized medicine (box A1) to out-of-pocket payment for private practitioners and hospitals (box C4).

The United States has neither an NHS nor an NHI system. Instead, the U.S. health care system relies on a patchwork of public and private insurance with large gaps in coverage (see Chapter 3). Its enormous pluralism exhibits components of its health system within each of the boxes in Table 4.1. It uses a social insurance system for older people and for those with permanent disabilities (Medicare: columns 1 and 2); a social welfare system for some people with low incomes (Medicaid, column 2); and an employer-based private health insurance system for a large percentage of salaried employees in the private and public sectors (column 3). Along with its public and private insurance programs, the United States also has elements of socialized medicine, such as the military health care system, the VHA system, and the Indian Health Service (IHS) for Native American and Alaskan Native people.

THE HEALTH SYSTEMS IN ENGLAND, CANADA, FRANCE, AND CHINA

Beyond the differences we have noted between NHI and NHS systems, these systems have evolved in similar directions. After World War II, governments have gradually extended their role in the financing and provision of health services. What was once largely the responsibility of the family,

> After World War II, governments have gradually extended their role in the financing and provision of health services.

philanthropy, religious institutions, employers, and local governments has largely been taken over by national and subnational governments—a trend that has accompanied the rise of the welfare state (de Kervasdoué, Kimberly, & Rodwin, 1984). This evolution has affected all wealthy OECD nations and, increasingly, BRIC and less developed nations. The U.S. reliance on employer-based private health insurance for many Americans is an important contrast to NHI and NHS systems. Yet even in the United States, recent decades have seen an expansion of public insurance and a decline in employer-based coverage.

The growth of government involvement in health systems has characterized OECD nations during the great boom years of health sector growth (1950s and 1960s) when governments encouraged hospital construction and modernization, workforce training, and biomedical research. It continued in the 1970s, when the goals of OECD countries shifted more in the direction of rationalization and cost containment (Rodwin, 1984). In the early 21st century, public and private health insurance has become the dominant source for funding health care, and public expenditure on health care services, along with education and Social Security, has become one of the largest categories of social expenditures as a share of gross domestic product (GDP).

In contrast to these trends in OECD nations, by the end of the 1970s, China moved from a health system dominated by public financing to one dominated by private, out-of-pocket payments. Between 1949 and the early 1980s, the Chinese health system was financed largely by the central government and state-owned enterprises (Valentine, 2005). In 1978, Deng Xiaoping called for market reforms. The central government reduced its share of national health care spending from 32% to 15% (Blumenthal & Hsiao, 2005). It slashed subsidies to public hospitals and introduced market mechanisms in health care, resulting in rapid growth of out-of-pocket payments and income-based inequities.

By the late 1990s, Chinese officials increased investment in public health to address growing disparities between rural and urban areas. Efforts to improve the public health and primary care systems accelerated after the outbreak of severe acute respiratory syndrome (SARS) in late 2002. By the end of 2003, more than 5,000 people were infected with SARS and 349 people died (Smith, 2006), thus exposing the weaknesses of the public health system. Since 2009, China has continued to expand the role of government through the creation of new public insurance schemes and the adoption of new public health regulations (Wang, Gusmano, & Cao, 2011).

In addition to the growth of government's role in health care, most OECD nations confront common challenges and exhibit distinct approaches for many issues. We illustrate how this is so by comparing the health systems of England, Canada, France, and China with respect to (a) provider payment, (b) coordination of care, (c) workforce and IT, and most important, (d) health system performance.

Provider Payment

All countries rely on multiple methods for paying physicians and hospitals. NHS systems traditionally have relied more on salaried and capitation forms of payment for physicians and budgets for hospitals. In the English system, about two-thirds of general practitioners (GPs) and dentists work as independent contractors reimbursed through a blended payment system, 75% from capitation payment and most of the rest (20%) from fee-for-service (FFS) payments based on performance. Since 2012, GPs have been placed in charge of clinical commissioning groups (CCGs), which control about 70% of the NHS budget (NHS Clinical Commissioners, 2018). CCGs are locally specific NHS bodies in charge of planning and commissioning health care for their area, including purchasing hospital and specialty medical care services for their patients. The NHS first introduced a prospective payment system for reimbursing public and private hospitals in 2003 and, in April 2004, phased in a new national tariff system. Since 2012, the NHS has adopted a Payment by Results (PbR) system based on the average cost of providing the procedure or the treatment across the NHS as a whole.

Historically, Canadian primary care physicians have been paid on an FFS basis. The Ministries of Health for all provinces and territories are responsible for negotiating an annual physician fee schedule based on a relative value scale (RVS) for each reimbursable procedure or code. The RVS may have developed from a resource-based fee schedule (RBFS), which tries to capture the inputs required to provide the service, or on historical charges. Studies have found wide variation in fee schedules across Canada (Roth & Adams, 2009). In more recent years, some provinces have experimented with blended capitation schemes in family health networks, family health teams, and family health organizations. Blended capitation relies on age- and gender-adjusted payments, coupled with financial incentives to follow "evidence-based" guidelines and FFS when physicians treat patients who are not enrolled in these schemes (HealthForceOntario, 2014).

In France, physicians in the ambulatory sector and in private hospitals are reimbursed largely on the basis of a fee schedule negotiated among physician associations, the central administration of NHI funds, and the government. Approximately 10% of GPs and 40% of specialists in private office-based practice have the option to extra-bill beyond the negotiated fees that represent payment in full for all other physicians. These figures vary by subspecialty and location. Physicians who have opted to extra-bill may do so as long as their charges are set with "tact and measure," a standard that has never been legally defined but which has been found, empirically, to represent a 50% to 100% increase to the negotiated fees. Physicians who "extra-bill" receive more revenue per patient seen but they need to recruit from a subset of patients able and willing to pay this extra out-of-pocket payment. Physicians based in public hospitals are remunerated on a part-time or full-time salaried basis, and those in private for-profit hospitals may bill NHI based on the negotiated fees.

Before 1984, public hospitals in France were reimbursed on the basis of a retrospective, cost-based, per diem fee; after that, they were placed on global budgets that were later gradually adjusted for patient case mix in the 1990s. Private for-profit hospitals used to be reimbursed on the basis of a negotiated per diem fee; in the 1990s, the per diem payments were also gradually adjusted for their case mix. The basis for case-based adjustment in France is an adaptation of the U.S. diagnosis-related group (DRG) categories known in France as GHM (groupes homogènes de malades). The most recent modification was introduced in 2004 (Schreyögg, Stargardt, Tiemann, & Busse, 2006) when activity-based payment (ABP) was introduced to create a level playing field for reimbursement of acute-care services among public and private hospitals. As of 2012, the reimbursement system for public and private hospitals has been completely aligned based on the national ABP tariffs that take into account each hospital's historical costs. This has resulted in expected activity growth, which in turn, results in downward price adjustments because annual hospital costs are constrained by national and regional hospital expenditure targets (Or, 2010).

In China, the expansion of health insurance is changing the nature of provider payment, but by the end of 2013 most physicians were still paid salaries. Subnational governments in China regulate prices in an effort to make health care affordable, and over the past two decades, with encouragement from the central government, they have introduced such incentives as pay-for-performance based on treatment protocols to improve quality (Yip, Hsiao, Meng, Chen, & Sun, 2010). Although the central government hopes the expansion of health insurance will limit hospital reliance on kickback payments from medical device and pharmaceutical companies, such payments continue to be an important source of revenue for Chinese health care providers (Wang et al., 2011; Shi et al., 2018).

> Two distinguishing characteristics of the U.S. health care system are that, in contrast to other OECD countries, there is neither a national budget cap nor a formal process of price negotiation between payers and representatives of physicians.

In comparison to England, Canada, France, and China, the United States pays significantly higher prices for medical care. Although there is some debate about the factors that drive U.S. health care spending, consensus has emerged that price is the most important factor in explaining why the United States spends so much more than any other health care system in the world (Papanicolas, Woskie, & Jha, 2018). Two distinguishing characteristics of the U.S. health care system are that, in contrast to other OECD countries, there is neither a national budget cap nor a formal process of price negotiation between payers and representatives of physicians.

Coordination of Care

All countries suffer from problems of coordination among hospitals and community-based services. They differ, nonetheless, with regard to the resources and organization of their delivery systems. France, for example, has more practicing doctors per 1,000 population (3.3) than the United Kingdom (2.8), the United States (2.6), Canada (2.7), or China (1.8) (OECD, 2015). France also has more acute hospital beds per 1,000 population (4.1) than the United States (2.5), the United Kingdom (3.0, 2013), Canada (2.0), or China (2.7, 2013) (OECD, 2013, 2015).

Since its creation in 1948, the NHS has been one of the largest public service organizations in Europe. With more than 1 million employees, more than 2,500 hospitals, and a host of intermediary health care organizations, the NHS poses an awesome managerial challenge (Klein, 2013, 2018). Perhaps because Britain has fewer health care resources than most OECD nations, the British have been more aggressive in efforts to reduce inefficiency than other wealthier countries. Because the NHS faces the same demands as other systems to make technology available and to care for an increasingly aged population, British policy makers recognize they must pursue innovations that improve efficiency in the allocation of limited resources. Such efforts, however, face numerous obstacles: opposition by professional bodies, difficulties in firing and redeploying health care personnel, and, not least, the tripartite structure of the NHS, which, since its inception, has created an institutional separation among hospitals, general practitioners, and community health programs. This separation is reinforced further by the fact that local authorities are responsible for a great deal of prevention and health promotion as well as social care, making it difficult to integrate hospital and community-based care.

In Canada, less separation exists between physicians and hospitals because specialists are paid FFS and work both in community-based practice as well as in hospitals. Hospitals are largely private nonprofit institutions with their own governing boards, but they are almost entirely publicly financed and subject to tight budget constraints. Most community-based physicians must refer their patients requiring diagnostic procedures and testing, as well as more specialized care, to local hospitals, which can lead to extended waiting times for elective procedures and problems in ensuring optimal coordination among hospital specialists and community-based providers.

France also faces problems with the coordination of care between hospitals and community-based providers. There is inadequate communication between full-time, salaried physicians in public hospitals and solo physicians working in private practice. Although GPs have informal referral networks to specialists and public hospitals, no formal institutional relationships exist to ensure continuity of medical care; disease prevention; health promotion services; posthospital follow-up care; or systematic linkages and referral patterns among primary-, secondary-, and tertiary-level services. Schoen et al. (2012) document that the French health care system is characterized by poor hospital discharge planning and a lack of coordination among medical providers.

In China, before 1978 the health care delivery system in rural areas was organized by communes, which provided housing, education, and social services as well as basic medical care. An important feature of the communes' Cooperative Medical System was the staff of paraprofessionals known as "barefoot doctors" (Rosenthal & Greiner, 1982). Most of the barefoot doctors were young peasants who received a few months of training and offered basic primary and preventive care, including health education. If the needs of patients were more complex, the barefoot doctors would refer them to physicians at the commune health centers or, if necessary, to the closest hospital. In urban areas, the health care delivery system relied heavily on so-called first-level hospitals, community clinics with a modest inpatient capacity, to provide ambulatory care.

With the introduction of market mechanisms in the health sector after 1978, the government ended its barefoot doctor program in rural areas, leaving the population in rural China without adequate access to health care services. It also reduced its subsidies to state-owned first-level hospitals; forced to become more self-reliant, these hospitals withdrew public health and primary health care services. Some first-level hospitals went bankrupt, and those that survived turned to profitable medical services rather than emphasizing primary care and prevention. Since the 2009 reform, the rapid increase in health insurance coverage brought nearly 1 billion people back under some form of financial protection. Service utilization has increased and hospital care has become more affordable, but there are still glaring disparities across regions and medical sectors (He & Meng, 2015). Moreover, a strong system of primary care is conspicuously absent, and coordination among primary care and hospitals remains an elusive goal.

Workforce and Information Technology

Primary care versus specialty care balance. Among OECD health care systems, an average of 31% of physicians are generalists. The United States stands out, in contrast, because about 90% of physicians are specialists, and only about 10% are generalists (Laugesen, 2018). Despite this difference, when adjustments are made, it turns out that one third of the physician workforce in the United States and other OECD nations works in primary care. The situation in China, however, presents a striking contrast because only 57% of cities have community-based primary care organization, and more than 40% of the population reports that it does not have convenient access to a primary care center (Wang et al., 2011). In addition, most general practitioners lack additional training after receiving their undergraduate medical education.

Primary care is important because systems with a higher concentration of primary care practitioners improve coordination and continuity of care. Access to an effective system of primary care appears to result in higher life expectancy at birth, lower infant mortality, lower mortality from all causes, lower disease-specific mortality, and higher self-reported health status (Starfield, Shi, & Macinko, 2005; World Health Organization [WHO], 2008).

Workforce shortages/surpluses. Concerns about the adequacy of primary care in the United States are reinforced by discussions about the adequacy of the health and social care workforce in the face of rapid population aging (Carrier, Yee, & Stark, 2011). Increases in Alzheimer's disease and other forms of dementia have raised concerns about the extent to which the health and long-term care systems will have a sufficient number of physicians, nurses, and other medical professionals to address the needs of an aging society (Warshaw & Bragg, 2014).

Although a shortage of clinicians, particularly in primary care, is the major concern in the United States, France, and China, some countries in Europe, particularly England, now wonder whether they may have too many doctors and nurses. Before the global economic crisis began in 2008, many OECD countries adopted policies designed to increase their supply of medical professionals. After the economic slowdown, many countries expressed concern about an "oversupply" of some health care workers (Ono, Lafortune, & Schoenstein, 2013).

Starting in 2000, for example, the English NHS adopted a workforce redesign initiative to increase the number of doctors and nurses in the system, expand the roles of existing professionals, and redistribute responsibilities to rely more on teams of health care professionals. As a result, there is now concern that the country may have too many hospital specialists, but there are persistent concerns that it still does not have a large enough supply of well-trained social care workers, particularly for providing home care to older patients (Bohmer & Imison, 2013). Similarly, a recent assessment of health care needs in Ontario, Canada, concluded that there will be an aggregate surplus of GPs and specialists in 20 years, even though some specialties and areas may experience shortages (Moat, Waddell, & Lavis, 2016).

The push for electronic medical records and other forms of health care IT. Throughout the world, policy makers are searching for ways to reduce health care spending while improving the quality of care. The use of electronic health records and other forms of health information technology (HIT) are often touted as solutions to these problems (see Chapter 14). Harvey Fineberg (2012), the president of the Institute of Medicine, argues that over the long term, HIT will improve the quality and efficiency of the health care system. Marmor and Oberlander (2012, p. 1217) dismiss the focus on HIT as a "fad" and suggest that the desire to find a "big fix" to the problems of cost and quality has led policy makers to embrace technical and managerial solutions, including the adoption of HIT, along with various forms of managed care, health planning, and payment reforms designed to align the incentives of providers and patients with public health goals.

This argument supports the classic James Morone (1993) thesis that the United States tends to search for a "painless prescription" to the major challenges in health care. Indeed, comparative analysis suggests that such technical solutions as HIT to the problems of cost and quality have had little effect on cost or quality in health care and that the United States should focus on more important structural features of other health care systems, such as global budgets, fee schedules, systemwide payment rules, and concentrated purchasing power.

Advocates of HIT argue that newer developments in the use of so-called big data are more likely to transform medical practice because of their capacity to link information among many institutions within a health care system. They also argue that the United States has never adopted HIT on a widespread basis, so the failure of previous efforts to improve quality or lower costs is not sufficient evidence that HIT cannot contribute to these goals in the future.

It seems plausible to suggest that HIT may be a valuable tool for addressing costs and quality in health care, but its value surely depends on the policy context in which it is used. For England, Canada, and France, HIT may further enhance the efficiency of resource allocation by providing administrators, providers, and patients with access to better information. In the United States, however, the effect of HIT within the context of a fragmented, open-ended financing system may be far more limited. Viewed from this perspective, it is easier to understand the arguments of those who remain skeptical of HIT's importance.

Health System Performance

Policy makers and researchers often want to compare the performance of different systems and identify lessons for health policy. Although these efforts have generated important information, they have often succumbed to the temptation of devising a composite indicator to rank health care systems against one another (Oliver, 2012). This practice encourages lavish attention from the media on the search for the best health care system, the new holy grail of performance assessments. Unfortunately, such an approach lacks any effort to understand, assess, and compare health care systems in relation to the cultural context, values, and institutions within which performance indicators are embedded.

The study of health system performance by the WHO is the most prominent example of the composite indicator approach to the comparative analysis of health systems (WHO, 2000). WHO ranked the health systems of 191 member states based on weighted measures of five objectives: (a) maximizing population health (as calculated by disability-adjusted life expectancy, or DALE); (b) reducing inequalities in population health; (c) maximizing health system responsiveness; (d) reducing inequalities in responsiveness; and (e) financing health care equitably.

Although controversial because of its many methodological flaws and missing data, the WHO report generated tremendous discussion about health system performance and the criteria that should be used to assess it (Musgrove, 2003). Some of the controversy generated by the report can be attributed to complaints from countries unhappy with their ranking, but prominent academics also criticized the study for relying on incomplete and inadequate data as well as on questionable methods (Williams, 2001).

WHO's use of DALE as a measure of health status illustrates the problem of using population health status to assess the performance of health care systems. DALE includes causes of death that are amenable to health care as well as a host of social determinants of health. As a result, this measure is not "related directly to the health care system" (Nolte & McKee, 2003, p. 1129). Using DALE, life expectancy at birth and infant mortality are inadequate measures of health system performance because the role of health care in improving population health is small compared with interventions aimed at social and environmental determinants.

As Bradley and Taylor (2013) argue, one reason the United States performs so poorly on such indicators is because we have failed to invest sufficiently in education, housing, employment, and other social programs that help to produce and sustain good health. Between those who emphasize the decisive effect of social determinants of health and those who focus on access to health care, there is a middle ground: attention not only to the consequences of poor social conditions, but also to barriers in access to what we have called effective health care services.

There is a vast literature that measures inequities in access to health care (see Chapter 2). Such studies rely either on comparisons of inputs (e.g., physicians, hospital beds) or on administrative or self-reported survey data to measure service utilization. An alternative approach attempts to capture the consequences of poor access to disease prevention, primary care, and specialty services—in other words, mortality amenable to health care (amenable mortality). Of course, few causes of death are entirely amenable, or not amenable to health care, and as medical therapies improve even more deaths may be classified as potentially avoidable. Nevertheless, based on an OECD study, this summary provides convincing evidence that the United States is not performing well in comparison to other wealthy nations (Mossialos, Wenzl, Obsorn, & Sarnak, 2016).

Cross-national analysis of trends in avoidable mortality indicates that amenable deaths have declined much faster over the last three decades than other causes of death (Nolte & McKee, 2012). This result lends further credence to the validity of amenable mortality as an indicator of the effectiveness of public health interventions and medical care. We have used this measure to compare the health systems in megacities located within four of the countries we highlight in this chapter: London, New York, Paris, and Shanghai (Gusmano, Weisz, & Rodwin, 2009).

Through ACOs in the United States (see Chapter 11) and various forms of disease management and integrated service delivery proposals in other countries, health care professionals are being encouraged to think about population as well as individual health. The effort to shift health systems in this direction is a positive development, but if we hope to understand the performance of health care systems and the relationship between health care inputs and health outputs, it is important to select such indicators as amenable mortality, which are more closely related to the performance of these systems than are broad measures of health such as life expectancy and DALEs.

The extensive criticism of WHO's effort to evaluate health system performance has not discouraged other groups from taking similar approaches. The Commonwealth Fund has a project designed to identify high-performing health systems within the United States and other wealthy nations. It also draws on more dependable data than WHO's for its assessments in part because its scope is more limited and focuses on nations for which population, health, and health system data are more readily available. For example, the Commonwealth Fund supplements many of the same data sources used by WHO with original surveys of patients and primary care providers fielded by Harris Interactive (Commonwealth Fund, 2014).

It then uses these survey results, along with a host of other data sources, to compare U.S. national averages on multiple criteria grouped by such categories as health outcomes, quality, access, efficiency, and equity (Schneider, Sarnak, Squires, Shah, & Doty, n.d.). The problem with such an approach, well summarized by Schneider and Squires (2017), is that little attention is paid to the validity of the multiple criteria measured and no rationale is provided for weighting the main categories equally and then ranking health systems on the basis of criteria on which diverse publics and policy makers rarely agree.

Access to services across income groups. An important dimension of health system performance is the extent to which a system provides access to health care services by income group. In contrast to the United States, countries with universal or near-universal coverage enjoy a relatively equitable distribution of primary care visits (van Doorslaer & Masseria, 2004). Lower-income residents of Australia, Canada, New Zealand, and the United Kingdom, for example, are less likely to report barriers to health care than people with below-median incomes in the United States (Blendon et al., 2002). A comparative study on hospitalizations for ambulatory care sensitive conditions (ACSCs), a measure of access to timely and effective primary care, finds that rates are much lower in England, France, and Germany than in the United States (Gusmano, Rodwin, & Weisz, 2014).

A concern often voiced by conservative analysts in the United States is that so-called "government-run" health care systems, by which they mean both NHS and NHI systems, "ration" care (Goodman, Musgrave, & Herrick, 2004). Because such systems operate within a budget, these analysts claim, they must limit access to specialty and surgical health care services in ways that are unacceptable. This claim is supported by studies that compare access to certain expensive health care services in England and the United States (Aaron, Schwartz, & Cox, 2005). Although there is evidence that some expensive technologies, including revascularization and kidney dialysis, are used less frequently in England than in the United States (Gusmano & Allin, 2011), this is not the case with respect to France or Germany. For example, after controlling for need, the use of revascularization (coronary artery bypass and angioplasty) is comparable in France, Germany, and the United States (Gusmano et al., 2014).

Even among countries that provide universal coverage, there are differences in access to specialty services by socioeconomic status. Residents of higher-income neighborhoods in Winnipeg, Canada, a country that strives to eliminate financial barriers to care, receive "substantially more" specialty and surgical care than lower-income residents of the city (Roos & Mustard, 1997). In France, Germany, and England, access to some specialty health care services is significantly worse among residents of lower-income neighborhoods (Gusmano et al., 2009). Inequalities in access to health care are even greater in BRIC countries and developing nations. Despite remarkable economic growth in recent decades, for example, there are flagrant disparities in access to health care within China.

Cost. As was evident during the debates over the ACA, there is a widely shared belief among American policy makers that a national program providing for universal entitlement to health care in the United States would result in runaway costs. In response to this presumption, nations that entitle all of their residents to a high level of medical care, while spending less on administration and on health care than the United States, are often held up as models. The Canadian health system is the most celebrated example. French NHI is another case in point. England's NHS, although typically considered a "painful prescription" for the United States (Aaron et al., 2005), nevertheless ensures first-dollar coverage for basic health services to its entire population and, as we have seen, spends less than half as much on health care, as a percentage of GDP, and significantly less on health care per capita as in the United States (Table 4.2). Huang (2011) expects that China's total health care expenditures will increase rapidly over the coming decade, but its current spending, as a percentage of GDP, is far below the OECD average.

Stories in the media often suggest that pressures from population aging will render existing welfare state commitments, including the Medicare and Medicaid programs in the United States, unsustainable. Despite these concerns, most studies conclude there is no correlation between the percentage of the older population (65 years and over) and health care expenditures as a percentage of GDP. The United States, which spends more on health care than any country in the world, is among the OECD countries with the youngest age cohorts. In contrast, Britain, Italy, Sweden, Germany, and France, with older populations than the United States, spend a far lower percentage of GDP on health care. Even if one excludes the United States and examines only the European Union, there is no correlation between population aging and health care spending.

Cross-national analysis of health care expenditure data indicates that, after controlling for income, age has little effect on national health care expenditures.

TABLE 4.2 HEALTH CARE EXPENDITURE AS A SHARE OF GDP: SELECTED COUNTRIES, 2016

United States	17.2%
France	11%
Canada	10.6%
United Kingdom	9.7%
OECD Average	8.9%
China	5.5%*

* Data only available up to 2014.

GDP, gross domestic product; OECD, Organisation for Economic Co-operation and Development.

Source: Organisation for Economic Co-operation and Development. (2017). *Health at a glance 2017: OECD indicators.* Paris, France: OECD Publishing.

Proximity to death, not age, leads to an increase in health spending (Moon, 1996). An analysis of health spending on older people in Switzerland found that expenditures are concentrated in the last few months of life (Zweifel, Felder, & Meiers, 1999). Although the OECD analysts project that "age-related spending for the average country will rise by around 6 to 7 percentage points of GDP between 2000 and 2050," they acknowledge that "part of this pressure is a result of cost pressures from advances in medical technologies, rather than ageing per se" (Australian Department of the Treasury, 2007).

Price, volume, and technology diffusion are the most important factors that drive health care costs; as noted earlier, however, high U.S. prices explain why the U.S. health care system is so expensive relative to other nations (Papanicolas et al., 2018). Although Americans spend more than any other nation, health service use in the United States is actually below the median for the OECD on most measures. A study for the McKinsey Global Institute (Angrisano, Farrell, Kocher, Laboissiere, & Parker, 2007), based on four diseases, provides further support for the role of prices in driving up U.S. health care costs. The study found that in 1990, Americans spent about 66% more per capita on health care than Germans but received 15% fewer real health care resources.

In addition to understanding the factors that drive health care spending, it is important to confront the question: How much spending on health care is too much? Most health economists argue that there is no right amount of money to spend on health care. Cutler (2007) argues that we should focus less on the level of health care expenditure and pay greater attention to whether the expenditures generate more benefits than costs. However, efforts to adopt explicit economic evaluation of health technology provoked controversy in the United States. The ACA forbids federal government agencies from using cost as a criterion for making coverage decisions. Among the countries compared in this chapter, France, Canada, and England, to varying degrees, all use economic evaluations of health technology to make coverage decisions. In France, economic evaluations of new drugs are recommended but not required (Sorenson, 2009). In Canada, these efforts are more decentralized than in England, and "only a handful" of technologies are subject to cost-effectiveness analysis (Menon & Stafinski, 2009). In England, the National Institute for Health and Care Excellence (NICE) focuses on new technologies only and is reputed to be the leading health technology assessment agency worldwide.

NICE, established in 1999 in response to growing concerns about variations in the use of new technology, is supposed to meet three primary objectives: (a) reduce unwarranted variation in prescribing patterns across England and Wales, principally through setting practice guidelines; (b) encourage the diffusion and uptake of effective health technologies; and (c) ensure value for money for NHS investment by assessing the cost-effectiveness of selected interventions. Record increases in NHS expenditures throughout the decade following 2000 were linked to meeting these objectives, particularly in terms of directing spending to facilitate widespread and uniform access to the most cost-effective treatments.

NICE prides itself on its transparency, methodological rigor, stakeholder inclusiveness, consistency, independence from government, and timeliness, all of which appear necessary to secure the legitimacy and effectiveness of its recommendations. Since 2003, it has been mandatory for local NHS purchasers and providers to act on all positive recommendations on technology appraisals (i.e., recommendations that specific health care interventions be made available in the NHS) within 3 months of their publication.

NICE arrives at conclusions about whether interventions are therapeutically beneficial and cost-effective compared with other relevant alternatives by reviewing a range of available evidence, assembled and synthesized by a publicly funded network of academic institutions. The role of social values in the appraisal process is increasingly apparent as NICE reviews complex cases, for instance, on whether select end-of-life cancer drugs be made available to NHS patients despite their offering insufficient value for money with respect to conventionally accepted thresholds of cost-effectiveness.

There is some evidence that widespread adoption of NICE recommendations for specific technologies, particularly cancer drugs and the use of varenicline for smoking cessation, has reduced geographic variations in access to the technologies (Chalkidou, 2009). Also, there is evidence that NICE guidance has increased costs to the NHS, which is not surprising because most cost-effective interventions are more expensive than the alternatives. This does not bode well for those in the United States who hope that economic evaluation of health technology will contain the growth of health care costs, particularly if assessment efforts are disproportionately focused on new, expensive technologies. Chalkidou (2009) estimates that since its creation, NICE's decisions have cost more than £1.5 billion a year. In this context, it should be noted that cost containment was never one of NICE's explicit objectives.

Quality. The focus on quality is a relatively recent phenomenon. For many years, the primary concern of most policy makers, particularly in developed countries, was on overcoming financial barriers to the health care system. In 2002, the OECD created the Health Care Quality Indicators (HCQI) project to develop and implement a set of international indicators. The project includes representatives from 23 of the 30 OECD nations, as well as a number of international partners, including the Commonwealth Fund, the Nordic Council of Ministers Quality Project, and the International Society for Quality in Health Care (ISQua). The project team identified five priority areas for monitoring quality: (a) cardiac care, (b) diabetes mellitus, (c) mental health, (d) patient safety, and (e) primary care and prevention/health promotion. The OECD secretariat asked participating countries to identify expert panelists to review potential indicators (Mattke, Epstein, & Leatherman, 2006). The panels were charged with reviewing existing indicators rather than developing entirely new measures. They used a consensus process and selected 86 indicators on the basis of relevance, including the extent to which the health system can influence the indicator, scientific soundness, and feasibility. Not surprisingly, the project has identified significant variation in quality as measured by these indicators (OECD, 2013).

Some quality indicators, such as leaving a foreign body inside patients during surgery, follow directly from the literature on medical errors that can be influenced by a health system. The relationships between health system quality and other indicators, however, are controversial. For example, higher rates of 5-year survival among patients diagnosed with breast or cervical cancer may reflect better access to high-quality cancer care. It is possible, however, that these outcomes may reflect more aggressive efforts to diagnose patients with cancer and have little to do with the quality of care patients receive. Beyond these conceptual issues, countries continue to struggle with a lack of relevant data for quality monitoring. Even in countries with relatively well developed health data systems, it is often difficult to link data with unique patient identifiers in ways that allow researchers and policy makers to understand quality of care across different episodes of care and different providers.

> Even in countries with relatively well developed health data systems, it is often difficult to link data with unique patient identifiers in ways that allow researchers and policy makers to understand quality of care across different episodes of care and different providers.

In 2010, the United Kingdom's coalition government published a white paper, *Equity and Excellence: Liberating the NHS,* which called for the measurement of health outcomes based on a number of specific indicators. To achieve this goal, England developed the NHS Outcomes Framework (Secretary of State for Health, 2014) with indicators to evaluate local health care arrangements across five different domains: (a) preventing people from dying prematurely; (b) enhancing the quality of life for people with long-term conditions; (c) helping people to recover from episodes of ill health or after injury; (d) ensuring that people have a positive experience of care; and (e) treating and caring for people in a safe environment and protecting them from avoidable harm.

In France, the Haute Autorité de Santé (HAS), or National Authority for Health, was established in 2004 as an independent public organization to promote quality of health services through accreditation, certification, and development of practice guidelines. Today, HAS leads the European Network for Patient Safety (EUNetPaS), which has developed a common agenda to promote patient safety. After a contaminated blood scandal in the early 1990s, the French government established new institutions to conduct disease surveillance and protect the population from unsafe foods, unsafe drugs, and unsafe blood. In addition, France's Ministry of Health recently initiated a small number of aggressive safety campaigns with strong patient involvement, such as one supported by TV spots to improve the use of antibiotics in preventing the appearance of resistant bacteria. Based on a risk-scoring system for surgical wound infections, national prevalence rates of methicillin-resistant *Staphylococcus aureus* (MRSA) in France declined from 2001 (33%) to 2006 (27%). These results are impressive in comparison with other European countries and the United States, where MRSA infections have increased (Degos & Rodwin, 2011).

In 1994, the Canadian government established the Canadian Institute for Health Information (CIHI) to improve its capacity to assess the health care system and to identify standards for health system performance. CIHI maintains 27 databases and clinical registries. The agency receives funding from the federal (80%) and provincial (20%) governments (Marchildon, 2013). In 2004, the federal government adopted a 10-year plan to strengthen health care. The plan increased federal health transfers to the provinces by 6%, and the provinces were supposed to place greater emphasis on reducing wait times and improving quality (Allin, 2012). Some of these funds have been used to track and reduce wait times. The federal government has also encouraged the use of health technology assessment, clinical guidelines, and best practices to enhance patient safety. Critics argue that despite the increase in attention to quality in individual provinces, problems of access, variation, and reform remain formidable (Lewis, 2015). Moreover, Canada lacks a "guiding framework that supports" quality improvement in primary care (Sibbald, McPherson, & Kothari, 2013, p. 2).

In China, the issue of quality is also central to recent policy debates, but their starting point is radically different. When the Chinese government reduced its subsidies for health care in the late 1970s, health care organizations and providers often turned to pharmaceutical companies to make up for these lost revenues. Rather than focus on providing primary and preventive care, for example, many first-level hospitals focused on selling drugs to patients (Wang et al., 2011). As a result, these institutions developed a reputation for poor quality, and patients were drawn to larger hospitals and academic medical centers, creating overcrowding problems. Part of the motivation for expanding health insurance in China was to improve the quality of care across the entire health care system, but this goal remains as elusive as the challenge of coordination (Wang et al., 2011).

Criteria used to evaluate the performance of health care systems—such as access to, cost of, and quality of health care—are often called the "three-legged stool" of health policy. Until recently, however, quality did not receive a great deal of attention. Since the 1970s, researchers, policy makers, and patients have been demanding better information about quality. In the late 1990s, the U.S. Institute of Medicine led the world in calling attention to the importance of this issue, based on a report that uncovered disturbing evidence of problems with safety and quality in the United States (Kohn, Corrigan, & Donaldson, 2000). In contrast, the SARS epidemic embarrassed the Chinese government and sparked efforts to improve access to and the quality of care. Finding solutions to such problems has been a challenge because stakeholders cling to existing practices and technologies, data limitations make it difficult to measure the quality of care, and fundamental disagreements remain about the meaning of quality and how to measure value for money in health care.

LESSONS

Based on the experience of NHI and NHS systems in the countries we have examined, we would highlight four lessons for policy makers in the United States:

- Achieving the goal of universal health coverage requires legislation to make such coverage compulsory.
- Financing broader insurance coverage in the United States—beyond Medicare and Medicaid—requires increasing government subsidies based on ability-to-pay criteria.
- Health care systems with universal coverage rely increasingly on economic evaluation of health technology as a criterion for making coverage decisions.
- Containing health care costs has not been achieved without greater reliance than in the United States on price regulation and systemwide budget targets.

The ACA represents the most significant health care reform since Medicare and Medicaid in 1965 because it has increased significantly the share of the population with health insurance coverage and redistributed the burden of health care financing from those who are wealthier, younger, and healthier toward those who are poorer, older, and sicker (see Chapter 3). We would argue that this legislation draws heavily on the first two lessons of comparative experience (the mandate and the move toward ability-to-pay criteria for financing health care) and less so on the third (economic evaluation of health technology), and it ignores the fourth (greater price regulation and budget targets). This will bring the United States closer to other wealthy nations in terms of population coverage. Yet the U.S. health care system continues to present some striking contrasts to most other wealthy nations. It remains a patchwork system characterized by a complex combination of institutions that include an enclave of socialized medicine such as the VHA, a social insurance program (Medicare), and social welfare programs (Medicaid and Children's Health Insurance Program [CHIP]); tax-subsidized employer-based private insurance for about half of the population; and heavy reliance on out-of-pocket payment for the population that remains uninsured, similar to the situation in China, India, and most developing nations.

The United States has the highest per capita expenditures; the highest salaries for physicians and other professionals making up the health care workforce; and the highest aggregate prices for hospitals, physicians' services, and pharmaceuticals. Despite our drive to innovate and invest in the latest medical technologies, access to high-technology services, as well as to basic primary care services, is highly inequitable compared with other OECD nations—but not with China, which faces not only the usual inequities among populations of different income and educational levels, but also massive inequities among its urban and rural residents and, within cities, among its registered and migrant populations.

Another way in which the U.S. health care system differs from that of wealthy OECD nations concerns the vast range of health insurance products we offer to our population, including the option (following the ACA) of not purchasing health insurance, albeit with a financial penalty. Despite the emphasis on choice of insurer, many people find themselves confined to obtaining health care within restricted provider networks outside which payment for services often becomes unaffordable. There is no parallel to this problem in wealthy OECD nations such as England, Canada, and France. In China, choice of too many insurance products is not the problem. The situation there is far worse than in the United States because a large part of the urban migrant population (about 250 million people) is typically excluded from decent health insurance coverage. The problem of internal migrants in China is substantial, but not surprising, for a system that spends only 5.5% of its GDP on health care and has only recently set the goal of providing universal coverage.

▶ CASE EXERCISE—EUROPEAN LESSONS LEARNED

You are an employee of a think tank in Washington, DC. The director has been asked to testify before a congressional committee on the following question: In reforming the ACA, what lessons should the United States learn from relevant experience abroad? Your job is to write a memorandum that will help the director answer this question. In writing this memo, you should address the following questions:

1. How can learning from abroad help policy makers engage in a process of self-examination of health policy at home?

2. Compare the NHS and NHI systems.

3. What should members of Congress know about China's problems and aspirations in health policy?

4. What lessons from abroad would be most relevant in reforming the U.S. health system?

DISCUSSION QUESTIONS

1. What are some reasons for studying health care systems abroad?
2. How do NHI and NHS systems compare with the health care system in the United States?
3. How do most countries with similar levels of per capita income differ from and resemble the United States with respect to cost, quality, and access to health care?
4. What can the United States learn from other OECD countries about how to extend health coverage while containing health care expenditures?
5. How can health system performance be measured? Compare the approaches adopted by WHO and the Commonwealth Fund.
6. How are the problems and opportunities different for China than for the United States and other OECD countries?

REFERENCES

Aaron, H., Schwartz, W., & Cox, M. (2005). *Can we say no? The challenge of rationing health care.* Washington, DC: Brookings Institution Press.

Allin, S. (2012). The Canadian health care system, 2012. In S. Thomson, R. Osborn, D. Squires, & M. Jun (Eds.), *International profiles of health care systems, 2012* (pp. 19–25). New York, NY: The Commonwealth Fund. Retrieved from http://apps.who.int/medicinedocs/documents/s19988en/s19988en.pdf

Angrisano, C., Farrell, D., Kocher, B., Laboissiere, M., & Parker, S. (2007, January). *Accounting for the cost of health care in the United States* (Report). Retrieved from http://www.mckinsey.com/insights/health_systems_and_services/accounting_for_the_cost_of_health_care_in_the_united_states

Australian Department of the Treasury. (2007). *Intergenerational report 2007.* Retrieved from http://archive.treasury.gov.au/documents/1239/PDF/IGR_2007_final_report.pdf

Blendon, R. J., Benson, J. M., & Hero, J. O. (2014). Public trust in physicians: U.S. medicine in international perspective. *New England Journal of Medicine, 371,* 1570–1572. doi:10.1056/NEJMp1407373

Blendon, R. J., Schoen, C., DesRoches, C. M., Osborn, R., Scoles, K. L., & Zapert, K. (2002). Inequities in health care: A five-country survey. *Health Affairs, 21*(3), 182–191. doi:10.1377/hlthaff.21.3.182

Blumenthal, D., & Hsiao, W. (2005). Privatization and its discontents—The evolving Chinese health care system. *New England Journal of Medicine, 353*(11), 1165–1170. doi:10.1056/NEJMhpr051133

Bohmer, R. M. J., & Imison, C. (2013). Lessons from England's health care workforce redesign: No quick fixes. *Health Affairs, 32*(11), 2025–2031. doi:10.1377/hlthaff.2013.0553

Bradley, E. H., & Taylor, L. A. (2013). *The American health care paradox: Why spending more is getting us less.* New York, NY: Public Affairs.

Carrier, E., Yee, T., & Stark, L. B. (2011). *Matching supply to demand: Address the U.S. primary care workforce shortage* (NIHCR Policy Analysis No. 7). Washington, DC: National Institute for Health Care Reform. Retrieved from https://nihcr.org/analysis/improving-care-delivery/prevention-improving-health/pcp-workforce/

Chalkidou, K. (2009). *Comparative effectiveness review within the U.K.'s National Institute for Health and Clinical Excellence* (Issue brief). New York, NY: The Commonwealth Fund. Retrieved from https://core.ac.uk/download/pdf/71350356.pdf

Commonwealth Fund. (2014). *Mirror, Mirror 2017: International Comparison Reflects Flaws and Opportunities for Better U.S. Health Care.* Retrieved from https://interactives.commonwealthfund.org/2017/july/mirror-mirror/

Cutler, D. M. (2007). The lifetime costs and benefits of medical technology. *Journal of Health Economics, 26*(6), 1081–1100. doi:10.1016/j.jhealeco.2007.09.003

de Kervasdoué, J., Kimberly, J., & Rodwin, V. G. (1984). *The end of an illusion: The future of health policy in western industrialized nations.* Berkeley: University of California Press.

Degos, L., & Rodwin, V. (2011). Two faces of patient safety and care quality: A Franco-American comparison. *Health Economics, Policy and Law, 6*(3), 287–294. doi:10.1017/S1744133111000107

Fineberg, H. (2012). A successful and sustainable health system—How to get there from here [Shattuck lecture]. *New England Journal of Medicine, 366*(11), 1020–1027. doi:10.1056/NEJMsa1114777

Goodman, J., Musgrave, G., & Herrick, D. (2004). *Lives at risk: Single-payer national health insurance around the world.* Lanham, MD: Rowman & Littlefield.

Gusmano, M. K., & Allin, S. (2011). Health care for older persons in England and the United States: A contrast of systems and values. *Journal of Health Politics, Policy and Law, 36*(1), 89–118. doi:10.1215/03616878-1191117

Gusmano, M. K., Rodwin, V. G., & Weisz, D. (2014). Using comparative analysis to address health system caricatures. *International Journal of Health Services, 44*(3), 547–559.

Gusmano, M. K., Weisz, D., & Rodwin, V. G. (2009). Achieving horizontal equity: Must we have a single-payer health care system? *Journal of Health Politics, Policy and Law, 34*(4), 617–633. doi:10.1215/03616878-2009-018

Hacker, J. (2006). *The great risk shift: The new economic insecurity and the decline of the American dream.* New York, NY: Oxford University Press.

Hargreaves, D. S., Greaves, F., Levay, C., Mitchell, I., Koch, U., Esch, T., … Sheikh, A. (2015). Comparison of health care experience and access between young and older adults in 11 high-income countries. *Journal of Adolescent Health, 57*, 413–420. doi:10.1016/j.jado-health.2015.05.015

He, A. J., & Meng, Q. (2015). An interim interdisciplinary evaluation of China's national healthcare reform: Emerging evidence and new perspectives. *Journal of Asian Public Policy, 8(1)*, 1–18. doi:10.1080/17516234.2015.1014299

HealthForceOntario. (2014). *Family practice compensation models* [Web page]. Retrieved from http://www.healthforceontario.ca/en/Home/Physicians/Training_%7C_Practising_Outside_Ontario/Physician_Roles/Family_Practice_Models/Family_Practice_Compensation_Models

Hipgrave, D., Guo, S., Mu, Y., Guo, Y., Yan, F., Scherpbier, R., & Brixi, H. (2012). Chinese-style decentralization and health system reform. *PLOS Medicine, 9*(11), 1–4. doi:10.1371/journal.pmed.1001337

Huang, Y. (2011, November 1). China's health costs outstrip G.D.P. growth. *The New York Times.* Retrieved from http://www.nytimes.com/roomfordebate/2011/11/01/is-china-facing-a-health-care-crisis/chinas-health-costs-outstrip-gdp-growth

Klein, R. (1997). Learning from others: Shall the last be the first? *Journal of Health Politics, Policy and Law, 22*(5), 1267–1278. doi:10.1215/03616878-22-5-1267

Klein, R. (2013). *The new politics of the NHS* (7th ed.). London, UK: Radcliffe.

Klein, R. (2018). The National Health Service (NHS) at 70: Bevan's double-edged legacy. *Health Economics, Policy and Law*, 1–10. doi:10.1017/S1744133117000354

Kohn, L. T., Corrigan, J. M., & Donaldson, M. S. (Eds.). (2000). *To err is human: Building a safer health system.* Washington, DC: National Academies Press.

Laugesen, M. (2018). Do other countries have a better mix of generalists and specialists? *Journal of Health Politics, Policy and Law, 43*(5), 853–872. doi:10.1215/03616878-6951199

Lewis, S. (2015). A system in name only: Access, variation, and reform in Canada's provinces. *New England Journal of Medicine, 372*, 497–500. doi:10.1056/NEJMp1414409

Marchildon, G. P. (2013). Canada: Health system review. *Health Systems in Transition, 15*(1), 1–179.

Marmor, T., Freeman, R., & Okma, K. (2005). Comparative perspectives and policy learning in the world of health care. *Journal of Comparative Policy Analysis: Research and Practice, 7*(4), 331–348. doi:10.1080/13876980500319253

Marmor, T., & Oberlander, J. (2012). From HMOs to ACOs: The quest for the holy grail in U.S. health policy. *Journal of General Internal Medicine, 27*(9), 1215–1218. doi:10.1007/s11606-012-2024-6

Mattke, S., Epstein, A. M., & Leatherman, S. (2006). The OECD health care quality indicators project: History and background. *International Journal for Quality in Health Care, 18*(Suppl. 1), 1–4. doi:10.1093/intqhc/mzl019

Menon, D., & Stafinski, T. (2009). Health technology assessment in Canada: 20 years strong? *Value in Health, 12*(Suppl. 2), S14–S19.

Moat, K. A., Waddell, K., & Lavis, J. N. (2016). *Evidence brief: Planning for the future health workforce of Ontario.* Hamilton, Canada: McMaster Health Forum. Retrieved from https://macsphere.mcmaster.ca/bitstream/11375/21003/1/workforce-planning-eb.pdf

Moon, M. (1996). *Medicare now and in the future* (2nd ed.). Washington, DC: The Urban Institute.

Morone, J. A. (1993). The health care bureaucracy: Small changes, big consequences. *Journal of Health Politics, Policy and Law, 18*(3), 723–739. doi:10.1215/03616878-18-3-723

Mossialos, E., Wenzl, M., Osborn, R., & Sarnak, D. (2016). *International profiles of health care systems, 2015.* New York, NY: Commonwealth Fund. Retrieved from http://www.commonwealthfund.org

Musgrove, P. (2003). Judging health systems: Reflections on WHO's methods. *The Lancet, 361,* 1817–1820. doi:10.1016/S0140-6736(03)13408-3

NHS Clinical Commissioners. (2018). About CCGs. London. Retrieved from https://www.nhscc.org/ccgs

Nolte, E., & McKee, M. (2003). Measuring the health of nations: Analysis of mortality amenable to health care. *British Medical Journal, 327,* 1129–1133. doi:10.1136/bmj.327.7424.1129

Nolte, E., & McKee, M. (2012). In amenable mortality—deaths avoidable through health care—progress in the U.S. lags that of three European countries. *Health Affairs, 31*(9), 2114–2122. doi:10.1377/hlthaff.2011.0851

Oliver, A. (2012). The folly of cross-country ranking exercises. *Health Economics, Policy and Law, 7*(1), 15–17. doi:10.1017/S1744133111000260

Ono, T., Lafortune, G., & Schoenstein, M. (2013). *Health workforce planning in OECD countries: A review of 26 projection models from 18 countries* (OECD Health Working Papers, No. 62). Ferney-Voltaire, France: Organisation for Economic Co-operation and Development. doi:10.1787/5k44t787zcwb-en

Or, Z. (2009). *Activity based payment in France. Euro Observer 11*(4). Retrieved from http://eurodrg.projects.tu-berlin.de/publications/Activity%20based%20payment%20in%20France%20-%20Zeynep%20Or.pdf

Organisation for Economic Co-operation and Development. (2013). *Health at a glance 2013: OECD indicators.* Paris, France: Author. doi:10.1787/health_glance-2013-en

Papanicolas, I., Woskie, L. R., & Jha, A. K. (2018). Health care spending in the United States and other high-income countries. *Journal of the American Medical Association, 319*(10), 1024–1039. doi:10.1001/jama.2018.1150

Qian, J. (2015). Reallocating authority in the Chinese health system: An institutional perspective. *Journal of Asian Public Policy, 8*(1), 19–35. doi:10.1080/17516234.2014.1003454

Rodwin, V. G. (1984). *The health planning predicament: France, Québec, England, and the United States.* Berkeley: University of California Press.

Rodwin, V. G. (2006). *Universal health insurance in France: How sustainable? Essays on the French health care system.* Washington, DC: Embassy of France. Retrieved from http://www.frenchamerican.org/sites/default/files/documents/media_reports/2006_fafreport_universalhealthinsurance.pdf

Rodwin, V. G. (2018). The French health care system. *World Hospitals and Health Services—Universal Health Coverage (UHC): Making Progress Towards the 2030 Targets* (special issue on universal coverage), *54*(1), 49–55. Retrieved from https://wagner.nyu.edu/impact/research/publications/french-health-care-system

Roos, N. P., & Mustard, C. (1997). Variation in health and health care use by socioeconomic status in Winnipeg, Canada: Does the system work well? Yes and no. *The Milbank Quarterly, 75*(1), 89–111. doi:10.1111/1468-0009.00045

Rosenthal, M. M., & Greiner, J. R. (1982). The barefoot doctors of China: From political creation to professionalization. *Human Organization, 41*(4), 330–341. Retrieved from https://www.jstor.org/stable/44126528

Roth, L. S., & Adams, P. C. (2009). Variation in physician reimbursement for endoscopy across Canada. *Canadian Journal of Gastroenterology, 23*(7), 503.

Schneider, E. C., Sarnak, D. O., Squires, D., Shah, A., & Doty, M. M. (n.d.). Mirror, mirror 2017: International comparison health reflects flaws and opportunities for better U.S. health care. Retrieved from http://www.commonwealthfund.org/interactives/2017/july/mirror-mirror

Schneider, E. C., & Squires, D. (2017). From last to first: Could the U.S. health care system become the best in the world? *New England Journal of Medicine, 377,* 901–904. doi:10.1056/NEJMp1708704

Schoen, C., Osborn, R., Squires, D., Doty, M., Rasmussen, P., Pierson, R., & Applebaum, S. (2012). A survey of primary care doctors in ten countries shows progress in use of health information technology, less in other areas. *Health Affairs, 31*(12), 2805–2816. doi:10.1377/hlthaff.2012.0884

Schreyögg, J., Stargardt, T., Tiemann, O., & Busse, R. (2006). Methods to determine reimbursement rates for diagnosis related groups (DRG): A comparison of nine European countries. *Health Care Management Science, 9*(3), 215–223. doi:10.1007/s10729-006-9040-1

Secretary of State for Health. (2014). *Equity and excellence: Liberating the NHS.* London, England: UK Department of Health.

Shi, J., Li, R., Jiang, H., Xiao, Y., Liu, N., Wang, Z., & Shi, L. (2018). Moving towards a better path? A mixed-method examination of China's reforms to remedy medical corruption from pharmaceutical firms. *BMJ Open, 8,* e018513. doi:10.1136/bmjopen-2017-018513

Sibbald, S. L., McPherson, C., & Kothari, A. (2013). Ontario primary care reform and quality improvement activities: An environmental scan. *BMC Health Services Research, 13,* 209. doi:10.1186/1472-6963-13-209

Smith, R. D. (2006). Responding to global infectious disease outbreaks: Lessons from SARS on the role of risk perception, communication and management. *Social Science and Medicine, 63,* 3113–3123. doi:10.1016/j.socscimed.2006.08.004

Sorenson, C. (2009). The role of HTA in coverage and pricing decisions: A cross-country comparison. *Euro Observer, 11*(1), 1–12.

Starfield, B., Shi, L., & Macinko, J. (2005). Contribution of primary care to health systems and health. *The Milbank Quarterly, 83*(3), 457–502. doi:10.1111/j.1468-0009.2005.00409.x

Thomson, S., Osborn, R., Squires, D., & Reed, S. J. (2012). *International profiles of health care systems.* New York, NY: The Commonwealth Fund.

Valentine, V. (2005, November 4). Health for the masses: China's "barefoot doctors" [Radio broadcast]. *National Public Radio.* Retrieved from https://www.npr.org/templates/story/story.php?storyId=4990242

van Doorslaer, E., & Masseria, C. (2004). *Income-related inequality in the use of medical care in 21 OECD countries* (OECD Health Working Papers, 14). Paris, France: Organisation for Economic Co-operation and Development. doi:10.1787/687501760705

Wang, H., Gusmano, M. K., & Cao, Q. (2011). Evaluation of the policy on community health organizations in China: Will the priority of new healthcare reform in China be a success? *Health Policy, 99*(1), 37–43. doi:10.1016/j.healthpol.2010.07.003

Warshaw, G. A., & Bragg, E. J. (2014). Preparing the health care workforce to care for adults with Alzheimer's disease and related dementias. *Health Affairs, 33*(4), 633–641. doi:10.1377/hlthaff.2013.1232

Williams, A. (2001). Science or marketing at WHO? A commentary on 'World Health 2000.' *Health Economics, 10,* 93–100. doi:10.1002/hec.594

World Health Organization. (2000). World health report 2000. Retrieved from http://www.who.int/whr/2001/archives/2000/en/index.htm

World Health Organization. (2008). *World health report 2000 – Health systems: improving performance.* Geneva, Switzerland: Author. Retrieved from https://www.who.int/whr/2000/en/

Yip, W. C. M., Hsiao, W., Meng, Q., Chen, W., & Sun, X. (2010). Realignment of incentives for health-care providers in China. *The Lancet, 375*(9720), 1120–1130. doi:10.1016/S0140-6736(10)60063-3

Zweifel, P., Felder, S., & Meiers, M. (1999). Ageing of population and health care expenditure: A red herring? *Health Economics, 8,* 485–496. doi:10.1002/(SICI)1099-1050(199909)8:6<485::AID-HEC461>3.0.CO;2-4

Keeping Americans Healthy

5

Population Health

Pamela G. Russo and Marc N. Gourevitch

LEARNING OBJECTIVES

▶ Understand the differences between the medical and population health models of producing health, including the difference between the concepts of health care and health

▶ Explain how the two models lead to different strategies for interventions to prevent disease and improve health

▶ Learn about the differential importance of various health determinants

▶ Review the evidence regarding social and physical environmental influences on behavior and on health outcomes

▶ Review the variation in health and life expectancy between counties and between countries

▶ Describe innovative synergistic approaches that integrate the clinical and population models

KEY TERMS

▶ cross-sectoral collaborative approaches

▶ determinants of health

▶ dose-response effect

▶ health care

▶ medical model

▶ medically indigent

▶ multiple determinants of health

▶ neighborhood effects

▶ reverse causality

▶ social determinants of health

TOPICAL OUTLINE

▶ The population health model

▶ The medical model

▶ Comparing the medical and population health models

▶ The influence of social determinants on health behavior and outcomes

▶ Leading determinants of health: weighting the different domains

▶ Health policy and return on investment

INTRODUCTION

Much of this book concerns what happens *within* the walls of health care institutions—hospitals, clinics, physician offices, and long-term care facilities.

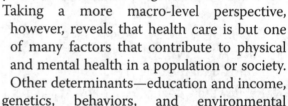

The physical and mental health of our communities is affected by more than just health care.*

Taking a more macro-level perspective, however, reveals that health care is but one of many factors that contribute to physical and mental health in a population or society. Other determinants—education and income, genetics, behaviors, and environmental exposures—are responsible for much of the health, or disease, in a population. In fact, the effects of the systematic differences in **health care** are far smaller than the effects of the nonrandom differences in other determinants of health on a population's overall health outcomes. These influences *outside* the health care system greatly influence which groups of people are more likely to become ill in the first place, to be injured, or to die early. These influences also help determine people's health care outcomes once they become sick, injured, or disabled. This chapter addresses the changes in health care and public policy emerging from the growing appreciation of the profound influences on the population's health that occur *outside* the health care system, where the vast majority of people—or patients, from a health care perspective—spend the overwhelming majority of their time.

The notion that health is influenced by factors outside the health care system is of course not new. Why, then, is it receiving renewed attention? More than anything else, growing attention to population health reflects widening acceptance of, and mounting frustration with, the poor performance of the United States on many indicators of health despite its excellence in many aspects of health care. Decades of studies and reports have documented conclusively that even in the face of unsustainably high spending on health care, the health of the U.S. population lags behind that of nearly every other peer country (National Research Council and Institute of Medicine, 2013). Armed with the more recent understanding that countries with a higher ratio of social service to health care spending have healthier populations (Bradley, Elkins, Herrin, & Elbel, 2011)

---

*To hear the podcast, go to https://bcove.video/2QEZxWe or access the ebook on Springer Publishing Connect™.

and that inadequately addressed social factors are significant drivers of health care spending, policy makers are coming around to the notion that addressing social determinants of health must be part of the solution to achieving national health goals and health care cost-savings goals. Should policy makers seeking to improve population health simply sidestep the health care sector if it contributes only modestly to health at a societal level? Doing so would likely be short-sighted, since health care is the sector in which resources earmarked for health are almost exclusively concentrated in the United States. How, then, are we to bridge the health care sector's focus on and resources for health, with an understanding of the broader societal factors that in fact determine so much of health and disease? Therein lies the core challenge of the emerging field of population health.

THE POPULATION HEALTH MODEL

Population health employs an integrative model in understanding and seeking to improve the health of groups of people, acknowledging that different factors intersect and combine to produce good or poor health. The population health model seeks to explain and intervene in the causes of the systematic differences in health between different groups (Kindig & Stoddart, 2003). To do so, it analyzes the patterns or distribution of health between different groups of people in order to identify and understand factors leading to differences in outcomes. These factors are often described as "upstream" causes in the sense that they influence health through a series of pathways that may not be immediately visible (see also Chapter 7).

Population health scientists use the term **determinants of health** rather than *factor* or *cause*, and they use the term **multiple determinants of health** to describe the determinants that arise from five important domains:

- The social and economic environment—factors such as income, education, employment, social support, and culture (often referred to as the **social determinants of health,** or SDOH)
- The physical environment, including urban design, housing, availability of healthy foods, air and water safety, exposure to environmental toxins
- Genetics (and, more recently, epigenetics—the study of gene–environment interactions)
- Medical care, including prevention, treatment, and disease management
- Health-related behaviors, such as smoking, exercise, and diet, which in turn are shaped by all of the preceding determinants

Health is therefore conceptualized as the result of exposure to different patterns of these multiple determinants (Figure 5.1). Over the past 40 years, a significant body of knowledge has developed that demonstrates the profound effects of multiple determinants from different domains as well as the interactions among

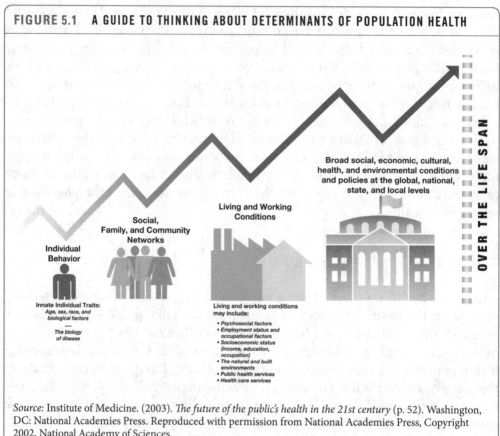

FIGURE 5.1 A GUIDE TO THINKING ABOUT DETERMINANTS OF POPULATION HEALTH

OVER THE LIFE SPAN

Broad social, economic, cultural, health, and environmental conditions and policies at the global, national, state, and local levels

Living and Working Conditions

Social, Family, and Community Networks

Individual Behavior

Innate Individual Traits: Age, sex, race, and biological factors
—
The biology of disease

Living and working conditions may include:

• Psychosocial factors
• Employment status and occupational factors
• Socioeconomic status (income, education, occupation)
• The natural and built environments
• Public health services
• Health care services

Source: Institute of Medicine. (2003). *The future of the public's health in the 21st century* (p. 52). Washington, DC: National Academies Press. Reproduced with permission from National Academies Press, Copyright 2002, National Academy of Sciences.

them, their effects at different stages in the life course from gestation to old age, and their cumulative effects. Although the determinant categories are listed independently, they have substantial and complex interactions over the life course of an individual or group.

Some health care outcomes can, in turn, affect the determinants; that is, they can have a **reverse causality** effect on determinants. For example, whereas social determinants such as income have an effect on outcomes, the outcome of being unhealthy also can have a negative effect on income (Kindig & Chin, 2009).

THE MEDICAL MODEL

In contrast to the population health model, the **medical model** hones in on individuals, focusing on the factors most immediately linked to the pathophysiology underlying a person's disease. It is a reductionist model in the sense that it searches for the molecular and physiological mechanisms that explain how specific factors produce illness or act as markers of incipient disease. In turn, the therapeutic ideal is to find the "silver bullet" that will stop or reverse those mechanisms and thus cure or prevent progression of the current medical problem.

The medical model frames risk factors as working through disease-specific pathways and typically analyzes risk factors as if they were independent in statistical modeling. The medical model considers how different biological systems within the individual interact—for example, the endocrine system and the cardiovascular system—but the lens remains focused on the body.

Health care is generally reactive, meaning that it responds to abnormality, disease, or injury, and as a result has been characterized as a "sickness care system" (Evans, Barer, & Marmor, 1994). Health care has traditionally been delivered (and reimbursed) in acute episodes and has placed less value on and provided less reimbursement for efforts to promote health or to prevent illness and injury. Although health care has achieved great strides in diagnosing, treating, and in some cases curing illness and injury, and although new knowledge and technology are constantly increasing the capacity to preserve life, relieve suffering, and maintain or restore function, Americans' chances for living long and healthy lives are not improving, despite ever-greater U.S. spending on health care (Figure 5.2).

The United States is the outlier point on the far right—the highest health care spending—yet Americans' probability of survival to age 80 is lower than that of other developed countries. This marked discrepancy between the highest

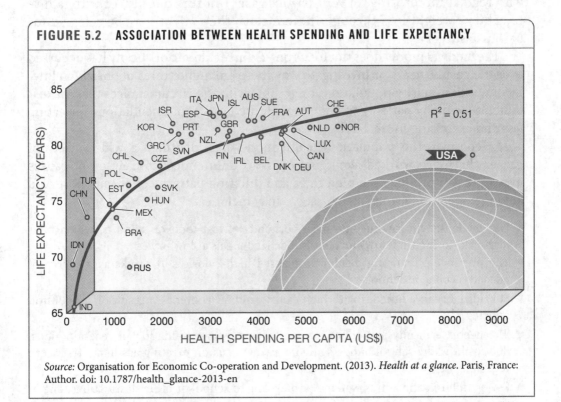

FIGURE 5.2   ASSOCIATION BETWEEN HEALTH SPENDING AND LIFE EXPECTANCY

Source: Organisation for Economic Co-operation and Development. (2013). *Health at a glance.* Paris, France: Author. doi: 10.1787/health_glance-2013-en

spending on health care and poorer survival rates is referred to as "the U.S. health disadvantage" (National Research Council and Institute of Medicine, 2013). The differences between the medical and population health models can help explain the reasons for the disparity between the United States and other developed countries as well as the severe disparities within the United States among different populations.

COMPARING THE MEDICAL AND POPULATION HEALTH MODELS

Consider two examples, obesity and tobacco use, that illustrate the different explanatory and intervention approaches of the medical model versus the population health model. In the medical model, when an adolescent with obesity visits a health care provider, the provider will likely assess the patient's family history, diet, and physical activity. These may be followed by laboratory tests to rule out hormonal or other physiological causes for obesity and to check for diabetes and other consequences of extreme overweight. Interventions are likely to include referrals to nutritionists and recommendations for decreasing calories and increasing physical activity, with regular monitoring. In very serious cases (morbid obesity) or with failure to achieve weight loss through these means, the patient may be referred for bariatric surgery.

> The medical model does not focus on *why* an epidemic of obesity has occurred over the past 30 years.

The medical model does not focus on *why* an epidemic of obesity has occurred over the past 30 years or investigate why there are higher rates of obesity in low-income and minority populations or grapple with the circumstances that make it difficult for many patients to comply with medical recommendations for eating less and exercising more.

In contrast, the population health model has identified a wide variety of causes that have worked synergistically—an unintended conspiracy of causes over time—to produce the high rates and differing patterns of obesity observed among population groups. Such causes may include:

- Higher density in low-income neighborhoods of fast-food restaurants, which offer high-calorie, high-fat, low-nutrient, supersized meals at low prices
- The presence of vending machines that sell high-calorie soft drinks as a source of needed revenue in schools
- Subsidized school lunches with high caloric and fat content—a result of agricultural policies
- The decrease in physical education classes and near-elimination of recess periods, due to shrinking school budgets and a narrow focus on meeting academic test score requirements
- Fewer children and adults walking or bicycling to school or other destinations, due in part to the lack of sidewalks, safe pedestrian crossings, and bicycle lanes

- Fewer safe places to play or walk in urban, low-income neighborhoods
- A lack of grocery stores with healthy food options such as fresh fruit and vegetables in many neighborhoods, due to the higher cost and lower profit margins of these foods
- Marketing obesogenic foods to children

These social and physical environmental determinants strongly limit people's behavioral choices. It is difficult to achieve lasting lifestyle behavioral changes among people who *do* have the economic resources to join gyms, have child care while they exercise, and afford healthier food choices. Such goals are more challenging still when healthy choices are largely beyond financial reach.

In a population health framework, relevant interventions could include zoning law changes; menu labeling; working with fast-food industries to provide healthier, but low-cost menu options; educational policies that encourage healthy food choices and increased physical activity in schools and after school; and so on. Such interventions are not traditionally considered part of the health care arena. Making the healthy choice the easier choice is not always sufficient; programs to change behavior boost the chances that people will make those healthy choices their default choices. Such programs might include workplace or community programs to encourage physical activity in the form of walking, bicycling, or other exercise or cooking classes using nutritious, affordable, noncalorie-dense foods.

Tobacco use offers a second example. In the medical model, the focus is on individual patients who smoke or chew tobacco. The solution is framed in individual terms and is geared toward behavioral change through cessation counseling and nicotine replacement options. Success requires having access to providers who support and encourage cessation (see Chapter 7).

In the population health model, the understanding of the problem includes the influences of tobacco production, advertising, distribution, and patterns of use in different groups, as well as the policies used to intervene include smoke-free laws, tobacco taxes, and regulation of advertising and marketing. These population-wide policy changes have changed U.S. social norms regarding the acceptability of tobacco use and led to dramatic decreases in the rate of smoking.

As with programs to increase physical activity and healthy eating, policy changes to reduce smoking are usually coupled with increases in access to cessation programs at the community level, such as free quitlines and free nicotine patches, which assist smokers in quitting. The population health model also enables targeting policies toward groups with the highest rates of tobacco use, and it responds to tobacco industry actions to redirect their advertising from the more affluent smokers who are able to access cessation programs to new, more susceptible markets, including youth, minorities, and people in developing countries (Kreuter & Lezin, 2001).

In short, key determinants of health are often shaped by policies and programs in sectors not traditionally considered as residing within the health care sector. In the obesity example above, the education sector is key to changes in school environments. Changes in zoning laws can alter the proximity of fast-food restaurants or liquor stores to schools or parks. **Cross-sectoral collaborative approaches** are essential to addressing underlying causes of poor health and therefore to improving health and health equity at the population level.

THE INFLUENCE OF SOCIAL DETERMINANTS ON HEALTH BEHAVIOR AND OUTCOMES

The medical model is well accepted and respected by health care providers and by basic science, clinical, and health services researchers. Indeed, medical knowledge is widely viewed as grounded in "hard science" and thus reflecting "truth" about the causes of disease. The population health model, conversely, with its inclusion of social science and diverse methods and data sources, is less widely perceived as scientifically rigorous. While few may doubt that poverty and lack of education are associated with worse health—as the Australian-born population health researcher John Lynch says, population health is the "science of the bleedin' obvious"—many are not aware of the magnitude and rigor of the scientific evidence underlying these findings or of the effectiveness of associated population-level interventions.

In fact, substantial advances have been made in defining the pathways by which social determinants influence health—in other words, how these factors "get under the skin"—using a wide variety of research methods, from experimental psychology and neuroimaging, to exploring the pathophysiology of how chronic stress causes inflammation, to epigenetics. For a comprehensive review of the research on the interaction between social determinants and human biology, see Adler and Stewart (2010).

Early and important research on health determinants was based on epidemiological findings linking morbidity and mortality to socioeconomic status, defined by education, income, or occupational status. One of the earliest studies to demonstrate the importance of such factors was Michael Marmot's Whitehall study, a longitudinal study conducted over two decades with results reported throughout the 1970s and 1980s (Evans et al., 1994). The British data were especially enlightening because they included a measure of social class, based on occupation.

The Whitehall study collected extensive information on more than 10,000 British civil servants, from the lowest rung of the income and rank hierarchy to the highest. Marmot found that the likelihood of death was about *three and a half times higher* for those in the lowest status rank (clerical and manual workers) than for those in the highest administrative jobs. Mortality rates increased steadily with every reduction in rank.

Such a steady increase is known as a gradient in the population health model and a **dose-response effect** in the medical model, where it is taken as evidence of a robust relationship between causal factor and outcome. All of the workers in this population had steady, paying jobs, and none had high exposure to work-related toxins or other risks in the physical environment. All had access to the British National Health System. The gradient in heart disease mortality continued to be present after adjusting the data for different rates of smoking, high blood pressure, and high cholesterol. In other words, after controlling for the traditional medical model risk factors, the 3:1 difference in death rate by social class could not be explained away. Marmot and others went on to investigate the role of stress associated with occupational rank.

Decades of study of the stress response have rigorously demonstrated its negative impact on health, mediated by multiple physiological pathways. A wide variety of stressful stimuli have been studied, including social subordination, lack of job control, discrimination, social isolation, economic insecurity, job loss, and bankruptcy. More recently, the impact of racism has also been studied in this framework. A proposed common pathway is that greater exposure to stress over time leads to chronic activation of physiological responses that, by virtue of resulting conditions (e.g., neurophysiological adaptations, elevated blood pressure, heightened inflammatory responses), result in elevated rates of morbidity and mortality. For example, babies born to mothers who fear targeting by immigration raids are more likely to be of low birth weight (Novak, Geronimus, & Martinez-Cardoso, 2017).

Scientists increasingly recognize that the mechanisms by which social determinants act depend on the context in which people encounter stressful events. One area of research focuses on **neighborhood effects**, which include the interaction of social and physical environmental determinants; for example, the negative interaction between the physical environment (poor housing, presence of crime and violence, absence of stores with healthy foods) and social determinants related to poverty.

Data on the links between social factors and health and the wide variations in health among groups can be found in a report from the Robert Wood Johnson Foundation Commission to Build a Healthier America (2014), a national, independent, nonpartisan group of leaders who investigated how factors outside the health care system shape and affect opportunities to live healthy lives. The Commission's team of researchers compared average life expectancy by county and found significant variations. For example, the average life expectancy in Wolfe County, Kentucky, is 70 years, compared with 78 years in nearby Fayette County— a difference of 8 years. Such findings of stark differences in life expectancy or other health outcome according to race/ethnicity, gender, sex, sexual orientation, place, and income have focused attention on the goal of achieving health equity. Health inequities "systematically put groups of people who are already socially disadvantaged (e.g., by virtue of being poor, female, and/or members of a disenfranchised racial, ethnic, or religious group) at further disadvantage with respect to their health" (Braveman & Gruskin, 2003). Building toward health equity, therefore, requires incorporating an intentional focus on combatting underlying causes of inequity—from structural racism to lack of parity in wages to underinvestment in early childhood education—into initiatives to improve population health.

Two of the most predictive factors of life expectancy are income and degree of education. Examination of the relationship between measures of education and income on U.S. life expectancy showed that:

- College graduates can expect to live at least 5 years longer than those who did not complete high school.
- The gap in life expectancy between the richest 1% and poorest 1% of individuals in the United States is 14.8 years for men and 10.2 years for women (Chetty et al., 2016). By way of context, in 2017, the federal poverty level (FPL) was $20,780 for a family of three.
- Even middle-income Americans can expect to live shorter lives than those with higher incomes, whether or not they have health insurance.

The Commission also examined the relationships among health status, educational attainment, and racial or ethnic group. The measure of health status was a self-reported assessment of one's own health as excellent, very good, good, fair, or poor. Self-reported health status corresponds closely with assessments made by health professionals. Indeed, among adults studied by the Commission's research team, those who reported being in less than very good health had rates of diabetes and cardiovascular disease more than five times as high as the rates for adults who reported being in very good or excellent health. Additional highlights of the Commission's results include:

- Overall, 45% of adults ages 25 to 74 reported being in less than very good health, with rates varying among states from 35% to 53%.
- Adults with less than high school degrees were more than *two to three times* as likely to be in less than very good health than college graduates. There was also a clear gradient in health by educational level.
- Health status varied across racial or ethnic groups; non-Hispanic Whites were more likely to be in very good or excellent health than other groups nationally and in almost every state. In some states, non-Hispanic Black and Hispanic adults were *more than twice* as likely as White adults to be in less than very good health.
- Analyzing both social factors simultaneously, non-Hispanic Whites had better health status than adults in any other racial or ethnic group *at every level* of education. The gradient in health by educational level within each racial or ethnic group is shown in Figure 5.3.

Educational attainment may influence healthy choices and better health via multiple pathways. For example, people with more schooling may have a better understanding of the importance of specific healthy behaviors, or higher educational attainment may lead to higher-paying jobs with greater economic security, healthier working conditions, better benefits, and greater ability to purchase more nutritious foods and live in a safe neighborhood with good schools and recreational facilities. Figure 5.4 demonstrates that behavior and education both

FIGURE 5.3   GRADIENTS WITHIN GRADIENTS

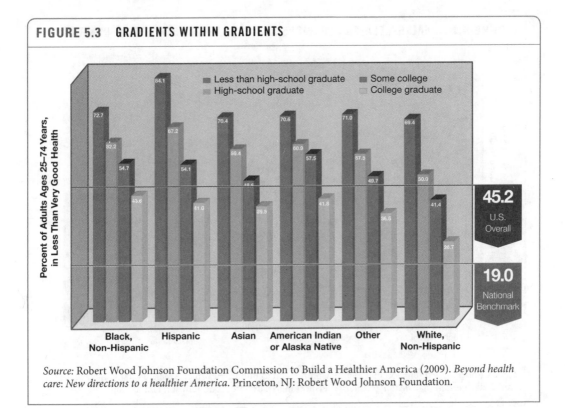

Source: Robert Wood Johnson Foundation Commission to Build a Healthier America (2009). *Beyond health care: New directions to a healthier America.* Princeton, NJ: Robert Wood Johnson Foundation.

affect health: At every level of educational attainment, adults who smoke and do not participate in leisure-time exercise are less likely to be in very good health than adults who do not smoke and do get exercise.

Similar to educational attainment, racial discrimination can affect health via multiple pathways. A substantial base of evidence exists regarding the effect of different policies on both discrimination and health. Exposure to discrimination in and of itself provokes a physiological stress response in the lab, and repeated or sustained exposure leads to chronic, unhealthful activation of the stress response. A variety of policies have combined to maintain or worsen Black–White segregation by neighborhood, despite the civil rights legislation of the 1960s. Residential segregation influences diverse social determinants of health, including educational and employment opportunities, access to safe and affordable housing, routine opportunities for physical activity, food "deserts" with scarce access to fresh healthy foods, and exposure to violence. There is strong evidence that reducing or eliminating residential segregation would substantially diminish Black–White differences in income, education, and unemployment, and in turn racial disparities in health (Williams & Collins, 2001).

As noted earlier, the population health model calls for integration of the multiple determinants of health, with consideration of both negative and positive interactions among different factors. The relationships between socioeconomic status and health are complicated, but the most persistent disparities in health between groups clearly involve the intersection of multiple types of social

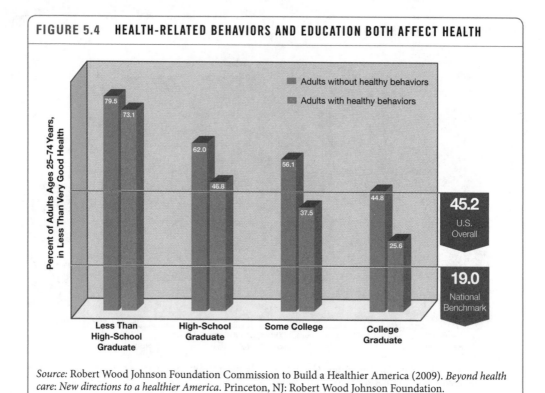

FIGURE 5.4 HEALTH-RELATED BEHAVIORS AND EDUCATION BOTH AFFECT HEALTH

Source: Robert Wood Johnson Foundation Commission to Build a Healthier America (2009). *Beyond health care: New directions to a healthier America.* Princeton, NJ: Robert Wood Johnson Foundation.

disadvantages (Adler & Stewart, 2010). The interconnected nature of social categorizations such as race, class, and gender as they apply to a given individual or group result in overlapping and interdependent systems of discrimination or disadvantage, as described by the concept of "intersectionality" (Schulz & Mullings, 2006).

LEADING DETERMINANTS OF HEALTH: WEIGHTING THE DIFFERENT DOMAINS

The five different domains or categories of health determinants, described earlier in this chapter, do not make equal contributions to the health outcomes of populations. This is not "new news." In the 1970s, Thomas McKeown (1976) concluded that improved health and longevity in England over the previous 200 years resulted from changes in food supplies, sanitary conditions, and smaller family sizes, rather than medical interventions. In the United States, John Bunker and colleagues (1995) estimated that during the 20th century, medical care explained only 5 of the 30-year increase in life expectancy

> During the 20th century, medical care explained only 5 of the 30-year increase in life expectancy.

and, between 1950 and 1990, when many new therapies were developed for infectious diseases and heart disease, medical care accounted for only 3 of the 7 years of life expectancy increase.

Medical care also can be responsible for *increasing* mortality rates. A 2000 Institute of Medicine (IOM) report publicized the startling finding that medical errors accounted for approximately 2% to 4% of U.S. deaths annually (Kohn, Corrigan, & Donaldson, 2000), placing medical error among the top causes of death (Bleich, 2005).

There was a period of time in the 1990s during which medical scientists expected that genetics could explain much of the variation in health between groups and individuals, yet the role of genetics in understanding such variation remains unresolved. Recent initiatives to study genetic factors at the population level, such as the National Institutes of Health (NIH) – sponsored All of Us project to enroll 1 million individuals in a cohort study collecting data on multiple domains of health, will deepen knowledge on this important front.

Health behaviors (e.g., smoking, physical activity, substance abuse, sexual activity, diet) are considered major determinants of health in both the medical and population health models. Analysis of data from 22 European countries showed that variations in health disparities could be attributed to variations in smoking, alcohol consumption, and access to care but that the patterns of determinants of inequality were different for men and women, by country, and by which outcome was measured (Mackenbach et al., 2008).

The best weighting scheme to determine the combined effects of determinants from different domains depends on the health outcome of interest. Some outcomes will be more dependent on certain determinants than on others. Researchers have therefore estimated the relative contributions of the multiple determinants of health through what are called *summary* measures of mortality and morbidity—that is, measures that summarize the length and quality of life. Significant progress has been made in accumulating the empirical data that can yield the best approximations of the relative weights of each domain on summary health outcomes.

McGinnis and Foege (1993) reviewed the relevant literature from 1977 to 1993 to analyze the leading causes of U.S. deaths. They concluded that approximately *half* of all deaths in 1990 were due to key behavioral factors, led by tobacco use and followed by diet and physical activity. Related estimates included that about 40% of deaths were caused by behavioral factors, 30% by genetics, 15% by social determinants, 10% by medical care, and 5% by physical environmental exposures. Ten years later, an IOM (2003) analysis revised the 1990 estimate of 50% of all deaths upward to 70% of all deaths being due to key behavioral and environmental factors. The Centers for Disease Control and Prevention (CDC) updated the McGinnis and Foege analysis and concluded that smoking remained the leading cause of preventable deaths, followed by poor diet and lack of physical activity (Mokdad, Marks, Stroup, & Gerberding, 2005).

The annual national *County Health Rankings* report, first launched in 2010, ranks the overall health of every county within each of the 50 states and reports the contribution of the multiple determinants of health on each county's overall health using a population health framework. Health outcomes are viewed as the result of a combined set of factors, and these factors are also affected by conditions, policies, and programs in their communities. The report is based on a model that compares overall rankings on health outcomes with rankings on different health factors (Figure 5.5).

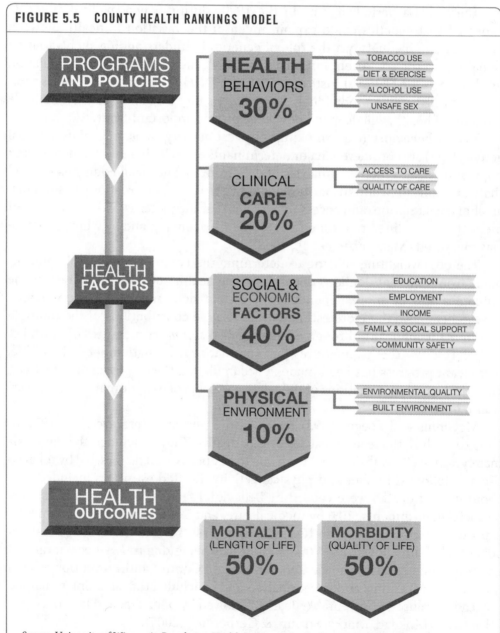

FIGURE 5.5   COUNTY HEALTH RANKINGS MODEL

Source: University of Wisconsin Population Health Institute (2010). County Health Rankings and Roadmaps 2018. Retrieved from http://www.countyhealthrankings.org/county-health-rankings-model

The *County Health Rankings* report estimates the influence on health and longevity of (a) health behaviors at 30%, (b) clinical care at 20%, (c) social and economic factors at 40%, and (d) physical environmental factors at 10%. Though there is a range of opinion on the merits of accounting for all causes of health and disease in such models (Krieger, 2017), the rankings have powerfully demonstrated dramatic variation between one county and another in health outcomes and in health determinants. This variation is even greater than the variation in health care expenditures and health care outcomes that has been demonstrated over many years by health service researchers. For example, the premature death rate in the least healthy counties was two and one half times greater than in the healthiest counties.

The bottom-line message of the *County Health Rankings* project is that *where* people live matters to their health. The population health framework enables communities to see which factors are contributing the most to their poor or good health outcomes, and thus choose to act to improve the factors affecting health, vitality, and productivity of all community residents.

HEALTH POLICY AND RETURNS ON INVESTMENT

In a logical world, the more that is known about the causes of a significant problem, the more resources would be allocated toward reducing the most important of those causes. In the United States, two-thirds of what we spend on health care is attributable to diseases that are preventable. But we invest less than 5% of our more than $3 trillion annual health spending on efforts to prevent these illnesses, whereas 95% goes to direct medical care. Yet, for the reasons set forth above, only perhaps 10% to 15% of preventable deaths could be avoided by increasing the availability or quality of medical care.

> The population health model suggests that investments and policy decisions in areas that are not traditionally considered the province of health care are more likely to have a significant effect on improving a population's health than increased spending on medical services.

The population health model suggests that investments and policy decisions in areas that are not traditionally considered the province of health care are more likely to have a significant effect on improving a population's health than increased spending on medical services. Indeed, the share of the U.S. GDP that is spent by the health care sector on processes, tests, and treatment of little value has been likened to theft from other sectors such as education, in which comparable investment could have a far more profound and enduring impact on health (Berwick & Hackbarth, 2012). An excellent review of the challenges and effect on health of policies in the areas of education, income transfer, civil rights, macroeconomics and employment, welfare, housing, and neighborhoods is provided in a comprehensive text by Schoeni, House, Kaplan, & Pollack (2008).

Researchers are only beginning to be able to provide the evidence to guide policy makers regarding the comparative effectiveness and costs of specific investment choices across the five categories of health determinants, reflecting in part methodologic challenges arising from interactions among determinants, the latency over time of their effects, and the sparsity of robust longitudinal data sets. Nevertheless, this evidence base is growing rapidly, as shown by research estimating that correcting disparities in education-associated mortality rates would have averted eight times more deaths than improvements attributable to medical advances between 1996 and 2002 (Woolf, Johnson, Phillips, & Philipsen, 2007). Another example comes from a study by the Urban Institute, which calculated the return on investment for prevention and concluded that an investment of $10 per person per year in proven community-based programs to increase physical activity, improve nutrition, and prevent smoking and other tobacco use could save the country more than $16 billion annually within five years. This is a return of $5.60 for every $1 invested (Trust for America's Health, 2008).

The Robert Wood Johnson Foundation Commission to Build a Healthier America delivered a series of evidence-based policy recommendations to improve health, including the following:

- Provide high-quality early developmental services and support for all children.
- Fund and design the Special Supplemental Nutrition Program for Women, Infants, and Children (WIC) and the Supplemental Nutrition Assistance Program (SNAP, also known as food stamps) programs to meet the need of hungry families for nutritious food.
- Eliminate so-called food deserts through public–private partnerships.
- Require healthy foods and physical activity in all schools (K–12).
- Ensure that decision makers in all sectors have the evidence they need to build health into public and private policies and practices.

The last strategy underscores the need to consider the health effects of policies, programs, and projects in sectors not traditionally thought of as affecting health. This can be achieved through the use of health impact assessments (HIAs; www .healthimpactproject.org), which have a long history of use in the same countries that have led the way in developing and acting upon the population health model. HIAs have been used in a wide variety of decisions regarding transportation, housing, zoning, and other aspects of the built environment and more recently have been used to address social policies related to education, labor, criminal justice, segregation, and other areas. HIAs are one of the tools that can be used to bring a health lens to policy, program, and project decisions made in nonhealth sectors, an approach known as health in all policies (HIAP).

While population health interventions have the potential to create much greater improvements in the health of Americans than further spending increases for medical services, a core challenge is to find sustainable approaches to financing them. Over the past 5 years, a number of innovative methods have been implemented to direct funding to community-level prevention initiatives addressing social, physical, and economic environments. One model is a wellness trust: a fund set aside specifically to support population-wide interventions or policies.

Funds for a wellness trust can come from a number of sources, such as a tax on insurers or hospitals, as was done in Massachusetts in 2013. Another innovation is a variation on social impact bonds as health impact bonds (also referred to as Pay for Success). Capital is raised from private investors to implement community or state prevention interventions, and the resulting health care cost savings are returned to the investors as break-even or profit. A number of health impact bonds are in progress, including home remediation of mold and other triggers of childhood asthma to reduce unnecessary hospitalizations and emergency room visits for asthma in multiple communities, or improving birth outcomes through the Nurse-Family Partnership in South Carolina.

Another potential source of funding is community benefit spending by nonprofit hospitals. Since the 1950s, to keep their tax-exempt status, nonprofit hospitals have owed certain duties to the community, largely focusing on providing charity care to the **medically indigent**. Concurrently with the passage of the Patient Protection and Affordable Care Act (ACA), amendments were made to the Internal Revenue Service code that increased the rigor and consistency of hospital reporting, requiring hospitals to perform a community health needs assessment every 3 years with collaboration from public health experts and the community and to use the resulting findings as the basis for conducting community health improvement activities. Such activities can include investments in community-based health services that are furnished outside of and are not billable by the hospital, as well as more upstream interventions addressing social and physical environmental determinants like investing in housing to improve health. These ACA-based changes have stimulated increased collaboration by many hospitals with public health and community partners, although the degree to which hospitals are committing funds to identified community priorities varies widely.

Other innovations include the concept of a "health dividend," which refers to the opportunity cost of waste in health care spending, estimated at $750 billion per year. If this waste could be eliminated and the funding recaptured, the money could be used to improve key determinants of population health—for example by investing in education, job training, or improving the built environment (McCullough, Zimmerman, Fielding, & Teutsch, 2012).

Additional potential population health financing innovations result from the implementation of the ACA. The Prevention and Public Health Fund, intended to provide stable funding for increased activities to improve community health, supported a number of programs to improve population health using place-based strategies, such as Community Transformation Grants. However, the fund was also used to fill gaps in the implementation of health care changes under the ACA and has been a continual target of those opposed to the health reform act.

Other opportunities have resulted from the ACA, including accountable care organizations (ACOs) and Medicaid waivers and innovation grants. ACOs are essentially networks of providers and hospitals that share responsibility for the health care and health outcomes of a set of patients. ACOs provide savings incentives by offering bonuses when providers keep costs down and meet specific quality benchmarks, focusing on prevention and carefully managing patients with chronic diseases. In other words, providers get paid more for keeping their patients healthy and out of the hospital. To do this well requires that providers and hospitals work in the community beyond the walls of their institutions to ensure better care coordination—and better social and physical conditions for promoting health. ACOs were designed to lay the foundation for the anticipated transition by the Center for Medicare and Medicaid Services (CMS) toward value-based payment. Another innovation opportunity came from state waivers for delivery of Medicaid. For example, the Texas Medicaid waiver was constructed such that 5% of the billions of dollars in the waiver was earmarked to support public health interventions that would prevent illness or injury and thus save Medicaid money. These payment model innovations, like those mentioned previously, require careful evaluation to document their ability to bring about population health improvements and to decrease health care costs. More recently, some Medicaid managed care organizations have begun to move toward global budgeting, freeing them to be able to consider funding community interventions like supportive housing if they led to better health outcomes (and lower total costs) for their capitated populations. Innovative variations on this approach to improving both health care delivery and the health of clinical populations care have been set in motion in numerous states through "accountable health communities" that take on responsibility for both health care and identifying and addressing social determinants of health among participants (Alley, Asomugha, Conway, & Sanghavi, 2016).

Recognizing the impact that factors outside the health care system can have on health care utilization and costs, the health care sector is beginning to screen patients for social determinants of health like housing, transportation, and food insecurity. A challenge to this approach is that while it may be relatively easy to identify a patient's social stressor (e.g., unstable housing), putting into place referral systems that are efficient and effective and generate feedback to the provider (as expected for other referrals made during the course of clinical care) can be a major challenge. Innovative solutions, such as local mapping of community health-related assets and social service referral software integrated with the electronic health record, are beginning to demonstrate promise toward this important goal (Lindau et al., 2016).

CONCLUSION

Recognition of the importance and value of population health science and of the population health model to advancing health in the United States has accelerated greatly in the last decade. Examples include:

- An extensive literature of high-quality publications in top U.S. medical, health care, and public health journals as well as books in multiple disciplines

- National Institutes of Health and CDC funding of multidisciplinary population health research and intervention programs
- Numerous National Academy of Medicine review committees and reports on the multiple determinants of health and its Roundtable on Population Health Improvement
- Interdisciplinary population health centers and training programs at premier universities across the country and the emergence of departments of population health at leading academic medical centers
- The MacArthur Research Network on Socioeconomic Status and Health, a research working group funded by the MacArthur Foundation, which operated from 1998 to 2010
- National commissions on population health and prevention, including the Robert Wood Johnson Foundation's two reports from the Commission to Build a Healthier America
- The annual national *County Health Rankings* report based on a multiple determinants of health framework as well as similar initiatives at the city level (e.g., the *City Health Dashboard*)

The population health model is increasingly accepted as a framework for understanding the multiple determinants of health, with an emphasis on prevention and a strong basis in scientific evidence. Importantly, the term "population health" also entered the lexicon of clinical practice in 2007 as part of the Institute for Healthcare Improvement's (IHI) Triple Aim initiative to (a) improve the health of the population, (b) enhance the experience and outcomes of the patient, and (c) reduce per capita cost of care for the benefit of communities. The Triple Aim initiative's use of the phrase "population health" has led to some confusion in terminology. Noting this, the IHI stated in 2014 that "population health" refers to the broader determinants of health, whereas the Triple Aim refers to "population medicine" as the management of a discrete population in a health care system, health plan, or ACO to improve outcomes.

There is great potential for population health strategies to aid medical care providers in improving the outcomes for their patients. As noted earlier in this chapter, population health is not only about primary prevention; the social, behavioral, and environmental determinants of health also strongly affect patients' ability and likelihood to carry out medical care providers' recommendations about changing lifestyle behaviors or preventing social crises (such as losing a job or becoming homeless) that in turn trigger serious health crises.

As envisaged in the 2003 IOM report on the future of the public's health, collaboration among those using the medical, governmental public health, and population health models would provide a more coherent national approach to health improvement. Such an approach would include a common, integrated set of metrics for determinants and outcomes, provide sustainable realigned funding, and result in more strategic and synergistic planning for the actions best suited for improving the conditions needed for all Americans to have the opportunity to lead healthy lives.

▶ CASE EXERCISE—SODIUM AND ITS EFFECTS ON OUR HEALTH

Recent data show that Americans consume, on average, more than three times the recommended level of sodium per day in their food and beverages. High salt intake contributes to high blood pressure and its complications—stroke, heart attack, congestive heart failure, and kidney failure. In fact, thousands of lives could be saved if sodium consumption were lowered in people with high blood pressure. Write a memo for the U.S. Secretary of Health and Human Services about what might be done to address concerns about the effect of high sodium intake on health. In preparing your memo, consider the following questions:

1. How might we address this problem in the patient population using the medical model that a health care provider might use versus a population health model that a public health official might use?

2. How far can and should governments go in attempting to create a more healthful environment? Intrinsic to many population health policies is the specter of the so-called nanny state. In this case, is it necessary for everyone to be exposed to lower sodium in their bread, in other common foods, and in restaurants, so as to protect people who have salt-sensitive illnesses?

3. Should manufacturers bear the costs of manufacturing different versions of foods in order to protect the public's health? Should they be required to manufacture healthier foods, even if customers prefer the less healthy versions? Or should they be liable if they don't manufacture healthier foods?

DISCUSSION QUESTIONS

1. The general public equates the word "health" with "health care." Polls asking people about their health typically result in responses about their health care experiences. How do you define health? How would you assess a population's health if you could ask the people in that population only one question on a survey?

2. Why do some people refer to the health care system as "the sickness care system"? Do you agree or disagree with this term?

3. Cross-sectional research shows that, on average, people with disabilities secondary to illness or injury have lower socioeconomic status than people without disabilities. How could longitudinal research help to explain whether this is because people of lower socioeconomic status are at higher risk of developing disabilities or because disability leads to loss of income and thus lower socioeconomic status? In a population health model, how might lower socioeconomic status increase the risk of disability secondary to illness or injury?

4. The Commission to Build a Healthier America found that non-Hispanic Whites were more likely to be in very good or excellent health than other groups nationally and in almost every state. In addition, non-Hispanic Whites had better health status than adults in any other racial or ethnic group at every level of education, but all groups showed a gradient in health by educational level. What are some of the determinants that are likely contributing to this disparity in health between non-Hispanic Whites and other groups after controlling for different educational levels?

5. It is possible that a community's *County Health Rankings* would suggest that the biggest driver of poor health in that community is unemployment. How would you present the case to your nonprofit hospital board that the biggest community benefit contribution the hospital could make would be to join and support an initiative to increase job openings in the community, rather than holding health fairs or offering educational lecture series?

REFERENCES

Adler, N. E., & Stewart, J. (Eds.). (2010). *The biology of disadvantage: Socioeconomic status and health. Annals of the New York Academy of Sciences* (Vol. 1186). San Francisco, CA: MacArthur Network for Socioeconomic Health.

Alley, D. E., Asomugha, C. N., Conway, P. H., & Sanghavi, D. M. (2016). Accountable health communities—Addressing social needs through Medicare and Medicaid. *New England Journal of Medicine, 374*, 8–11. doi:10.1056/NEJMp1512532

Berwick, D. M., & Hackbarth, A. D. (2012). Eliminating waste in U.S. health care. *Journal of the American Medical Association, 307*, 1513–1516. doi:10.1001/jama.2012.362

Bleich, S. (2005, July). Medical errors: Five years after the IOM report. *Issue Brief (The Commonwealth Fund), 830*, 1–15. Retrieved from https://pdfs.semanticscholar.org/b132/d78f82d6a8f8f724069f6fbe4bdb85181b2e.pdf

Bradley, E. H., Elkins, B. R., Herrin, J., & Elbel, B. D. (2011). Health and social service expenditures: Associations with health outcomes. *BMJ Quality & Safety, 20*, 826–831. doi:10.1136/bmjqs.2010.048363

Braveman, P., & Gruskin, S. (2003). Defining equity in health. *Journal of Epidemiology and Community Health, 57*, 254–258. doi:10.1136/jech.57.4.254

Bunker, J. P., Frazier, H. S., & Mosteller, F. (1995). The role of medical care in determining health: Creating an inventory of benefits. In B. C. Amick III, S. Levine, A. R. Tarlov, & D. C. Walsh (Eds.), *Society and health* (pp. 304–341). New York, NY: Oxford University Press.

Chetty, R., Stepner, M., Abraham, S., Lin, S., Scuderi, B., Turner, N., ... Cutler, D. (2016). The association between income and life expectancy in the United States, 2001–2014. *Journal of the American Medical Association, 315*, 1750–1766. doi:10.1001/jama.2016.4226

Evans, R. G., Barer, M. L., & Marmor, T. R. (Eds.). (1994). *Why are some people healthy and others not? The determinants of health of populations.* New York, NY: Walter de Gruyter.

Institute of Medicine. (2003). *The future of the public's health in the 21st century.* Washington, DC: National Academies Press.

Kindig, D., & Chin, S. (2009, June 18). Achieving "a culture of health": What would it mean for costs and our health status? *Innovation, health, and equity: Taking a systems approach to health and economic vitality.* Presentation sponsored by Altarum Institute, Ann Arbor, MI.

Kindig, D., & Stoddart, G. (2003). What is population health? *American Journal of Public Health, 93*, 380–383. doi:10.2105/AJPH.93.3.380

Kohn, L. T., Corrigan, J. M., & Donaldson, M. S. (Eds.). (2000). *To err is human: Building a safer health system.* Washington, DC: National Academies Press.

Kreuter, M., & Lezin, N. (2001). *Improving everyone's quality of life: A primer on population health.* Seattle, WA: Group Health Community Foundation.

Krieger, N. (2017). Health equity and the fallacy of treating causes of population health as if they sum to 100%. *American Journal of Public Health, 107*, 541–549. doi:10.2105/AJPH.2017.303655

Lindau, S. T., Makelarski, J., Abramsohn, E., Beiser, D. G., Escamilla, V., Jerome, J., ... Miller, D. C. (2016). Community Rx: A population health improvement innovation that connects clinics to communities. *Health Affairs, 35,* 2020–2029. doi:10.1377/hlthaff.2016.0694

Mackenbach, J. P., Stirbu, I., Roskam, A. R., Schaap, M. M., Menvielle, G., Leinsalu, M., & Kunst, A. E. (2008). Socioeconomic inequalities in health in 22 European countries [Special article]. *New England Journal of Medicine, 358,* 2468–2481. doi:10.1056/NEJMsa0707519

McCullough, J. C., Zimmerman, F. J., Fielding, J. E., & Teutsch, S. M. (2012). A health dividend for America: The opportunity cost of excess medical expenditures. *American Journal of Preventive Medicine, 43,* 650–654. doi:10.1016/j.amepre.2012.08.013

McGinnis, J. M., & Foege, W. H. (1993). Actual causes of death in the United States. *Journal of the American Medical Association, 270,* 2207–2212. Retrieved from https://pdfs.semanticscholar.org/7e7b/c02006a12833c8f164c38d0074a59e0469e6.pdf

McKeown, T. (1976). *The role of medicine: Dream, mirage, or nemesis?* London: Nuffield Provincial Hospitals Trust.

Mokdad, A. H., Marks, J. S., Stroup, D. F., & Gerberding, J. L. (2005). Actual causes of death in the United States, 2000: Corrected version. *Journal of the American Medical Association, 293,* 293–294. doi:10.1001/jama.293.3.293

Novak, N. L., Geronimus, A. T., & Martinez-Cardoso, A. M. (2017). Change in birth outcomes among infants born to Latina mothers after a major immigration raid. *International Journal of Epidemiology, 46,* 839–849. doi:10.1093/ije/dyw346

Organisation for Economic Co-operation and Development. (2013). *Health at a glance.* Paris, France: Author. doi: 10.1787/health_glance-2013-en

Robert Wood Johnson Foundation Commission to Build a Healthier America. (2009). *Beyond health care: New directions to a healthier America.* Princeton, NJ: Robert Wood Johnson Foundation.

Robert Wood Johnson Foundation Commission to Build a Healthier America. (2014). *Time to act: Investing in the health of our children and communities.* Princeton, NJ: Robert Wood Johnson Foundation.

Schoeni, R. F., House, J. S., Kaplan, G. A., & Pollack, H. (Eds.). (2008). *Making Americans healthier: Social and economic policy as health policy.* New York, NY: Russell Sage Foundation.

Schulz, A. J., & Mullings, L. (Eds.). (2006). *Gender, race, class & health: Intersectional approaches.* San Francisco CA: Jossey-Bass.

Trust for America's Health. (2008). *Prevention for a healthier America: Investments in disease prevention yield significant savings, stronger communities.* Washington, DC: Trust for America's Health. Retrieved from http://healthyamericans.org/reports/prevention08

University of Wisconsin Population Health Institute. (2010). County Health Rankings and Roadmaps 2018. Retrieved from http://www.countyhealthrankings.org/county-health-rankings-model

Williams, D., & Collins, C. (2001). Racial residential segregation: A fundamental cause of racial disparities in health. *Public Health Reports, 116,* 404–416. doi:10.1093/phr/116.5.404

Woolf, S. H., & Aron, L. (Eds.). (2013). *U.S. health in international perspective: Shorter lives, poorer health.* Washington, DC: National Academies Press.

Woolf, S. H., Johnson, R. E., Phillips, R. L., & Philipsen, M. (2007). Giving everyone the health of the educated: An examination of whether social change would save more lives than medical advances. *American Journal of Public Health, 97,* 679–683. doi:10.2105/AJPH.2005.084848

6

Public Health: A Transformation in the 21st Century

Laura C. Leviton, Paul L. Kuehnert, and Kathryn E. Wehr

LEARNING OBJECTIVES

▶ Discuss why a healthy population is in the public interest
▶ Contrast defining characteristics of prevention-oriented public health and treatment-oriented health care
▶ Identify the core functions of public health
▶ Define essential public health activities
▶ Describe state, federal, tribal, and local authority for public health laws, regulations, and services
▶ Identify how challenges and opportunities are transforming public health

KEY TERMS

▶ Association of State and Territorial Health Officers (ASTHO)
▶ health (World Health Organization definition)
▶ health impact assessments (HIAs)
▶ health promotion
▶ health status of entire populations
▶ multisectoral collaborations
▶ National Association of County and City Health Officials (NACCHO)
▶ nongovernmental organizations
▶ policy development

- ▶ population health
- ▶ primary prevention
- ▶ Public Health Accreditation Board (PHAB)
- ▶ secondary prevention

TOPICAL OUTLINE

- ▶ Overview of a complex infrastructure
- ▶ Public health requires a collective response from society
- ▶ Public health is different from individual health care
- ▶ The core functions of public health define essential public health activities
- ▶ Governmental agencies have legal authority for the core functions
- ▶ Various social, economic, and political forces are transforming public health

OVERVIEW OF A COMPLEX INFRASTRUCTURE

This chapter introduces the policies, programs, and practices that constitute public health in the United States. Public health is "what society does collectively to assure the conditions for people to be healthy" (Institute of Medicine, 2002). It is the science, practice, and art of protecting and improving the health of populations (Kindig, 2015). We first describe the goals and characteristics of public health that differentiate it from health care treatment, and we outline the core functions of public health. We then describe the complex network of laws, regulations, authorities, and services involved. Federal, tribal, state, and local government agencies, often called the infrastructure, have legal authority for the core functions. At the same time, champions of public health span many public, private, and nonprofit organizations. In the concluding section, we describe forces at work to transform public health in the 21st century.

> Public health focuses on entire populations and the design of policies, systems, services, and environments to achieve not just the absence of disease, but a collective sense of well-being.*

Historically, public health emphasized regulating and improving community sanitation, monitoring environmental hazards, and care of poor mothers and children. Over time, it greatly expanded its role in documenting and controlling communicable diseases and encouraging health promoting behavior. In the late 20th century, many local health departments were the provider of last resort for indigent health care. With passage

> Public health is "what society does collectively to assure the conditions for people to be healthy" (Institute of Medicine, 2002).

---

*To hear the podcast, go to https://bcove.video/2DY99Vw or access the ebook on Springer Publishing Connect™.

of the Patient Protection and Affordable Care Act (ACA) in 2010, health departments began to reorganize and direct more resources to prevention as more people received health insurance. The ACA included an unprecedented single investment in its Prevention and Public Health Fund, which also enabled this shift. However, federal funding for prevention has since declined, the ACA is in jeopardy, state funding has been level since 2010, and state and local health departments have seen a 20% drop in personnel since 2008 due to budget cuts (see the following). It is too soon to predict a long-term trend of support for government-funded public health, given political volatility in 2018. What is certain is that the principles and services we describe in this chapter are quite simply necessary to ensure the health of populations. Public health activity only accounts for an estimated 1% to 3% of national spending (Leider et al., 2016), yet greater spending per capita is linked to decline in preventable deaths (Mays & Smith, 2011). And despite politics, there is growing recognition that public health in the United States needs to move away from piecemeal responses to health problems toward a more coherent and comprehensive approach. Public health champions are also working far beyond the conventional health sector to advocate for a broader set of policies and systems changes that improve and protect health.

Public Health Every Day

Public health activities affect the lives of Americans profoundly, but more often than not these activities are invisible. A thought experiment shows how this works. Imagine waking up and going through your morning routine. You slept 8 hours for a change because health experts claim that lack of sleep causes stress and other health problems. You wander into the bathroom and brush your teeth—teeth that are still in your mouth and pain free thanks to regular brushing and flossing, adequate nutrition, and routine dental visits. You feel that good habits are your personal responsibility, but you take for granted the

> Public health activities affect the lives of Americans profoundly, but more often than not these activities are invisible.

services and policies that made these choices possible. You also take for granted that your environment keeps you healthy. Fluoride in your local water supply helps strengthen your tooth enamel and prevents cavities. You rinse your mouth with water that is safe to drink. Before it ever reached your faucet, it was checked for sickness-causing bacteria, heavy metals such as lead (which harm children's brains and nervous systems), and chemicals such as polychlorinated biphenyls (which cause cancer). When you flushed the toilet, the waste did not get into the water supply where it could kill you.

You get your children ready for school; so far, they have all survived, never having had measles, diphtheria, polio, or other diseases that killed and maimed so many children in bygone days. Thank goodness for immunizations. The kids' breakfast includes cereal and pure pasteurized milk. You looked at the nutritional label on their cereal and saw whole grains and not too much sugar—some food companies are feeling the pressure and voluntarily offering healthier kids' cereals these days.

The news feed warns that a new influenza strain is spreading, and the authorities have renewed their advisory for hand washing and travel precautions. Your sister calls to announce she is going to have a baby! She is not aware that the toast she is eating is fortified with folic acid, the B vitamin that prevents birth defects. Thanks to comprehensive sex education and family planning, the couple never had (or were quickly treated for) gonorrhea and chlamydia infection, which can cause infertility.

The two of you also discuss your father. He's over 70 and not in the best health, so he needs to get his flu and pneumonia shots right away! The last time he had flu, it turned into pneumonia; he went to the hospital and could have died. Both of you are worried about him because he is overweight, still smokes, and never exercises. Is a heart attack, diabetes, or stroke in his future? The odds are not in Dad's favor. Programs to quit smoking are available in the community without charge, so you agree that Dad's doctor should try suggesting them again. Too bad there are no sidewalks in Dad's neighborhood; he loves to walk, but there is too much traffic. Does the senior center have an exercise program that might appeal to him? You buckle the kids into their safety belts. When you get to your job, you see signs that read: "607 days without an accident at this worksite" and "proud to be tobacco free since 2008." These everyday experiences are not just about making healthier choices on your own, but about public health giving the opportunities for healthier choices and making healthier choices the easy choices.

Divided Responsibilities and Issue-Specific Organizations

The responsibility for the public's health and the infrastructure to make it work are divided among many agencies across all levels of government and many nongovernmental organizations, professional associations, and businesses (see Figure 6.1). In our thought experiment, for example, municipal authorities handle waste water, but the federal government regulates chemicals in the water supply. The federal government recommends physical activity for older adults, but local organizations like senior centers, YMCAs, private gyms, and city departments of transportation, parks and recreation, and public safety all make it possible to be physically active. The federal government requires seat belts and air bags in cars, but state laws mandate seat belt use and the penalties for violation, and local police generally enforce the laws.

At least four factors account for the complexity and diffuse responsibility for public health in the United States. The first factor is that the U.S. Constitution calls for decentralized government; states have authority for public health, except where specified by federal and tribal law. How much authority the states in turn share with local government varies a great deal and rests with diverse agencies, boards of health, and municipal and tribal codes (Hodge, 2012; Institute of Medicine, 2011).

Second is the distinctive American tendency, first recognized by Alexis de Tocqueville in the 1830s, to design laws, policies, and organizations that are problem-specific, rather than general. For example, individual diseases receive special legal recognition, and new federal programs, policies, and categorical funding streams are created to deal with them. As seen in the following, such

FIGURE 6.1   THE PUBLIC HEALTH SYSTEM AT THE LOCAL LEVEL

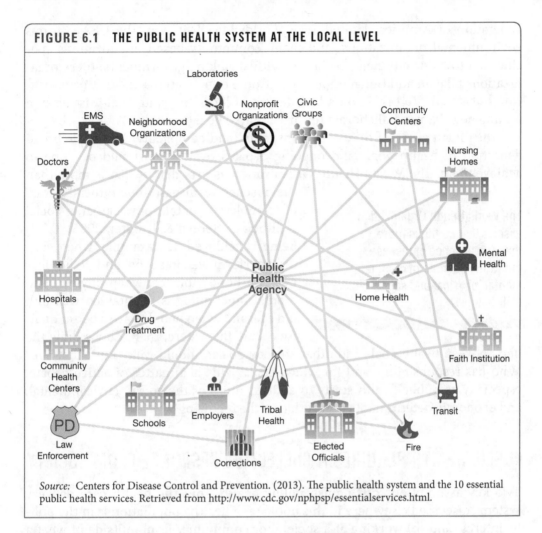

Source: Centers for Disease Control and Prevention. (2013). The public health system and the 10 essential public health services. Retrieved from http://www.cdc.gov/nphpsp/essentialservices.html.

problem-specific policies get in the way of comprehensive policies and systems to prevent and treat disease and respond to health hazards. Diverse federal departments deal with such health problems as assuring pure food and drugs (Food and Drug Administration [FDA] and United States Department of Agriculture [USDA]), monitoring and controlling infectious diseases (Centers for Disease Control and Prevention [CDC]), providing guidance to prevent chronic diseases (CDC, National Institutes of Health [NIH]), improving traffic safety (Department of Transportation [DOT], National Highway Traffic Safety Administration [NHTSA]), maternal and child health care (Centers for Medicare & Medicaid Services [CMS], Health Resources and Services Administration [HRSA]), and ensuring a healthy and safe place to work (Occupational Safety and Health Administration [OSHA], Mine Safety and Health Administration [MSHA], National Institute for Occupational Safety and Health [NIOSH]).

A third distinctively American approach is the heavy reliance on nongovernmental organizations to achieve public health goals. Yet these organizations also tend to be issue-specific: national organizations and their local affiliates such as the American Red Cross, American Heart Association, the Planned Parenthood

Federation of America, United Way Worldwide, YMCA of the USA, various environmental organizations, and many community-based organizations specific to a town or city neighborhood. With shrinking governments, these organizations take on additional importance. Some organizations and **multisectoral collaborations** are taking on a broader set of local and state health issues and finding new ways to collaborate toward a shared goal (see below).

The fourth cause of diffuse responsibility (and complexity) lies in the broad definition of health goals and ongoing debates over what should be done to achieve them. The World Health Organization asserts that **health** is more than the absence of disease, but rather "a state of complete mental, physical and social well-being" (Green & Kreuter, 2005). Well-being is achieved, for example, when children perform well in school and do not fear neighborhood violence, when physical and mental functioning is maintained well into old age, and when people have a better quality of life. But where, then, do we draw the line between health goals and other societal goals? Should we draw such a line? Who has responsibility, and for which goals? This is a matter of active debate, especially as public health starts to address more of the social, environmental, and economic determinants of health (see the following).

> The World Health Organization asserts that health is more than the absence of disease, but rather "a state of complete mental, physical and social well-being."

PUBLIC HEALTH REQUIRES A COLLECTIVE RESPONSE FROM SOCIETY

Two key assumptions distinguish public health from the health care delivery systems discussed elsewhere in this book: (a) a healthy population is in the public interest and (b) working at a societal or community level (outside of what a clinician can do in a health care setting), we can improve an entire population's health.

The Health of Populations Is in the Public Interest

The goal of public health is to improve the **health status of entire populations**, not just individuals. It is concerned with the incidence, prevalence, and distribution of health problems and differences by places and populations. In using these indicators, public health aims to identify health problems and improve them through action at a community, state, or other collective level. This aim is well justified by past successes. Between 1900 and 2015, average life expectancy increased from 47.3 to 78.8 years (National Center for Health Statistics, 2017). Medical care treatment did not accomplish this change. Rather, society made pervasive improvements in 10 public health arenas (see Exhibit 6.1). In the present day, health still is most strongly determined by behavioral, community, environmental, and societal forces, not by health care (see Chapter 7).

EXHIBIT 6.1 10 GREAT PUBLIC HEALTH ACHIEVEMENTS—UNITED STATES, 1900–1999

- Vaccination
- Motor vehicle safety
- Safer workplaces
- Control of infectious diseases
- Decline in deaths from coronary heart disease and stroke
- Safer and healthier foods
- Healthier mothers and babies
- Family planning
- Fluoridation of drinking water
- Recognition of tobacco use as a health hazard

Note: Based on the impact on death, illness, and disability in the United States and not ranked by order of importance.
Source: US Centers for Disease Control and Prevention. (1999). Ten great public health achievements— United States, 1900–1999. *Morbidity and Mortality Weekly Report, 48*(12), 241–243. Retrieved from https:// www.cdc.gov/mmwr/preview/mmwrhtml/00056796.htm

The Public Interest Justifies a Collective Response

Public health is necessary because neither individual behaviors, nor medicine, nor the private sector are enough to keep people healthy. Thus, the public interest requires government services, or at least some form of effective collective action. Since ancient times, people have taken collective action to protect themselves from disease and environmental disaster. In the 19th century, public health was justified on utilitarian grounds: the greatest good for the greatest number. Healthy people are a more productive workforce and better able to defend the nation. The utilitarian argument is still compelling: For example, a high childhood obesity rate impairs America's economic competitiveness and the combat readiness of youth (Institute of Medicine, 2012). However, public health today is also justified as a human right, and public health is seen as a means to achieve social justice by addressing social and economic disparities that contribute to health inequities (Beauchamp & Steinbock, 1999).

Not everyone agrees with this rationale. Conservatives often reject social justice as a reason for collective action. In truth, most public health services serve both utilitarian and social justice aims. For example, many publicly funded prevention efforts are targeted to poor children, but these efforts also help produce a healthier workforce. Also, libertarians believe public health limits individual liberty (Leviton, Needleman, & Shapiro, 1997). Indeed, public health policy and practice usually balance individual freedoms and collective benefits. For example, health departments have police powers to control infectious disease as a "clear and present danger," but they need to do so without appearing to abuse this power. Some legal decisions have, in fact, limited public health activities where they infringed on individual liberty.

Finally, some Americans may question whether government should be involved in public health: Can't private or nonprofit organizations play the role that government plays now? In fact, private and nonprofit organizations do play important roles, but without government there is no way to address what economists term "market failures" of health care. For example, private physicians lack the health department's legal authority to monitor, reach people, and intervene, and disrupt the spread of sexually transmitted infections, food-borne disease outbreaks, rat infestations, lead poisoning among children, and other many other problems. In the same way, free markets will not assure adequate water sanitation systems or housing conditions.

PUBLIC HEALTH IS DIFFERENT FROM INDIVIDUAL HEALTH CARE

Prevention and Health Promotion at a Population Level

Public health works on prevention at a collective level through health promotion, changes in policy or law, professional and scientific consensus about prevention efforts, and recently, by incorporating health considerations in decisions of sectors outside the health care system. **Health promotion** addresses behavior and lifestyle: "the combination of educational and environmental supports for actions and conditions of living conducive to health" (Green & Kreuter, 2005). Health promotion often works through schools, businesses, recreational facilities, community associations, and health care settings.

The U.S. Preventive Services Task Force (2018) uses three long-accepted categories to describe the full array of potential preventive interventions:

- **Primary prevention**, helping people avoid the onset of a health condition, including injuries
- **Secondary prevention**, identifying and treating people who have risk factors or preclinical disease
- Tertiary prevention, treating people with an established disease in order to restore their highest functioning, minimize negative impact, and prevent complications

These categories, especially tertiary prevention, obviously spill over into the medical treatment of individuals, but at a systems or community level, they are public health issues. Providers need guidance and support to carry them out. In Table 6.1, we can see the differences between individual and collective prevention for heart disease and stroke. Notice that successful prevention for an individual (in this case, a person who might have a heart attack or stroke) depends on the widespread availability of prevention services at a *population* level. To understand more about how medical care and public health can support each other, see the Surgeon General's National Prevention Strategy: www.surgeongeneral.gov/priorities/prevention/strategy/index.html.

Planning and Policy at a Population Level

An important U.S. Department of Health and Human Services (DHHS, 2013) effort, *Healthy People 2020*, provides a comprehensive review of priority health

TABLE 6.1 DIFFERENCES BETWEEN THE ROLES OF INDIVIDUAL MEDICAL CARE AND PUBLIC HEALTH

	INDIVIDUAL MEDICAL CARE	PUBLIC HEALTH
Primary Prevention	Encourages patients to maintain healthy weight, be physically active, and not smoke	Works to establish bike and walking paths and to eliminate trans-fats from foods, offers smoking quit-lines, advocates for smoke-free public spaces and higher cigarette taxes, provides prevention guidelines to medical care providers
Secondary Prevention	Encourages regular checkups for detecting and treating high blood pressure, elevated cholesterol, and other risk factors	Mounts public service campaigns about the importance of controlling blood pressure and "knowing your number" for cholesterol, provides guidelines to medical care providers on diagnosis of blood pressure and hypercholesterolemia
Tertiary Prevention	Treats heart attack to save the heart muscle, treats stroke to minimize nervous system damage, treats atherosclerosis, restores function, and prevents recurrence through cardiac rehabilitation and medication	Provides guidelines on treatment to medical care providers, creates widespread awareness of the symptoms of heart attack and stroke and the need to seek help quickly to save the heart muscle, teaches CPR, locates automated external defibrillators in public places and worksites, establishes effective emergency systems, sponsors patient support groups

risks, effective strategies, and public health focus areas for the nation, each with many specific objectives. These areas are updated every 10 years. Progress in meeting the Healthy People objectives has been very uneven; many of the objectives are quite ambitious (Sondik, Huang, Klein, & Satcher, 2010). Disease prevention and health promotion are rarely completely effective because there are no "magic bullets" that can prevent 100% of people from becoming sick or being injured. For example, prevention has greatly reduced the rate of heart attacks, but some heart attacks still occur. People die in car crashes in spite of safety improvements that have resulted in lower fatalities overall. Not only is there no magic bullet, but public health efforts can't be "one shot," either. Efforts need to be maintained over time. Otherwise, the nation tends to lose some of its health gains. For example 2018 saw increased sexually transmitted infections, likely due in part to pervasive cuts in health department staff (see below). Forty-five years ago Congress passed the Safe Drinking Water Act, yet the aging water systems of inner cities contaminate children's drinking water with lead. Public health problems are not simple and they adapt over time. For example, we have not "solved" the tobacco problem if young people use e-cigarettes and then turn to smoking. Such problems need a combination of activities, so the reader will see lists of activities and responsibilities throughout this chapter. Each activity holds a story in itself.

Universal prevention means that everyone receives an intervention equally, while targeted prevention involves identifying and serving people at higher risk. When they are possible, universal approaches are often more effective in improving the health of populations. The case of traffic safety illustrates these approaches. People who drive while intoxicated are clearly at high risk of injury to themselves and others, and targeting drunk drivers improves road safety for everyone. However, universal protections, such as seat belts, air bags, and safer vehicles, contribute much more to reducing traffic fatalities and injuries because they help everyone, even those who never encounter a drunk driver (NHTSA, 2017).

Targeted prevention is an important focus for public health when the risk is prevalent and when there are effective means to identify and treat it. For example, a national campaign in the 1970s led to improved identification and treatment of people with high blood pressure. This in turn greatly reduced premature death and disability from cardiovascular disease (CDC, 2011). However, an initial goal was to make sure that providers screened *all* their patients for high blood pressure, a universal strategy with a population focus. Combining both universal and targeted strategies can have a cumulative benefit. A balance of targeted and universal approaches is important to avoid stigma or victim blaming of people at risk and to address health equity.

Increasing Focus on Health Equity

A term related to targeted prevention is health equity, meaning actions to eliminate health disparities or inequalities. As seen in Chapter 8, health disparity "is a difference in which disadvantaged social groups—such as the poor, racial/ethnic minorities, women, or other groups who have persistently experienced social disadvantage or discrimination—systematically experience worse health or greater health risks than more advantaged social groups" (Braveman, 2006, p. 167). In order to increase consensus about health equity, the Robert Wood Johnson Foundation provided this definition: "Health equity means that everyone has a fair and just opportunity to be healthier. This requires removing obstacles to health such as poverty, discrimination, and their consequences, including powerlessness and lack of access to good jobs with fair pay, quality education and housing, safe environments, and health care" (as cited in Braveman, Orleans, Proctor, & Plough, 2017, para. 1). Health equity may address immediate and concrete issues, like safe traffic crossings in poor neighborhoods, or it may address "upstream" social determinants of health, like affordable housing and minimum wage. Health equity appeals to social justice, but also supports the utilitarian focus on a healthier workforce. Health equity is not a zero sum game with winners and losers, however. Disparities are sometimes reduced when the majority population gets sicker—for example the reduced life expectancy of middle-age Whites in recent years. But health equity is never intended to impair other people's opportunities to be healthy.

THE CORE FUNCTIONS OF PUBLIC HEALTH DEFINE ESSENTIAL PUBLIC HEALTH ACTIVITIES

Definition of Core Functions

Public health serves three core functions, as seen in Figure 6.2, to solve health problems at a population level (Institute of Medicine, 2002). Assessment of public health problems involves understanding their prevalence, severity, and causes, using various well-tested statistical tools. While private and nonprofit organizations often do such assessments, public health agencies have the primary responsibility for surveillance of **population health** status, monitoring of disease

FIGURE 6.2   THE CIRCLE OF PUBLIC HEALTH ACTIVITIES AND 10 ESSENTIAL SERVICES

The 10 Essential Public Health Services describe the public health activities that all communities should undertake and serve as the framework for the National Public Health Performance Standards (NPHPS) instruments. Public health systems should:

ASSESSMENT

1 Monitor health status to identify and solve community health problems.

2 Diagnose and investigate health problems and health hazards in the community.

POLICY DEVELOPMENT

3 Inform, educate, and empower people about health issues.

4 Mobilize community partnerships and action to identify and solve health problems.

5 Develop policies and plans that support individual and community health efforts.

ASSURANCE

6 Enforce laws and regulations that protect health and ensure safety.

7 Link people to needed personal health services and ensure the provision of health care when otherwise unavailable.

8 Ensure competent public and personal health care workforce.

9 Evaluate effectiveness, accessibility, and quality of personal and population-based health services.

10 Research for new insights and innovative solutions to health problems.

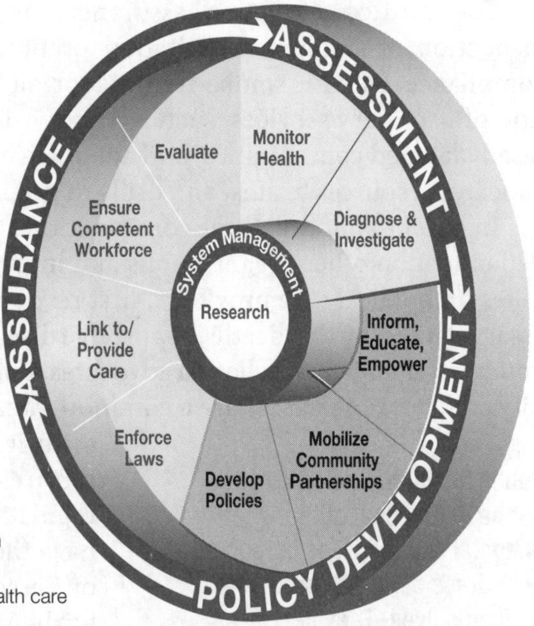

Source: Centers for Disease Control and Prevention. (2013). The public health system and the 10 essential public health services. Retrieved from https://www.cdc.gov/stltpublichealth/publichealthservices/essentialhealthservices .html

trends, and analysis of the causes of those trends and points for intervention. As seen in the final section, the assessment function is undergoing dramatic changes in resources, technology, and even reframing of public health problems as direct action on the social determinants of health.

The second core function, **policy development**, is to create and advocate for solutions to achieve public health goals. Formal policy development includes devising laws and regulations to protect the public, as in the case of environmental protection; funding and reimbursement for specific services such as child immunizations; prohibiting smoking in public places; voluntary agreements, such as businesses taking excess sugar out of the food supply; and setting guidelines or standards for services or practices, such as laboratory testing for infectious diseases. However, policy development can also involve multisectoral changes and agreements in communities, business, health care, or nonprofit organizations. For example, tax credits may help to finance a new supermarket in an underserved area so that people have access to fresh fruits and vegetables. However, the community still needs to find an operator who understands the business and will take the risk of opening the supermarket, the city needs to facilitate through zoning, the extension service may put on cooking demonstrations to familiarize people with the produce, the Supplemental Nutrition Assistance Program (SNAP) may provide two-for-one offers on produce, faith-based organizations may publicize the new market, and so on.

The third core function, assurance, involves enforcement of policy, as with inspection of restaurant sanitation or nursing home safety; monitoring legal compliance, as with smoke-free indoor air laws; ensuring proper implementation of necessary services, such as supervision of home visits to new mothers in disadvantaged communities; and adequate crisis response, as when public health allocates resources, trains, and drills to prepare for natural disasters.

In order to fulfill all three core functions, public health departments are highly dependent on other organizations and individuals. For *assessment*, public health relies on medical care providers, first responders, and others to provide the necessary data on births, deaths, reportable diseases, and environmental hazards. For *policy development*, it relies on advocates, policy makers, businesses, and community collaborators who share a common interest in public health goals. For *assurance*, it relies on complementary health care services and compliance with standards and regulations. Public health agencies do not have the legal authority, financial capability, or personnel to address all health problems by themselves. They need to collaborate with other organizations that have the power, influence, and resources to achieve better population health outcomes, for example, in promoting worker safety, assuring safe food, or building bicycle and pedestrian-friendly streets for physical activity.

> Public health agencies do not have the legal authority, financial capability, or personnel to address all health problems by themselves. They need to collaborate with other organizations that have the power, influence, and resources to achieve better population health outcomes.

Core Functions: An Example

The following example, concerning the birth defect spina bifida, illustrates the cyclical problem-solving approach used in public health (see Figure 6.2 and www.cdc.gov/ncbddd/spinabifida/data.html). Different types of assessment, policy development, and assurance issues emerge during this cycle.

1. *Monitor the problem:* Spina bifida is a neural tube defect that develops in the first 3 to 4 weeks of pregnancy, when the "neural tube" that will form the spine does not close properly. In its most severe form, spina bifida leads to leg paralysis, bowel and bladder control problems, and, without treatment, mental retardation. Spina bifida affects 3.05 out of every 10,000 live births *(assessment)*.

2. *Diagnose and investigate causes:* The CDC projects that 50% to 70% of spina bifida cases can be prevented if women take enough folic acid (a B vitamin) before and during pregnancy. Folic acid is most effective in promoting healthy neural tube development

when taken before pregnancy and during the critical first weeks. For this reason, CDC recommends that, even *before they become pregnant*, women take a multivitamin with 400 mg of folic acid every day and eat foods rich in folic acids *(policy development)*.

3. *Develop policies:* Unfortunately, women may not know they are pregnant until the defect has developed, as roughly half of all pregnancies are unintended. Also, foods that naturally contain folic acid may not be readily available to the poor or to individuals eating certain diets *assessment*. One alternative is to fortify common foods with folic acid. Since 1998, the government has required that enriched cereal, pasta, flour, and bread products include folic acid *(policy development)*.

4. *Enforce laws and regulations:* The USDA enforces folic acid requirements. WIC centers must give pregnant women nutrition education and provide the enriched foods (see www.fns.usda.gov/wic/about-wic-how-wic-helps#ImprovedDiet and Diet-Related; Outcomes); *(assurance)*.

5. *Evaluate effectiveness:* After the fortification requirement began, the rate of spina bifida in the United States declined by 31% from the rate before the policy *(assessment)*.

6. *Diagnose and investigate:* Many scientists believe we could prevent more cases of spina bifida if new regulations increased the amount of folic acid in grain products. The USDA now requires folic acid in corn masa (for tortillas); *(policy development, assessment)*.

GOVERNMENTAL AGENCIES HAVE LEGAL AUTHORITY FOR THE CORE FUNCTIONS

If people think about public health at all, they often think of federal agencies such as the CDC, which issues public guidance on prevention and warnings about the flu season. They might also think about the Environmental Protection Agency (EPA) for hazardous waste cleanup or NIH for the basic science, as in the case of folic acid. However, it is the states that have primary authority for public health, under the 10th Amendment to the U.S. Constitution. In contrast, the Constitution recognizes tribes as sovereign nations and designates federal responsibility for their health. Thus, we begin with state and tribal law and state health departments.

State Authority for Public Health

State law. The 50 states vary greatly on how they define and delegate public health authority and responsibility. States enacted public health statutes over time to respond to specific diseases or health threats. These laws are fragmented and often have not kept up with developments in science, practice, or societal change, so public health law has become a powerful force to improve effectiveness (Institute of Medicine, 2011). For example, some state laws have separate sections for specific communicable diseases, instead of standard approaches to address infectious disease in general. This fragmentation leaves them with no standards for addressing new infectious diseases, advances in public health practice, and changes in constitutional law. State laws need updating to permit new multisectoral health promotion efforts—for example, collaborations among public health, transportation, and parks and recreation to encourage more physical activity. State laws may also neglect important safeguards for privacy, due process, and protection from discrimination. One proposal, the Model State Public Health Act, was to modernize the entire body of states' public health laws. While the Model Act itself did not have much uptake, parts of its subject matter have been featured in many new state bills and laws (Hodge, 2012; Institute of Medicine, 2011). This kind of incremental policy change is typical in the United States. The Network for Public Health Law provides states with legal technical assistance that is usually more topical and less comprehensive than the Model Act (www.networkforphl.org).

Other improvements are needed for problems that cross state lines. Chief among these are problems arising from human-made and naturally occurring events such as the anthrax attacks in the fall of 2001, the increase in devastating hurricanes and other severe weather events since 2005, the 2009 H1N1 influenza pandemic, and the 2014 Ebola outbreak. These events underscored the need for legal reforms to enhance public health emergency preparedness by addressing a variety of issues, including (a) declaring public health emergencies separate from other types of disasters; (b) expediting public health powers such as those needed to collect health data, to screen, vaccinate, or treat exposed people, to seize property to abate hazards, or to isolate or quarantine residents; (c) recruiting and deploying trained health professional volunteers; and (d) providing liability protections to health professionals and entities, among others (Hodge, 2012). As of 2015, 34 states and Washington, DC, incorporated "public health emergencies" or similar terms in their statutes (Network for Public Health Law, 2015).

State health departments. In 2016, 29 state health departments were freestanding as separate agencies, while 21 states combined public health into umbrella agencies with related programs, such as Medicaid, human services and welfare, mental health and substance abuse, or environmental management. The website of the **Association of State and Territorial Health Officers** (ASTHO, www.astho.org) provides a wealth of detail on the characteristics and financing of state health departments.

A state's chief health official directs the department of public health and may report directly to the governor or to an officer in the governor's cabinet. The state health department's position in the chain of command and the governor's priorities affect the authority and power of its director. Medicaid and other state public assistance programs tend to garner most of a governor's attention because of their cost—sometimes Medicaid is part of the state health officer's authority, but usually not. These other programs can affect public health drastically given the social, economic, and environmental determinants of health. The ways various health-related functions and programs are organized affects how well public health activities can be coordinated. For example, environmental protection is often located in another agency outside the health department, in which case conservation, wilderness preservation, or litigation around toxic spills may head that agency's agenda. This situation often leaves less opportunity for effective interaction with the health department, even though it must monitor potential health consequences of environmental exposures.

Tribal public health. There are 565 federally recognized tribes, with additional tribes recognized by state governments. Each tribe has a distinct language, culture, and governance structure. Tribal governments are sovereign nations and have a government-to-government relationship with the federal government that the U.S. Constitution, Supreme Court decisions, treaties, and legislation established. Tribes gave their land and natural resources to the federal government in exchange for education, health care, and other services.

Since 1955, the Indian Health Service supports and delivers health care and public health services to American Indians and Alaska Natives. Tribes may provide public health services together with federal agencies, local and state health departments, Tribal Epidemiology Centers, and other private or public third parties. The nature and extent of these partnerships vary by tribe, region, and type of service.[1]

Tribal sovereignty and federal, state, and local agreements with tribes are particularly important when it comes to understanding policy and law across a wide range of public health issues—from injury and harm prevention, to environmental health, to animal control, to health services—and why tribal public health codes are important to recognizing tribal authority, honoring tribal culture, coordinating public health responses across jurisdictions, and ensuring adequate resources.[2]

Intergovernmental Relations

Federal–state relations. Although the states have constitutional authority to implement public health, a wide variety of federal programs and laws affect their work. Federal law relating to public health preempts state laws, just as state law preempts local laws. However, tribal governments are sovereign nations so that tribal law supersedes all but federal laws. Preemption affects public health because the federal government can require minimum protections below which states cannot go—a "floor preemption." For example, the Clean Water Act requires a minimum standard for water in all states, although states are allowed to have more stringent standards. But "ceiling preemption" can pose an obstacle to prevention when states and localities are more aggressive than the federal government. For example, the tobacco industry challenged state and local regulation of tobacco in the courts citing less stringent federal regulations. Preemption of local law plays out the same way, as in recent local efforts to prevent childhood obesity by limiting junk food and sugar-sweetened beverages. Ten states have passed preemption laws to prohibit such local efforts at the behest of food and beverage companies (Dana & Nadler, 2018).

---

[1] For more information on the organization of tribal public health, see https://www.nihb.org/docs/07012010/NIHB_HealthProfile%202010.pdf and http://www.norc.org/Research/Projects/Pages/national-profile-of-tribal-public-health-agencies.aspx

[2] For more information on policies relating to tribal public health, see http://www.ncai.org/policy-research-center/initiatives/projects/tribal-public-health-law

The federal agencies working in public health are described in Chapter 3. States must constantly interact with these federal agencies. For example, DHHS supports state health departments with grants and technical assistance for maternal and child health and preventive services, child welfare services, substance abuse treatment and prevention, and mental health services. DHHS also funds the states to train the public health workforce. CDC provides grants and cooperative agreements to states, cities, and community-based organizations for HIV prevention, chronic disease control, and improving state and local infrastructure (see below). USDA provides health departments with direct support for food assistance and nutrition education. EPA provides direct resources to the states for environmental management. Most of these funding streams are categorical—that is, the funding is intended for specific categories of people or special purposes. Congress authorizes categorical funding to address a specific health problem, such as preventing AIDS or addressing bioterrorism. However, categorical funding limits states' flexibility to deliver a range of relevant services with available resources. Block grants offer greater flexibility to states; however, Congress often reduces block grant funding over time.

Delegation of state authority to local health departments. States vary in terms of the authority they give to local governments and local public health departments. In 2016, 14 states had centralized public health departments, meaning that employees of the state led the local health units, and the state retained authority over many decisions relating to the budget, public health orders, and the selection of local health officials. Health departments were decentralized in 27 states: Local governments made many decisions and staffed the local health units. Four states shared authority, decision making, and employment with local governments. The remaining five states were mixed, meaning that some features were centralized while others were shared or decentralized.

The **National Association of County and City Health Officials** (NACCHO) website (www.naccho.org) offers further detail on the wide variety of organizational arrangements, responsibilities, financing, staffing, and authority of the estimated 2,533 local health departments. One reason for this variety is simply historical. The first public health agencies were formed in the early 1800s and were primarily city based. Later in the 19th century, state health agencies began to form. Throughout the 20th century, county health departments developed. One can see the effects by comparing older states to states admitted to the union more recently: Massachusetts had 328 local boards of health in 2016,[3] while Oregon[4] had 34 county health departments (NACCHO, 2017b).

Collaboration among federal, tribal, state, and local health departments. Health departments are exploring ways to coordinate public health responses and share services, functions, and staff across jurisdictional boundaries. From "handshake agreements" to more formal memoranda of understanding

---

[3] A 2016 Massachusetts law may lead to consolidation of local health departments over time.
[4] Oregon has about half the population of Massachusetts but almost 10 times the land area.

to consolidations and mergers, these sharing arrangements often seek to bal-ance effectiveness and efficiency in assuring the core public health functions (NACCHO, 2017b).

Local, state, tribal, and federal agencies all have strengths and resources for public health. States, tribes, and localities usually understand their own prob-lems best and how their context affects services. Meanwhile, the federal govern-ment has greater resources and scientific expertise for tackling large and complex health threats. The CDC, for example, leads the investigation of serious disease outbreaks, such as influenza, and makes recommendations for both clinical and community prevention. The federal government also steps in when health threats cross state borders, or when states cannot comply with federal regulations, offer-ing technical assistance and financial support.

Public Health Services

State responsibilities. These generally include disease and injury prevention, sanitation, controlling water and air pollution, vaccination, isolation and quaran-tine, inspection of commercial and residential premises, food and drinking water standards, extermination of vermin, fluoridation of municipal water supplies, and licensure of physicians and other health care professionals. However, the specific activities and services provided vary widely across states and localities. For exam-ple, tribal, state, and local health departments work to prevent chronic disease, but their approaches focus to varying degrees on education, social marketing, or policy and environmental changes (see Chapter 7).

10 essential services. In the face of this variation, most public health profes-sionals agree that all health departments should provide the 10 essential services listed in Figure 6.2. Many health departments are challenged to provide these ser-vices on their own, given their resource and staffing limitations. For example, most local health departments are small and rural, with 62% serving fewer than 50,000 people, and usually have 15 or fewer full-time staff. Many health departments have weak staff capacity in some of the 10 essential services, and higher education is not providing the appropriate training. Many experienced professionals are on the verge of retirement, and replacements are in short supply given the low salaries and rural location of many local health departments. Many health departments are thinking creatively about how to meet these challenges, the topic of the final section.

Public health emergencies. Since the 2001 anthrax attacks, public health agencies have faced the added responsibility of protecting the public against bio-terrorism threats and other communicable disease emergencies. The 2018 flu season was severe, and experts believe that we may soon experience one like the 1918 pandemic that killed an estimated 675,000 U.S. residents. Diseases spread much more quickly than they did in the past because of international travel, urban overcrowding and poverty, climate change, and misuse of antibiotics that pro-duce multiple drug-resistant infections. Interventions include global surveillance networks, stockpiles of vaccines, and better communications and data sharing to deal with outbreaks. Although preparedness is much better than in 2001, a recent study found that 28 states had inadequate policies and capabilities to protect against threats from communicable diseases (Trust for America's Health, 2015).

New training, competencies, and accreditation. In 2011, national voluntary performance standards were created for public health agencies, with development, refinement, and review by the **Public Health Accreditation Board** (PHAB). Among departments that had been accredited for at least 1 year, a recent survey found that over 90% believed that their departments had better opportunities for quality and performance improvement, were better able to identify strengths and weaknesses, had better accountability and transparency, and had better management practices (Kronstadt et al., 2016). At the end of 2017, 31 states, 1 statewide system of many local departments, 1 tribal, and 179 (7%) local health departments were accredited, while 158 were seeking accreditation. Accredited departments serve about 66% of the U.S. population. The PHAB website gives updates on progress and details of the accreditation standards (www.phaboard.org). PHAB also developed a consensus set of core competencies for public health practice at entry, supervisory, and executive levels. Movement to upgrade the competence of individual public health workers is seen in new management academies, continuing education, and certificate programs (Schaeffer, Schultz, & Salerno, 2009).

SOCIAL, ECONOMIC, AND POLITICAL FORCES ARE TRANSFORMING PUBLIC HEALTH

Challenges

Government agencies are important, but they are really only part of the public health infrastructure. Moreover, government is shrinking in the early 21st century. Champions of the public's health are meeting this challenge by working in new ways, communicating more effectively with the public, advocating for a wider variety of policies that affect health, and engaging new partners that are vital to achieving public health goals.

> Champions of the public's health are meeting this challenge by working in new ways, communicating more effectively with the public, advocating for a wider variety of policies that affect health, and engaging new partners that are vital to achieving public health goals.

Shrinking government. According to ASTHO and NACCHO, state and local health departments were hit hard by the recession of 2008–2010, with job losses totaling about 20% of the total public health workforce. During the recession, nearly every health department reported making cuts to programs and services, and the following decade saw continued, severe cuts in staffing and programs. State public health spending has been mostly level since 2010, with median spending of $31.62 per capita (Segal & Martin, 2017). Yet in the future, these agencies will need to do even more to manage new disasters and epidemics, meet the standards of accreditation, and achieve health equity. Both national developments and creative partnerships at the regional, state, and local level may help to meet this challenge.

Wide swings in federal support. Under the Obama administration, the American Recovery and Reinvestment Act of 2009 provided $650 million for prevention activities, and ACA authorized $15 billion over 10 years for the Prevention and Public Health Fund. Almost from its inception, however, Congress reduced the Prevention Fund to pay for various offsets in the federal budget, and the February 2018 budget deal cut $1.36 billion from the fund. Although there have been a few budget victories, current debates continue to challenge public investments in public health. The American Public Health Association (APHA) website (www.apha .org) gives updates on the Fund and other federal support for public health.

The Obama administration aimed to augment planning and coordination of prevention across sectors. For example, childhood obesity prevention efforts spanned the USDA, CDC, NIH, and Department of Education (Institute of Medicine, 2012). All cabinet-level agencies came together to develop and execute the National Prevention Strategy through the National Prevention Council. A Surgeon General's report outlined how medical care and public health could support each other (www.surgeongeneral.gov/priorities/prevention/strategy/index.html). Only time will tell how political changes will alter these and other federal coordination efforts. At the state and local levels, however, there is a growing realization that public health must rely on the range of partners with power and resources and across a variety of sectors to bring about needed changes in the conditions that affect the quality and length of people's lives.

Opportunities

Public health institutes. As defined by the National Network of Public Health Institutes (www.nnphi.org), these institutes are "nonprofit organizations dedicated to advancing public health practice and making systematic improvements in population health ... [they] emerged as a complement to governmental public health systems for addressing the most pressing current and emerging public health issues." The website for the National Network provides details on the 44 institutes and related services in all 50 states as well as tribal communities (www .nnphi.org). As **nongovernmental organizations**, they can accept private funds, leverage funding from multiple sources, and serve as fiscal intermediaries for health departments to speed the delivery of services and processes (e.g., hiring staff and buying supplies or equipment). Institute staff can advocate vigorously for public health programs and funding, whereas government employees have restrictions. Institutes can offer a credible, neutral, third-party voice on issues and can convene all the interested parties to address a broad health problem and implement a multisector strategy.

A new role for the health care sector. For more than 40 years, many local health departments provided direct health care services, leaving fewer resources to improve the health of *populations.* The ACA aimed to free up these resources by insuring many more people, who may choose providers other than the health department. Some health departments explored ways to divest their primary care services to other community providers while still fulfilling their duties to assure health care in their jurisdictions, especially for vulnerable populations (Kuehnert & McConnaughay, 2012). Where they continue to provide health care services, health departments are now able to collect third-party reimbursements, collections they have not had to do or been able to do historically. ACA also alleviated pressure on health departments by giving incentives for providers to work in underserved areas and by reimbursing private plans for essential prevention services, such as vaccinations and screening, if the plans meet federal standards.

At the same time, hospitals and health care systems have started to develop strategies for population health, often in collaboration with health departments and other community organizations. Hospitals' interest extends to the whole sector, including for-profit hospitals like Humana. Nonprofit hospitals are required to satisfy their community benefit obligations under the ACA by conducting a Community Health Improvement Plan and aligning their community investments to this plan. Safety-net hospitals have incentives to keep their populations well, given new reimbursement models, such as those that limit reimbursement of preventable readmissions to the hospital. An American Hospital Association survey (Health Research & Educational Trust, 2016) documented its members' interest in better prevention as well as the highest priority needs their communities were experiencing. The American Hospital Association also reported on actions that leading hospitals were taking to address community health needs beyond their walls, such as Sitka, Alaska's work to become nationally recognized as a walk-and-bike friendly community, and Fort Worth, Texas's efforts to improve parenting skills and reduce family violence (Health Research & Educational Trust, 2016, 2017).

New resources for assessment. As part of their federal community benefit requirements, nonprofit hospitals must conduct community health needs assessments once every 3 years. These assessments aim to engage multisectoral community coalitions to identify priority needs (www.cdc.gov/policy/chna). Some states require additional activity. Also, PHAB accreditation sets health department standards for more consistent and high-quality assessment. New data sources such as electronic health records, shared and linked databases, "big data" analytics, and techniques like geographic information systems (GIS), allow rapid response to potential public health emergencies. Equally important, however, they help policy makers and community coalitions to understand health differently, including opportunities to promote health and reduce health disparities. For example, GIS makes it possible to design communities proactively to prevent obesity (Institute of Medicine, 2012) or reduce triggers for asthma (e.g., Propeller Health at www.propellerhealth.com).

Effective Communication and Advocacy

Putting the public back in public health. Champions of the public's health need to build a constituency that understands public health's value, in order to create coalitions, gain allies to solve public health problems, and advocate effectively for solutions to improve health and achieve health equity. The general public does not understand public health, often supposing it refers solely to programs for the poor. The public—and policy makers—react to specific problems and crises. They do not see the disease cases, injuries, disabilities, and deaths that have been prevented. When an eroded infrastructure hinders crisis response—such as when the 2001 anthrax episode overwhelmed many public health laboratories or after Hurricane Katrina, when even such a basic function as handling the dead broke down—they do not understand why the problem is not solved quickly. In reality, public health is often invisible because it is generally so effective. With this in mind, how can public health develop an effective public constituency?

> How can public health develop an effective public constituency?

Building and maintaining trust. Public health practitioners sometimes can be seen as authoritarian or paternalistic, especially when they stress science and technology ("what's good for you because science says so") while ignoring collaboration, community history, democratic processes, and people's preferences. This tendency weakens their connections to grassroots groups and local leadership and limits input from (and active listening to) their constituents. The last years of the 20th century heightened public awareness of the need for a new form of leadership in public health—one that engages people on their own terms, in order to engender trust and cooperation. For example, the EPA learned to work with communities affected by toxic contaminants. But in the early days, it did not listen to the public about their concerns, did not provide the information they needed, or gave them incomprehensible "techno-babble" that enraged community leaders (Leviton et al., 1997). The old bureaucratic ways of doing business were simply not effective when people had legitimate concerns.

The most difficult lesson for public health came from the Tuskegee Syphilis Experiment (Jones, 1993). In 1932, 600 poor African American men in Macon County, Alabama, unknowingly became syphilis research subjects when the Public Health Service and the Tuskegee Institute began a study of the natural course of syphilis and offered the men "free medical care." Of 600 subjects, 339 had syphilis but were left untreated for up to 40 years, even though a penicillin cure became available in 1947. As many as 100 of the men died of syphilis, and many more suffered long-term disabilities before a public outcry and a federal advisory panel's recommendations halted the study in 1972. Along with the Nuremberg Code on medical experiments, this episode led Congress to require new protections for participants in human research. In 1997, President Bill Clinton offered an official public apology to the Tuskegee Study's eight survivors and participants' families. However, public health—and the health care system more generally—never fully regained African Americans' trust.

More effective voices. ASTHO, NACCHO, and APHA offer important communication tools to increase effectiveness in advocating for policies and resources at state and local levels. Public health also has advocates such as the Trust for America's Health (www.healthyamericans.org), which draws attention to specific health problems—what Americans generally respond to—and ties these issues to the need for better public health infrastructure and investment. The Trust has also been able to bring together diverse constituencies interested in similar kinds of health protections to amplify the collective message about these issues. The County Health Rankings and Roadmaps (www.countyhealthrankings.org) convey a snapshot of the health and well-being of counties within each state. These rankings have been found to attract the interest of policy makers and the public, and stimulate community discussions and collaborations to improve health (Wandersman, Osher, Winfrey, et al, 2018).

Advocacy in public health generally has a two fold purpose. It aims to strengthen public health resources and infrastructure, but also to make changes that health departments cannot make on their own. For example, advocates outside government have worked for many years to strengthen laws and regulations on issues such as newborn screening and lead remediation. Nongovernmental advocacy led to increased taxes on cigarettes and smoke-free indoor air laws, both of which discourage smoking (Center for Public Program Evaluation, 2011). To help prevent childhood obesity, public health advocates work to change state and local policies to require healthier foods and beverages in school and childcare, offer more opportunities for physical activity, and finance new supermarkets in underserved areas (Robert Wood Johnson Foundation, 2017).

Public health advocacy deals with a wider range of topics today than ever before. Because health is rooted in a wide variety of social and economic conditions, the field advocates for the principle of "health in all policies." In this approach, health advocates engage policy makers across various sectors to make sure that decisions will promote, or at least not adversely affect, health. The state of California, for example, has established a Health in All Policies Task Force (Caplan et al., 2017) to help the state's Strategic Growth Council achieve its goals, including "improving air and water quality, protecting natural resources and agricultural lands, increasing the availability of affordable housing, improving infrastructure systems, promoting public health, planning sustainable communities, and meeting the state's climate change goals"—all tied to the health of the state's residents.

Health impact assessments (HIAs) help policy makers and community leaders to identify the health impacts of decisions about nonhealth issues, such as economic development, housing, and transportation plans. The HIA is a structured process to gather, analyze, and present scientific data, health expertise, and public input to a public policy body so that policy choices can be made that will protect or promote health. HIAs have been used effectively around the world and have become more widespread in the United States over the past nine years with the development of the Health Impact Project (www.pewtrusts.org/en/projects/health-impact-project).

The Case for Multisector Collaboration

Throughout this chapter, we have attempted to show the many ways in which a wide variety of organizations take on the public health role when they focus on populations. This approach means that other interests can align with the public health mission. For example, walkable communities can appeal to real estate developers, city planners, public health practitioners, and advocates—all for somewhat different reasons. Across the nation, community coalitions are reframing suburban sprawl as something that discourages physical activity and therefore has consequences for people's health. Likewise, community violence is framed as a public health problem as well as a problem for community and child well-being, business development, public safety first responders, and hospitals. And employers and public health advocates alike see advantages to workplace health promotion, smoke-free campuses, and employment policies such as paid family and sick leave.

Profile data from 600 health department managers indicate that managers are more effective when they know how to collaborate across sectors (Altman, 2007). Collaboration means they can access other organizations' power, connections and resources. Given its importance, PHAB is developing standards for multisector collaboration. Tribal, state, and local public health departments have always connected to grassroots leadership and other public services in order to solve collective problems. However, their leadership abilities for multisector collaboration are now being cultivated as never before in what has become known as the collaborative leadership approach or collective impact. Collaborative leadership means understanding where public health shares common goals with other interest groups and building coalitions based on those common interests. In the same way, public health organizations are now participating more effectively in emergency preparedness and in health care reform because they can show where the public health interest is aligned with national defense and preparation for natural disasters, on the one hand, and health care quality and cost containment, on the other.

The leadership of coalitions cannot simply be left to health departments, however. In underresourced communities, leadership may come from hospitals, nongovernmental organizations, or even business. An important vehicle for coalition building is the 100 Million Healthier Lives Campaign (www.100mlives .org), which strives to achieve the Triple Aim: maximizing population health and patients' experience of care while reducing the per capita cost of care.

Conditions in our communities, our homes, and our workplaces affect our health and determine whether all people have a fair opportunity to achieve their best possible health. Enabling these conditions is just too big for governmental public health to take on alone and certainly too big for health care service providers. Instead, across sectors like housing, transportation, education, and economic development, we need to consider the health effects of our decisions. There are glimmers where this is already happening, for example, with the Culture of Health Prize (www.rwjf .org/prize). But the glimmers need to become beacons if we as a nation are going to shift from focusing on treating people who are sick to keeping people well.

CONCLUSION

Public health differs from individual health care by focusing on entire populations and designing policies, systems, services, and environments to achieve not only the absence of disease, but a complete sense of well-being. If public health goals are to be met, however, some changes are needed: (a) a greater consensus that the health of the individual is important to the community and society, (b) more effective ways to address the upstream social determinants that are at the root of today's health problems and disparities in health outcomes, (c) more comprehensive approaches to addressing population health problems, and (d) a focus on multisectoral collaborations because government cannot do it all. Sometimes government must lead, and sometimes it must follow, but in the future, we will find governmental public health departments walking hand in hand with their many partners and building on the assets of the communities it serves to preserve and protect the public's health.

▶ CASE EXERCISE—CURE FOR BIRTH DEFECTS POLICY OPTIONS

You are an analyst for a federal agency. Congress has ordered your agency to come up with policy options to find a cure for birth defects. You recognize that (a) birth defects have many causes, (b) some can be treated, (c) some can also be prevented, but (d) not all of them can be "cured." You analyze this issue using the core functions of public health and the problem-solving process outlined under Core Functions of Public Health.

Based on the information about spina bifida in this chapter, you decide it should be the focus for policymaking on birth defects. You decide to propose four options to Congress: more research on treatment of spina bifida, more health education for women about folic acid, more promotion of birth control to reduce the proportion of unplanned pregnancies in the country, and new regulations to increase the amount of folic acid in grain products. You may also see other options, so be sure to discuss them!

1. For each option, what would you need to know to determine effectiveness? Cost-effectiveness?

2. What are the tradeoffs in each course of action?

3. Who would support this option, who would be opposed, and does it matter?

4. Is there a single best option? Why?

DISCUSSION QUESTIONS

1. What examples of public health and prevention can you identify in your daily life? How do you believe they have affected your health?

2. Pick two such examples in either your own life or the text; then research which federal laws and agencies, state laws and agencies, local health departments, nonprofit organizations, or city and county government units affect this aspect of your health. The more complete your answer, the better your answer is!

3. What is the difference between individual- and population-based prevention efforts? For population-based prevention, what is the difference between universal and targeted strategies?

4. What does a population focus take in terms of planning, consensus building, and resources for implementation? In the case of safety belts? Heart attack prevention?

5. Why can't public health do more to achieve its goals? Name some of the political, legal, logistical, and resource challenges.

6. What should be left to the public sector to do, to achieve public health goals? Where could the private sector do more to help? Why?

7. Give some examples of the constituencies that public health will have to reach in order to implement its goals in the case of chronic disease prevention and in the case of childhood immunizations. How are the constituencies similar or different for these goals?

8. How would you personally balance individual liberty, the common good, and social justice in public health? What would have to change to achieve this balance? Give specific examples in the area of public health you are best acquainted with.

9. In what ways might public health build a stronger constituency?

REFERENCES

Altman, D. (2007). Leadership training for DrPH students. Greensboro, NC: Center for Creative Leadership, November 2007 (unpublished).

Beauchamp, D. E., & Steinbock, B. (1999). *New ethics for the public's health*. New York: Oxford University Press.

Braveman, P. (2006). Health disparities and health equity: Concepts and measurement. *Annual Review of Public Health, 27*, 167–194.

Braveman, P. Arkin, E., Proctor, D., & Plough, A. (2017). What is health equity? Retrieved from https://www.rwjf.org/en/library/research/2017/05/what-is-health-equity-.html

Caplan, J., Ben-Moshe, K., Dillon, L., Gould, S., Lee, M., Lyles, K., … Rudolph, L. (2017). California health in all policies task force. Retrieved from http://sgc.ca.gov/programs/hiap/

Centers for Disease Control and Prevention. (1999). Ten great public health achievements—United States, 1900–1999. *Morbidity and Mortality Weekly Report, 48*(12), 241–243. Retrieved from http://www.cdc.gov/mmwr/preview/mmwrhtml/00056796. htm

Centers for Disease Control and Prevention. (2011). Ten great public health achievements: United States, 2001–2010. *Morbidity and Mortality Weekly Report, 60*, 619–623. Retrieved from http://www.cdc.gov/mmwr/preview/mmwrhtml/mm6019a5.htm

Centers for Disease Control and Prevention. (2013). The public health system and the 10 essential public health services. Retrieved from https://www.cdc.gov/stltpublichealth/publichealthservices/essentialhealthservices.html

Center for Public Program Evaluation. (2011). *The tobacco campaigns*. Princeton, NJ: Robert Wood Johnson Foundation. Retrieved from https://www.rwjf.org/en/library/research/2011/04/the-tobacco-campaigns-.html

Dana, D. A., & Nadler, J. (2018). Soda taxes as a legal and social movement. *Northwestern Journal of Law and Social Policy, 13*(2), Article 3. Retrieved from https://scholarlycommons.law.northwestern.edu/cgi/viewcontent.cgi?article=1167&amp=&context=njlsp&amp=&sei-redir=1&referer=https%253A%252F%252Fwww.bing.com%252Fs

earch%253Fq%253DSoda%252Btaxes%252Bas%252Ba%252Blegal%252Band%252B
social%252Bmovement%2526src%253DIE-TopResult%2526FORM%253DIETR02%
2526conversationid%253D#search=%22Soda%20taxes%20as%20legal%20social%20
movement%22

Green, L. W., & Kreuter, M. (2005). *Health promotion planning: An educational and ecological approach*. (4th ed.). St. Louis, MO: McGraw-Hill.

Health Research & Educational Trust. (2016). *Creating effective hospital-community partnerships to build a culture of health*. Chicago, IL: Author. Retrieved from http://www.hpoe.org/Reports-HPOE/2016/creating-effective-hospital-community-partnerships.pdf

Health Research & Educational Trust. (2017). *A playbook for fostering hospital-community partnerships to build a Culture of Health*. Chicago, IL: Author. Retrieved from https://www.aha.org/system/files/hpoe/Reports-HPOE/2017/A-playbook-for-fostering-hospital-community-partnerships.pdf

Hodge, J. (2012). The evolution of law in biopreparedness. *Biosecurity and Bioterrorism: Biodefense Strategy, Practice, and Science, 10*(1), 38–48. doi:10.1089/bsp.2011.0094

Institute of Medicine. (2002). *The future of the public's health in the 21st century*. Washington, DC: National Academies Press.

Institute of Medicine. (2011). *For the public's health: Revitalizing law and policy to meet new challenges*. Washington, DC: National Academies Press.

Institute of Medicine (2012). *Accelerating progress in obesity prevention: Solving the weight of the nation*. Washington, DC: National Academies Press.

Jones, J. H. (1993). *Bad blood: The Tuskegee syphilis experiment*. (new and expanded edition). New York: Free Press.

Kindig, D. (2015). What are we talking about when we talk about population health? *Health Affairs Blog*. doi:10.1377/hblog20150406.046151

Kronstadt, J., Meit, M., Siegfried, A., Nicolaus, T., Bender, K., & Corso, L. (2016). Evaluating the impact of national public health department accreditation—United States, 2016. *Morbidity and Mortality Weekly Report, 65*(31), 803–806. doi:10.15585/mmwr.mm6531a3

Kuehnert, P. L., & McConnaughay, K. S. (2012). Tough choices in tough times: Enhancing public health value in an era of declining resources. *Journal of Public Health Management and Practice, 18*(2), 115–125. doi:10.1097/PHH.0b013e3182303616

Leider, J. P., Resnick, B. A., Sensenig, A. L., Alfonso, N., Brady, E., Colrick, I. P., & Bishai, D. M. (2016). Assessing the public health activity estimate from the National Health Expenditure Accounts: Why public health expenditure definitions matter. *Journal of Health Care Finance, 43*(2), 226–240.

Leviton, L. C., Needleman, C. E., & Shapiro, M. (1997). *Confronting public health risks: A decision maker's guide*. Thousand Oaks, CA: Sage.

Mays, G. P., & Smith, S. A. (2011). Evidence links increases in public health spending to declines in preventable deaths. *Health Affairs, 30*(8), 1585–1593. doi:10.1377/hlthaff.2011.0196

National Association of County and City Health Officials. (2017b). *2016 national profile of local health departments*. Washington, DC: Author. Retrieved from https://nacchovoice.naccho.org/2017/01/25/2016-national-profile-of-local-health-departments

National Center for Health Statistics. (2017). *Health, United States, 2016: With chartbook on long-term trends in health*. Hyattsville, MD: U.S. Department of Health and Human Services. Retrieved from https://www.cdc.gov/nchs/data/hus/hus16.pdf

National Highway Traffic Safety Administration (2017). Traffic safety facts: Occupant protection in passenger vehicles. Washington, DC: U.S. Department of Transportation. Retrieved from https://crashstats.nhtsa.dot.gov/Api/Public/ViewPublication/812374

National Network of Public Health Institutes (2018). Network Engagement. Retrieved from https://nnphi.org/network-engagement/

Network for Public Health Law. (2015). *Emergency declaration authorities across all states and DC.* Retrieved from https://www.networkforphl.org/_asset/gxrdwm/Emergency -Declaration-Authorities.pdf

Robert Wood Johnson Foundation. (2017). *Evaluation of Voices for Healthy Kids program.* Retrieved from https://www.rwjf.org/en/library/research/2017/06/evaluation-of -voices-for-healthy-kids-program.html

Schaeffer, L. D., Schultz, A. M., & Salerno, J. A. (Eds.). (2009). *HHS in the 21st Century.* Washington, DC: National Academies Press.

Segal, L. M., & Martin, A. (2017). A funding crisis for public health and safety: State-by-state public health funding and key health facts. Washington, DC: Trust for America's Health. Retrieved from https://www.tfah.org/report-details/a-funding-crisis-for -public-health-and-safety-state-by-state-public-health-funding-and-key-health-facts -2017/

Sondik, E. J., Huang, D. T., Klein, R. J., & Satcher, D. (2010). Progress toward meeting the Healthy People 2010 goals and objectives. *Annual Review of Public Health, 31,* 271–281. doi:10.1146/annurev.publhealth.012809.103613

Trust for America's Health. (2015). *Outbreaks: Protecting Americans from infectious disease.* Retrieved from: https://www.tfah.org/report-details/outbreaks

U.S. Department of Health and Human Services. (2013). *Healthy People 2020.* Retrieved from https://www.healthypeople.gov

U.S. Preventive Services Task Force. (2018). *Recommendations for primary care practice.* Retrieved from https://www.uspreventiveservicestaskforce.org/BrowseRec/Index/ browse-recommendations

Wandersman, A., Osher, D., Winfrey, K., Scardaville, M., Berg, J. & Pan, J. (2018). County Health Rankings and Roadmaps: Findings from a national study of county health officials. Washington, DC: American Institutes for Research.

7

Health and Behavior

Brian Elbel, Elaine F. Cassidy, Matthew D. Trujillo,
and C. Tracy Orleans

LEARNING OBJECTIVES

▶ Learn about the contributions of personal health practices (e.g., tobacco use, risky drinking, physical activity, diet, obesity) to individual and population health status

▶ Understand how strategies for changing individual and population health behavior have evolved, and identify the targets and characteristics of effective interventions

▶ Learn about the social, policy, and environmental determinants of healthy and unhealthy behaviors and the disparities and inequities in exposure to them

▶ Understand models and prospects for addressing behavioral risk factors through national health care quality improvement efforts and health reform

▶ Describe provider-oriented interventions for changing individual and population health behavior and their influence in achieving national health care quality objectives

KEY TERMS

▶ behavioral risk factors

▶ chronic care model

▶ energy balance equation

▶ practice ecology model

▶ quality improvement

▶ social determinants of health

▶ social ecological models

▶ social marketing strategies

TOPICAL OUTLINE

▶ Behavioral risk factors: overview and national goals

▶ Changing health behavior: closing the gap between recommended and actual health lifestyle practices

▶ The role and impact of primary care interventions

▶ Multilevel models for population-based health behavior change

▶ Changing provider behavior: closing the gap between best practice and usual care

INTRODUCTION

Health care professionals, who live in a world in which often heroic efforts are needed to save lives, can easily believe that medical care is the most important instrument for maintaining and ensuring health. This chapter explains, however, that behavioral choices—and the social, environmental, and policy factors that influence them—are key determinants of Americans' health and well-being.

> Chronic diseases such as cancer and heart and lung disease have now replaced acute and infectious diseases as the major causes of death in the United States. Yet a large part of the burden these illnesses cause is actually preventable.*

To some extent, the task of helping people adopt healthy lifestyles falls into multiple realms, including behavioral psychology, public health, and even social marketing. However, current models for shaping healthy lifestyles include major roles for medical providers and the health care systems in which they practice. Therefore, clinicians, health care payers, managers of provider organizations, and health care policy makers need to understand and address the powerful behavioral determinants of health and illness.

This chapter begins with a brief overview of the major **behavioral risk factors** that contribute to the growing burden of preventable chronic disease in the United States—tobacco use; alcohol abuse; and sedentary lifestyle and unhealthy diet, including the joint effects sedentary lifestyle and unhealthy diet have on adult and childhood obesity and overweight. There is now voluminous and incontrovertible evidence for the roles these behaviors and risk factors play in shaping public health, along with growing knowledge of the power of **social determinants of health** and health outcomes: education; income; access to safe places to walk, bike, and play; and healthy affordable foods (as noted in Chapters 5 and 6).

The chapter then describes the progress that has been made over the past four decades to help adults modify these risk factors by intervening both at the individual level—with behavioral and clinical treatments that can be delivered in health care settings—and at the broader population level—with public health environmental and policy changes and social marketing and media strategies that

---

*To hear the podcast, go to https://bcove.video/2PfVAmp or access the ebook on Springer Publishing Connect™.

can prompt and support the development and maintenance of healthy behavior. Theoretical advances (e.g., social learning theory and stage-based and social ecological models) have led to a clear understanding of the need for broad-spectrum, multilevel ecological approaches, and new science-based clinical and community practice guidelines have been developed to guide them.

While it is increasingly widely understood that social determinants play a major role in shaping health and health outcomes multifaceted efforts have been successful in encouraging clinicians to use proven health behavior change protocols in their interactions with patients. Many parallels can be drawn between what we have learned about ways to promote health through individual behavior change and what we have learned about strategies to improve health care quality through provider behavior change. Health reform legislation at the local, state, and national levels increasingly recognizes that the significant progress in both areas holds unprecedented potential for breakthrough improvements in national health status and health care quality.

BEHAVIORAL RISK FACTORS: OVERVIEW AND NATIONAL GOALS

Acute and infectious diseases are no longer the major causes of death, disease, and disability in the United States. Today, chronic diseases—cancer, heart, and lung disease—are the nation's leading causes of illness and death (Mokdad et al., 2018). Given the continued aging of the population, both the prevalence and the costs of chronic illness care will continue to rise. Yet, much of the growing burden of chronic disease is preventable.

More than two decades ago, McGinnis and Foege (1993) estimated that 50% of the mortality from the 10 leading causes of death could be attributed to personal behavior. A more recent analysis by Mokdad and colleagues (2018) reinforced this estimate, finding that tobacco use, high body mass index (BMI), dietary risk, and alcohol and drug abuse are the four largest risk factors for mortality in the United States. Moreover, research findings over the past two decades have established that modifying these behavioral risk factors leads to improved health and quality of life and to reduced health care costs and burden (Orleans, Ulmer, & Gruman, 2004).

Almost 90% of Americans have reported they have at least one of these risk factors, and 52% have reported having two or more, with the highest prevalence of individual and multiple behavioral risks occurring in low-income and racial and ethnic minority groups (Coups, Gaba, & Orleans, 2004). Given these statistics, it is not surprising that many of the leading health indicators tracked by *Healthy People 2020* (U.S. Department of Health and Human Services, 2011)—which updates the nation's primary objectives for promoting longer, healthier lives and eliminating health disparities—relate to healthy lifestyles. Although recent analyses suggest that our nation had an uneven record in achieving *Healthy People 2010* (U.S. Department of Health and Human Services, 2000) targets in previous years (see Chapter 6), more well-rounded improvements across multiple health indicators are needed in order to advance quality of life and significantly reduce health disparities (Koh, 2010). Selected indicators for tobacco use, alcohol abuse, physical activity, diet, and obesity are shown in Table 7.1.

TABLE 7.1 SELECTED *HEALTHY PEOPLE 2020* OBJECTIVES: BEHAVIORAL RISK FACTORS

	BASELINE[a] (%)	2020 GOALS (%)
Tobacco Use		
Cigarette smoking		
▪ Adults (18 years and older)	24	12
▪ Adolescents (grades 9 through 12)	35	16
Exposure to secondhand smoke		
▪ Children (6 years and younger)	27	10
Alcohol Misuse/Risky Drinking		
Proportion of adults who drank excessively during past 30 days	28	25
Binge drinking		
▪ Adults (18 years and older)	27	24
▪ Adolescents (12 to 17 years old)	10	9
Deaths from alcohol-related auto crashes[b]	.39	.38
Physical Activity		
Regular moderate physical activity		
▪ Adults (18 years and older)[c]	15	30
▪ Adolescents (grades 9 through 12)[d]	27	35
Vigorous physical activity (at least 3 days per week for 20 minutes)		
▪ Adults (18 years and older)[c]	23	30
▪ Adolescents (grades 9 through 12)[d]	65	85
Diet and Overweight (Older Than Age 2)		
▪ Proportion of people eating at least two servings of fruit daily	28	75
▪ Proportion of people eating at least three servings of vegetables (at least one of which is dark green or orange) daily	3	50
▪ Proportion of people eating at least six servings of grain products (at least three being whole grains) daily	7	50
Overweight and obesity		
▪ Obesity among adults (aged 20 years and older)	23	15
▪ Overweight and obesity among children and adolescents (aged 6 to 19)	11	5

[a] Baseline data extracted from sources between 1988 and 1999.
[b] Per 100 million vehicle miles traveled.
[c] At least 30 minutes per day.
[d] At least 30 minutes 5 or more days per week.

Source: U.S. Department of Health and Human Services. (2011). Healthy People 2020: Understanding and improving health. Washington, DC: Author.

The past decade of social science, behavior change, and population health research also has revealed the profound sociodemographic inequities in access to community-level and health care supports for healthy behavior and health behavior change (Adler, Bachrach, Daley, & Frisco, 2013). These inequities are powerful drivers of health disparities and threats to the health of the nation. In fact, the Robert Wood Johnson Foundation's Commission for a Healthier America convened in 2013 to emphasize that the nation's health depends fundamentally on ensuring equitable access to the supports and resources needed for making healthy choices in the environments where people live, learn, work, and play.

Tobacco Use

Tobacco use causes more preventable deaths and diseases than any other behavioral risk factor, including at least 480,000 premature deaths from several forms of cancer, heart, and lung disease (U.S. Department of Health and Human Services [DHHS], 2014). It accounts for annual health care costs of $170 billion, in addition to an estimated $156 billion in lost productivity costs (Xu, 2014; DHHS, 2014).

Smoking remains the single most important modifiable cause of poor pregnancy outcomes, accounting for 20% of low birth weight deliveries, 8% of preterm births, and 5% of perinatal deaths. For infants and young children, parental smoking is linked to sudden infant death syndrome (SIDS), respiratory illnesses, middle ear infections, and decreased lung function, with annual direct medical costs estimated at $4.6 billion. Quitting, even after 50 years of smoking, can produce significant improvements in health and less use of health care services.

Although the adult smoking prevalence rate decreased to 15.5% in 2016 (Jamal et al., 2018), smoking prevalence among adults remains well above the *Healthy People 2020* target of 12% (Ward, Barnes, Freeman, & Schiller, 2012). Nearly one in five adults still smokes, with the highest rates (29%) among members of low-income populations (Centers for Disease Control and Prevention [CDC], 2018). And even though rates of smoking during pregnancy also have dropped in the past decade, 10% of women reported in 2011 that they smoked during pregnancy (CDC, 2017). Vaping and e-cigarette use is also a broad concern, particularly among youth, with controversy over its potential for harm reduction at the same time (as noted below).

Each day, more than 3,200 children and teens become new smokers, and 30% of those young people will become addicted to tobacco (DHHS, 2014). Some 18% of high school students smoke cigarettes, and more than 8 million Americans, mostly adolescent and young adult males, report using smokeless tobacco, which is linked to oral cancer, gum disease, and tooth loss (American Cancer Society, 2012; CDC, 2013d). Furthermore, public health and tobacco control experts are concerned that the availability and marketing of electronic cigarettes (e-cigarettes) may reverse recent declines in youth tobacco use initiation and tobacco addiction by re-glamorizing smoking and igniting lifelong nicotine addiction (Richtel, 2013). In addition, the most recent survey data from 2009 and 2010 suggest that 42% of children ages 3 to 11 and 28% of adult nonsmokers were exposed to secondhand smoke. Socioeconomics may play an important role in influencing smoking behaviors and exposure to tobacco-control policies. A study by Giovino and colleagues (2009) revealed that increasing median household income was associated with decreasing prevalence of smoking, higher cessation rates among smokers, higher state cigarette excise tax rates, and stronger legal protections from tobacco smoke pollution.

Alcohol Use and Misuse

The millions of Americans who abuse or misuse alcohol include those who are alcohol dependent as well as those who engage in drinking behavior that is risky (e.g., because they drive after drinking alcohol) or harmful (e.g., because they suffer the effects of episodic binge drinking). About 5% of the U.S. adult population meets the criteria for alcoholism or alcohol dependence, and another 20% engages in harmful or risky drinking, defined as drinking more than 1 drink per day or 7 drinks per week for women, more than 2 drinks per day or 14 drinks per week for men; periodic binge drinking (5 or more drinks on a single occasion for men; 4 or more for women); drinking and driving; or drinking during pregnancy.

The 2017 Monitoring the Future Survey indicated that 16.6% of high school seniors reported that they engaged in binge drinking in the two weeks before the survey (Miech et al., 2018). Alcohol misuse is most common in young adults, particularly among White and Native American men. And excessive alcohol use among U.S. college students remains a problem with college students, compared with their noncollege peers, reporting more instances of heavy drinking and being drunk (Johnston, O'Malley, Bachman, & Schulenberg, 2013a). It should be noted, however, that low and moderate levels of alcohol use in adults (below those defined as risky) have been linked to modest health benefits, such as lowered risk for heart disease.

Alcohol misuse accounts for approximately 80,000 deaths and more than 2 million years of potential life lost a year (CDC, n.d.). The estimated cost of excessive alcohol use was recently estimated at $249 billion (CDC, 2016). Of this $249 billion, $191 billion was attributed to binge drinking, $24 billion to underage drinking, and $5.5 billion to drinking during pregnancy (Sacks, Gonzalez, Bouchery, Tomedi, & Brewer, 2015).

Factors associated with alcohol access, such as alcohol retail density and alcohol-related advertising, can vary by certain neighborhood sociodemographic characteristics. For instance, compared with individuals living in high-income, high-education, mostly White neighborhoods, those living in low-income, low-education, predominantly minority neighborhoods have relatively higher densities of alcohol retail outlets available to them (Berke et al., 2010). Disparities also exist in completion rates for alcohol treatment, with people from minority backgrounds having significantly lower completion rates than their White counterparts (Saloner & LêCook, 2013).

The health benefits of treating alcohol dependence are well established, and the U.S. Preventive Services Task Force (USPSTF) found that brief behavior change interventions to modify risky drinking levels and practices produced positive health outcomes detectable 4 or more years later.

Physical Activity and Sedentary Lifestyle

The health risks associated with physical inactivity and sedentary lifestyle are numerous. They include heart disease, type 2 diabetes, stroke, hypertension, osteoarthritis, colon cancer, depression, and obesity (Micha et al., 2017; Yu et al., 2016). Engagement in physical activity helps to maintain healthy bones, muscles, joints, and weight, and it is also associated with positive psychological benefits. Physical activity has been shown to reduce feelings of anxiety and depression and promote feelings of well-being.

In 2011, 48% of adults engaged in at least 75 minutes per week of moderate-to-vigorous aerobic exercise, a proportion that met the *Healthy People 2020* guideline for recommended physical activity among adults. In comparison, national guidelines recommend at least 60 minutes of moderate-to-vigorous physical activity every day for children and teens, but the majority of young people do not meet this goal (Troiano et al., 2008). Sedentary behavior also has risen for U.S. youth, with the amount of time young people spend in sedentary behaviors, including all forms of screen time, increasing dramatically in recent years (Rideout, Foehr, & Roberts, 2010). Sedentary behaviors are independently linked to a higher risk for obesity, diabetes, and other chronic health problems among adults, even those who are physically active and consume healthy diets (Hamilton, Hamilton, & Zedric, 2007).

Reflecting the power of social determinants of health, the adults, youth, and families most at risk for inactivity include those with lower income and education levels, those living below the poverty line in all racial and ethnic groups, members of several racial/ethnic minority groups (e.g., African Americans, Hispanics), and those with disabilities. Sallis and colleagues (2011) found neighborhood-level income disparities for numerous variables affecting everyday physical activity. For instance, residents of high-income neighborhoods reported more favorable pedestrian and building facilities, safety from traffic, safety from crime, and access to recreation facilities than residents of low-income areas. Furthermore, growing evidence shows that within the United States, African American and Latino youth, and youth living in lower-income communities, do not have as many built and social environmental supports for physical activity as White children or those living in middle- and higher-income communities (Taylor & Lou, 2012).

Although the societal costs of physical inactivity are difficult to quantify, the CDC has estimated that nearly $95 billion (adjusted to 2009 dollars) would be saved if all inactive American adults were to become active (CDC, 2013c). In addition to providing objectives for physical activity behaviors, *Healthy People 2020* includes objectives for policies that facilitate physical activity, particularly for children. These policy objectives focus on policies that promote physical activity in childcare settings as well as during recess and physical education classes in schools.

Diet and Nutrition

Approximately 45% of deaths from heart disease, stroke, and type 2 diabetes in 2012 can be attributed to poor diet (Micha et al., 2017). Poor diet and nutrition also has contributed to a surge in overweight and obesity that has reached epidemic proportions over the last 20 years, particularly within low-income and minority populations with limited access to healthy affordable foods and greater advertising for unhealthy foods.

Four of the 10 leading causes of death—coronary heart disease, some cancers, stroke, and type 2 diabetes—are associated with an unhealthy diet. The relationships between dietary patterns and health outcomes have been examined in a wide range of observational studies and randomized trials with patients at risk for diet-related chronic diseases. The majority of studies suggest that people consuming diets that are low in fat, saturated fat, trans fatty acids, and cholesterol and high in fruits, vegetables, and whole grain products containing fiber have lower rates of morbidity and mortality from coronary artery disease and several forms of cancer (Micha et al., 2017; Yu et al., 2016). Moreover, dietary change has been found to reduce risks for many chronic diseases as well as for overweight and obesity.

> Four of the 10 leading causes of death—coronary heart disease, some cancers, stroke, and type 2 diabetes—are associated with an unhealthy diet.

The 2010 Dietary Guidelines for Americans recommended that Americans reduce their caloric intake from solid fats and added sugars and increase the amount of fruits, vegetables, and whole grains in their diets. Again, as Table 7.1 shows, gaps exist between the recommended guidelines and actual diets of American children and adults. Numerous studies have documented wide racial, ethnic, and socioeconomic inequalities in access to healthy food outlets, particularly chain supermarkets (Powell, Han, & Chaloupka, 2010), and that access to healthy food is associated with lower risks of obesity and diet-related chronic diseases. In 2010, PolicyLink and the Food Trust published "The Grocery Gap: Who Has Access to Healthy Food and Why It Matters," a comprehensive review of two decades of food access research (Treuhaft & Karpyn, 2010). This review found evidence that access to healthy food was particularly limited for low-income communities, communities of color, and rural communities.

> The 2010 Dietary Guidelines for Americans recommended that Americans reduce their caloric intake from solid fats and added sugars and increase the amount of fruits, vegetables, and whole grains in their diets.

Obesity

As poor dietary habits and physical inactivity have become endemic, national obesity rates have soared. Nearly 70% of all American adults are overweight or obese—up almost 10% from just one decade ago. This trend is alarming, given the strong links between obesity and many chronic diseases. Total global expenditures related to overweight- and obesity-related problems were estimated at nearly $2 trillion—a number that will continue to increase without effective interventions to teach and reinforce healthy behavior and change the physical and media environments and economic incentives that enable, promote, and supply healthy diets. Even modest weight loss (e.g., 5% to 10% of body weight) over a period of 12 to 24 months can reduce these risks and prevent the onset of diabetes among adults with impaired glucose tolerance.

More alarming is the prevalence of overweight and obesity among children and adolescents (ages 6 to 19), which has increased significantly over the past three decades. Like adults, overweight youth are at risk for coronary heart disease, hypertension, certain cancers, and even type 2 diabetes early in life. The highest and fastest-rising rates of childhood obesity are seen among children and adolescents of African American or Latino descent and children (particularly girls) from low-income backgrounds and residing in communities with historically limited access to the resources and opportunities for physical activity and healthy diets—making efforts to reach these groups a public health priority (White House Task Force on Childhood Obesity, 2010).

Reducing obesity among adults, adolescents, and children are leading health goals for *Healthy People 2020*, which set the target rates of adult and child and adolescent obesity at 31% and 15%, respectively. In 2012, the Institute of Medicine (IOM) released the report *Accelerating Progress in Obesity Prevention: Solving the Weight of the Nation*, which identified five critical environments in which reform was urgently needed to prevent obesity: (a) environments for physical activity, (b) food and beverage environments, (c) message environments, (d) health care and work environments, and (e) school environments. In a 2013 follow-up report, *Creating Equal Opportunities for a Healthy Weight*, the IOM focused on the research, policies, and actions most needed to ensure greater equity in opportunities to achieve a healthy weight and address the pervasive disparities in obesity prevalence and health and economic tolls in the United States.

CHANGING HEALTH BEHAVIOR: CLOSING THE GAP BETWEEN RECOMMENDED AND ACTUAL HEALTH LIFESTYLE PRACTICES

In 1982, the IOM published *Health and Behavior*, one of the first scientific documents to establish convincingly the links between behavioral risk factors and disease, and to identify the basic biopsychosocial mechanisms underlying them. The IOM recommended intensified social and behavioral science research to develop interventions that could help people change their unhealthy behaviors and improve their health prospects. This section presents a broad overview of the ensuing research—research that has attempted to close the gap between what we know and what we do when it comes to adopting and fostering healthy lifestyles.

A Brief History of Behavior Change Interventions

Early behavior change efforts in the 1970s and 1980s relied primarily on public education campaigns and individually oriented health education interventions. They were guided by the health belief model and similar theories (the theory of reasoned action, the theory of planned behavior), which emphasized the cognitive and motivational influences on health behavior change and recommended raising awareness of the harms of unhealthy behavior versus the benefits of behavior change as a primary intervention. These cognitive/decisional theories were based on an underlying premise that people's intentions and motivations to engage in behavior strongly predict their actually doing so (i.e., "if you tell them, they will change"). Because raising health risk awareness and motivation was a primary goal, the doctor–patient relationship was seen as a unique and powerful context for effective health education.

Both population-level and individual clinical health education efforts based on these theories achieved initial success. For instance, tens of thousands of smokers quit in response to the publication of the first U.S. Surgeon General's *Report on Smoking and Health* in 1964 and the multiple public education campaigns that followed.

By 2000, hundreds of studies had confirmed that even brief physician advice could be an important catalyst for health behavior change—boosting the number of patients who quit smoking for at least 24 hours or who made some changes in their diet and activity levels. But a growing body of research found these successes to be modest—the interventions were important and perhaps *necessary* for changing people's health knowledge, attitudes, and beliefs, as well as broader social norms, but *not sufficient* to produce lasting behavior change. Cumulative findings made it clear that people needed not only motivation, but also new skills and supports to succeed in changing deeply ingrained health habits, including supportive community, social, and media environments.

These findings spurred the development and testing of expanded multicomponent, cognitive behavioral treatments designed not only to (a) raise perceptions of susceptibility to poor health outcomes and benefits of behavior change, but also to (b) teach the skills required to replace ingrained unhealthy habits with healthy alternatives and to (c) help people make changes in their natural (home, work, social) environments to assist them in successfully establishing and maintaining new behaviors. Social learning theory, which emphasized interactions between internal and external environmental influences on behavior, provided the primary theoretical basis for this evolution, and it remains the dominant model for effective cognitive behavioral health behavior change interventions.

Lifestyle change interventions derived from social learning theory combined education and skills development. They included techniques such as modeling and behavioral practice to help people learn not just *why*, but *how*, to change unhealthy habits. For instance, they taught effective self-management and behavior change skills, such as goal-setting, self-monitoring, and stress management skills for people who had relied on smoking, eating, or drinking as coping tactics. They taught skills for reengineering the person's immediate environments, replacing environmental cues and supports for unhealthy behavior with new cues and supports for healthy ones (e.g., removing ashtrays; replacing unhealthy high-calorie foods with healthy alternatives; finding exercise buddies; and avoiding high-risk events, such as office parties at which risky drinking was expected).

The "nudge" principles of modern behavioral economics that, for instance, are used to advocate for replacing soda with water and French fries with apple slices in fast-food children's meals have their roots in these approaches. Another principle was that problem solving should start with helping people set realistic, personal behavior change goals and go on to address the unique barriers and relapse temptations they face. Finally, new social learning theory treatments taught patients to take a long-range perspective, viewing repeated attempts over time as part of a cumulative learning process rather than as signs of failure.

Effective multicomponent treatments were initially delivered and tested in multisession, face-to-face group or individual clinic-based programs, typically offered in clinical or medical settings and usually led by highly trained (e.g., MD, PhD) professionals. Results were extremely encouraging, with substantial behavior change—for example, smoking quit rates as high as 40%—maintained 6 to 12 months after treatment. However, participants were typically self-referred or recruited based on high readiness or motivation for change and thus represented a small fraction of those who could benefit.

The next push was to distill core elements of this treatment approach into lower-cost formats with much wider reach. These formats included paraprofessional-led worksite clinics, self-help manuals and programs, and brief primary care counseling. Absolute treatment effects were smaller—for example, 20% long-term smoking quit rates—but potential population effects were much greater. Only 5% to 10% of smokers might ever attend intensive clinics, whereas 70% of U.S. smokers might receive brief, effective tobacco interventions during visits with their primary care physicians, introducing a context that could double the nation's annual quit rate. Access to telephone quitlines providing free or no-cost counseling and medication proved equally effective and had the benefit of better reaching smokers in sociodemographic populations with limited access to high-quality health care (Schlam & Baker, 2013).

Development of the stages-of-change model in the mid-1980s accelerated the shift from individual to population intervention models and has had a profound, lasting effect on the design and delivery of health behavior change programs. Studying how people went about changing on their own, Prochaska and DiClemente (1983) discovered that health behavior change was a multistage process:

- *Precontemplation:* no plans to change behavior; behavior is not seen as a problem
- *Contemplation:* serious plans to change behavior within the next 6 months, weighing the pros and cons, and building supports and confidence

- *Preparation:* plans to change are imminent; small initial steps are taken
- *Action:* active attempts are made to quit smoking, drink less, become more active, or change to a healthier diet and to sustain changes for up to 6 months
- *Maintenance:* change is sustained beyond 6 months
- *Relapse:* the individual returns to any earlier stage and begins to recycle through the earlier stages

Based on these findings, different skills, knowledge, and types of treatment were recommended to help people in each stage; motivational and educational interventions were helpful to people in the precontemplation and contemplation stages, and active cognitive behavioral interventions were needed for those in the preparation, action, and maintenance stages. Many population surveys found that, at any given time, the vast majority of people (80%) are in the precontemplation and contemplation stages, which helped to explain why so few enrolled in weight-loss or quit-smoking clinics, even when these were free and accessible.

The stages-of-change model has been successfully applied to numerous behavioral health risks and has helped people with multiple risk factors make progress in changing several at the same time. One of the greatest effects of this model was to propel a dramatic shift away from one-size-fits-all approaches to individualized, stage-tailored strategies that could be applied effectively to entire populations—in communities, worksites, and health care settings—assisting people at *all* stages of change, not just the motivated volunteers in action stages, but also those needing motivation and support to reach action stages. The model stimulated the development and wider use of effective motivational interventions for clinical settings, especially motivational interviewing, which seeks to help people strengthen their determination to change behavior (Emmons & Rollnick, 2001).

Originating as they did in the study of successful self-change, stages-of-change models fueled a burgeoning movement toward low-cost self-help tools and treatment formats. Some tools capitalized on computer-based and interactive communication technologies to design and deliver print and web-based materials, interactive video, and telephone interventions geared to the individual's stage of change. These treatments also addressed many other variables important for tailoring treatment methods and improving treatment outcomes—for example, degree of nicotine addiction, unique behavior change assets, barriers, and cultural norms.

A final force in the evolution from individual to population-based approaches was the emergence of **social marketing strategies**, which apply the concepts and tools of successful commercial marketing to the challenge of health behavior change. Basic marketing principles and methods—including market analysis, audience segmentation, and a new focus on consumer wants and needs—catalyzed the development of culturally appropriate communication and intervention strategies for reaching underserved, high-risk, low-income, and racial/ethnic minority populations for whom the prevalence of behavioral health risks is often highest and access to health-promoting environments and resources is often lowest. For instance, one model program employed social marketing strategies to tailor a no-cost smoking cessation intervention to the needs of African American smokers, using messages on Black-format radio stations to promote culturally tailored quitline counseling and materials. Results included a higher quitline call rate and a higher quit rate among African Americans receiving the tailored intervention versus a generic one.

> Social marketing strategies apply the concepts and tools of successful commercial marketing to the challenge of health behavior change.

Social networks have been found to help motivate and support health behavior change in multiple areas—including weight loss, alcohol use, and smoking cessation (Volpp & Mohta, 2017). Through the Internet, individuals can share and receive health information through open forums, such as those provided through Facebook or Twitter. They can upload health-related apps or access online communities intentionally designed to promote good health. Additionally, social media platforms can provide a more stable source of support as individuals switch social media user names less frequently than they do cell phone numbers (Volpp & Mohta, 2017). These social media tools have made health interventions more accessible than ever before by delivering strategic, effective, user-friendly messages directly to target audiences, even right into people's hands via their hand-held mobile devices.

The use of using social media tools to promote health has become so widespread in the past decade that the CDC now offers communication guidelines and a social media toolkit for creating social messages in health communications and activities (CDC, 2013a). Similarly, in 2013, the National Library of Medicine, a division of the DHHS, announced its plan to install software that will mine Facebook and Twitter to assess how Tweets and Facebook posts can be used as change agents for health behaviors. Still, more research is needed to assess the effect of social media on health behavior.

THE ROLE AND IMPACT OF PRIMARY CARE INTERVENTIONS

The progress in health behavior change research and treatment set the stage for the development of brief, individually oriented, primary care health interventions that could be offered and tailored to all members of a practice, health plan, or patient population.

These efforts were based on a strong rationale for primary care interventions to address behavioral health risks. Patient surveys have repeatedly found that patients expect and value advice from their providers about diet, exercise, and substance use and are motivated to act on this advice. Most primary care providers describe health behavior change advice and counseling as an essential part of their role and responsibilities.

The unique extended relationship that is the hallmark of primary care affords multiple opportunities, over time, to address healthy behavior in a "string of pearls" approach, capitalizing both on teachable moments—for example, introducing physical activity or diet counseling when test results show elevated cholesterol levels—and on a therapeutic alliance that often extends beyond the patient to include key family members. Moreover, evidence suggests that the health benefits and cost-effectiveness of evidence-based preventive health behavior change interventions rival, and frequently surpass, those of remedial disease treatments (Maciosek et al., 2006).

In the minimal contact primary care counseling interventions that were distilled from the successful multicomponent models, the physician was seen as the initial catalyst for change, providing brief motivational advice, social support, and follow-up, with referral to other staff members or community resources for more intensive assistance. Stage-based and social marketing approaches held the potential to reach and assist entire populations of patients, including those not yet motivated for change and those in underserved and high-risk groups. As social media introduced innovative options to promote health information, computer-based, patient-tailored, and population-targeted interventions provided new ways to reduce provider burden. In fact, in 2013, the Community Preventive Services Task Force added mobile phone–based quit smoking counseling to its roster of recommended tobacco control interventions.

Progress in developing effective minimal-contact, primary care interventions occurred first in the area of smoking cessation, culminating in the development of an evidence-based, practice-friendly intervention model now known as the 5 A's: Ask, Advise, Agree, Assist, Arrange follow-up. The 5 A's model was found to be effective when used by a variety of health care providers (physicians, nurses, dentists, dental hygienists), with as few as two to three minutes of in-office provider time.

The model starts with *asking* about tobacco use, leading to clear and personal *advice* to quit for smokers (or congratulations for quitters), and the offer of help. The *agree* step starts with assessing patient readiness to quit and goes on to establish a goal and quitting plan. For those not ready to quit, *assistance* includes a recommended motivational intervention; for those who are ready to quit, *assistance* combines brief face-to-face or telephone-based behavior change counseling with Food and Drug Administration (FDA)–approved pharmacotherapy, such as nicotine gum, patch, nasal spray or inhaler; bupropion hydrochloride (Zyban); varenicline (Chantix); or some combination of these, unless medically contraindicated (e.g., in pregnancy).

Behavioral counseling was effective when provided through multiple formats— self-help materials *and* face-to-face or telephone counseling—and there is a clear dose-response relationship between the amount of counseling and quit rates. Effective follow-up *arrangements* include planned visits, calls, or contacts to reinforce progress, adjust the quitting plan to better meet individual needs, or refer for more intensive help. One-year quit rates for patients receiving these interventions are typically two to three times higher than the 5% to 7% quit rates among people who try quitting on their own. In fact, the CDC and Prevention and Partnership for Prevention found the 5A's intervention to be one of the most effective and cost-effective of all evidence-based clinical preventive services (Maciosek et al., 2006).

The 5 A's model has been formally adopted by the USPSTF as a unifying conceptual framework or guideline applicable to addressing *all* behavioral health risks, including risky drinking, physical activity, diet, and obesity. In most cases, the USPSTF found that counseling interventions could produce clinically meaningful, populationwide health improvements that were sustained for at least 6 to 12 months. Although there are many common elements, the specific intervention components and intensity of recommended strategies vary from behavior to behavior, as does their effectiveness with unselected versus high-risk patients. Primary care providers may intervene more forcefully with healthy patients when they are known to be at high risk for a particular chronic disease, and patients at high risk may feel more vulnerable and motivated to act on the advice and assistance they receive.

The first step is always to *assess* not only the relevant behavior (using a standard health-risk appraisal or brief screening that can easily be administered in a busy practice setting), but also the individual factors that are helpful in tailoring the intervention, such as medical and physiologic factors, motives, barriers, patient's stage of change, social support, and cultural values. Based on this information, and with reference to the patient's immediate health concerns and symptoms, the clinician provides brief, personalized *advice*, expressing confidence in the patient's ability to change and soliciting the patient's thoughts about the recommended changes.

The next critical step is to negotiate and *agree* on a collaboratively defined behavior change goal and treatment plan, which commonly includes practical problem solving to *assist* the patient in addressing personal change barriers, building social support, developing a more supportive immediate social and physical environment, and securing adjunctive behavior change resources and pharmacologic aids, such as nicotine replacement. Adjunctive resources can include evidence-based face-to-face, telephone, or mobile phone counseling; targeted or generic self-help materials; and interactive Internet-based tools that are tailored to a patient's gender, age, racial/ethnic or cultural group, health status or condition, stage of change, and other relevant variables. These resources can be used before, during, and after the office visit.

The final step is to *arrange* follow-up support and assistance, including referral to more intensive or customized help, or to online tools and supports to help the patient maintain behavior change maintenance.

These new guidelines provided unprecedented scientific support for the USPSTF assertion that "the most effective interventions available to clinicians for reducing the incidence and severity of the leading causes of disease and disability in the United States are those that address patients' personal health practices" (USPSTF, 1996, p. iv).

However, several important limitations and gaps remain. The greatest limitation is the lack of long-term maintenance after successful behavior change for 12 months or longer. This is not surprising, given that patients return to the environments that shaped and supported their unhealthy lifestyles and choices. Higher maintenance rates are achieved in clinic-based programs that offered extended booster or maintenance sessions, providing ongoing social support and behavior change assistance, or in those that helped patients to create an enduring "therapeutic microenvironment" to shield them from unhealthy influences—for example, implementing an in-home smoking ban, arranging for the delivery of recommended diet foods, or arranging ongoing behavior change buddies.

Researchers and policy makers agree that current research and evidence gaps are the result of too few studies that have developed and tested primary care interventions for children, adolescents, and underserved populations.

MULTILEVEL MODELS FOR POPULATION-BASED HEALTH BEHAVIOR CHANGE

The shift to population-based models of health promotion and disease prevention was prompted by several factors:

- The success of effective, brief, and intensive interventions based on social learning theory, which gave greater prominence to environmental factors in behavior
- The emergence of new stage-based and social marketing models for populationwide interventions
- The disappointing reach and long-term effectiveness of even the most successful cognitive behavioral treatments

The lackluster performance of individual treatment approaches was especially apparent when contrasted with new evidence from public health research showing far-reaching and lasting health effects from environmental and policy changes that eliminated the need for individual decision making. A prime example is the development of safer roads and more crashworthy automobiles, combined with shifts in laws and norms regarding seat belt use and drinking and driving, which collectively produced a dramatic decline in auto-related deaths and injuries.

With the stage well set, the final push for a change in approach came in the 1990s with the development of **social ecological models** of health behavior. These models integrate behavioral science with clinical and public health approaches. They redefined what the targets of successful health interventions need to be—not just individuals but also the powerful social contexts in which they live and work. And they emphasized that a person's health behavior is affected by multiple levels of influence: interpersonal factors (e.g., physiologic factors, knowledge, skill, motivation), social factors (e.g., social–cultural norms, supports, and networks), organizational and community factors, broader environmental influences, and public policies.

Proponents of the ecological model recommend multilevel strategies that address all these levels of influence (Glickman, Parker, Sim, Del Valle Cook, & Miller, 2012; IOM, 2000, 2013; Koh, 2010). Specifically, they propose that educational and clinical interventions to improve the motivation, skills, and supports for individual behavior change (e.g., for permanently quitting smoking or risky drinking, or for adopting and maintaining healthier activity and eating patterns) would be more successful when policies and influences in the wider environment prompt and reinforce healthy behavior through, for example, clean indoor air laws and access to safe and attractive places to walk or bike and obtain healthy, affordable foods.

A strong, early proponent of the ecological approach to prevention, McKinlay (1995) proposed a template for more effective population health promotion strategies that linked individual-level, clinical health behavior change strategies with broader, population-level health promotion efforts, including upstream policy and environmental interventions. The model McKinlay proposed (see Table 7.2) recommended interventions across a broad spectrum of factors, linking *downstream* individual clinical approaches with *midstream* interventions aimed at health plans, schools, worksites, and communities with *upstream* macro-level public policy and environmental interventions strong enough to subvert or redirect countervailing societal, economic, and industry forces. In essence, McKinlay was one of the first to argue that success in achieving lasting populationwide health behavior change required a "full court press."

In its landmark review of the past three decades of progress in population health promotion, the IOM's (2000) report, *Promoting Health: Intervention Strategies from Social and Behavioral Research*, recommended individual-level interventions aimed at those who possess a behavioral risk factor or suffer from risk-related disease. For these groups, the emphasis is on changing rather than preventing risky behavior. Population-level interventions that target defined populations in order to change and/or prevent behavioral risk factors may involve

TABLE 7.2 THE POPULATION-BASED INTERVENTION MODEL

DOWNSTREAM INTERVENTIONS	MIDSTREAM INTERVENTIONS	UPSTREAM INTERVENTIONS
Individual-level interventions aimed at those who possess a behavioral risk factor or suffer from risk-related disease; emphasis on changing rather than preventing risky behavior	Population-level interventions that target defined populations in order to change and/or prevent behavioral risk factors; may involve mediation through important organizational channels or natural environments	State and national public policy/environmental interventions that aim to strengthen social norms and supports for healthy behavior and redirect unhealthy behavior
▪ Group and individual counseling	▪ Worksite and community-based health promotion/disease prevention programs	▪ National public education/media campaigns
▪ Patient health education/cognitive behavioral interventions	▪ Health plan–based primary care screening/intervention	▪ Economic incentives (e.g., excise taxes on tobacco products; reimbursement for effective primary care, diets, and extensive counseling)
▪ Self-help programs and tailored communications	▪ School-based youth prevention activities	▪ Policies reducing access to unhealthy products (e.g., pricing, access, labeling)
▪ Pharmacologic treatments	▪ Community-based interventions focused on defined at-risk populations	▪ Policies reducing the advertising and promotion of unhealthy products and behavior

Source: From McKinlay, J. B. (1995). The new public health approach to improving physical activity and autonomy in older populations. In E. Heikkinen, J. Kuusinen, & I. Ruoppila (Eds.), *Preparation for aging* (pp. 87–102). New York, NY: Plenum.

> It is unreasonable to expect that people will change their behavior easily when so many forces in the social, cultural, and physical environment conspire against such change (Institute of Medicine, 2000).

mediation through important organizational channels or natural environments. State and national public policy/environmental interventions aim to strengthen social norms and supports for healthy behavior and redirect unhealthy behavior.

The IOM used McKinlay's broad-spectrum, multilevel model for describing the balance needed between the dominant clinical and individually oriented approaches to disease prevention on the one hand and the population-level approaches addressing the generic social and behavioral factors linked to disease, injury, and disability on the other. Observing that many forces in the social, cultural, and physical environment often constitute enormous barriers to health behavior change (IOM, 2000, p. 2), the authors recommended population-based health promotion efforts that:

- Use multiple approaches (e.g., education, social support, laws, incentives, behavior change programs) and address multiple levels of influence simultaneously (i.e., individuals, families, communities, nations)
- Take account of the special needs of target groups (e.g., based on age, gender, race, ethnicity, and social class)
- Apply a long view of health outcomes because changes often take many years to become established
- Involve a variety of sectors in society that have not traditionally been associated with health promotion efforts, including law, business, education, social services, and the media

Examples From Tobacco Control

The last three decades of progress in national tobacco control, hailed by some as one of the greatest public health successes of the second half of the 20th century, is the example most often used to illustrate the power and promise of ecological approaches for health intervention.

Although major disparities in tobacco use and its addiction remain, regressive tobacco tax and price increases have proved especially effective in certain high-risk and underserved populations—including adolescents, pregnant women, and low-income smokers. State telephone quitlines (1-800-QUIT-NOW) offering cost-free counseling and medication have greatly expanded the reach of evidence-based individual cessation treatments to traditionally underserved low-income and minority populations.

Reflecting the growth in research evaluating the population effects of midstream and upstream interventions for tobacco control, the CDC's Task Force for Community Preventive Services was launched in 1996 to conduct systematic reviews of community-based and policy interventions to change health behavior, similar to the reviews conducted by the USPSTF of downstream clinical preventive interventions. Based on its review of evidence for 14 different tobacco control interventions, the CDC makes these recommendations:

- Smoking bans and restrictions to reduce exposure to environmental tobacco smoke
- Tax and price increases and mass media campaigns to reduce the number of youth who start smoking and to promote cessation
- Telephone quitline and mobile phone-based support, as well as a number of health care system interventions, also to increase cessation

Similar ecological models have been described and proposed for each of the other major behavioral risk factors discussed in this chapter—risky drinking, physical inactivity, dietary behavior change, and obesity. These are summarized on the CDC's Community Preventive Services Task Force Community Guide website (CDC, 2013b) and in the Task Force's 2013 *Third Annual Report to Congress* (CDC, 2013), presenting more than 200 evidence-based recommendations for promoting better health among community members.

Examples From Childhood Obesity Prevention

A great sense of urgency surrounds the need to identify evidence-based "full-court press" strategies that can halt the nation's current obesity epidemic, especially among children (Glickman et al., 2012; Kumanyika, Parker, & Sim, 2010; White House Task Force on Childhood Obesity, 2010). The dramatic rise in the prevalence of overweight and obesity among youth and adults over the past several decades is primarily due to environmental and economic changes affecting behavior on both sides of the **energy balance equation**; that is, the amount of energy (calories) used versus the amount consumed.

The cumulative effects of technology—such as automobile-dependent transportation and more sedentary jobs—along with changes in lifestyles in typical suburban environments, which limit the places to which adults and children can walk, have reduced the amount of physical activity in everyday life.

At the same time, increased access to low-cost, sugar-laden, and high-fat foods and beverages; increased exposure to marketing for these unhealthy products; larger portion sizes; increased restaurant use; an exodus of grocery stores and other sources of fresh fruits and vegetables from cities to suburbs; and the rising cost of fresh produce relative to soda and snack foods have all played a critical role in promoting excessive caloric intake, especially for low-income and racial/ethnic minority populations facing inequalities in access to healthy affordable foods. Pervasive racial/ethnic disparities in access to safe places to walk, bike, and play have sparked numerous studies documenting socioeconomic differences in access to community sports areas, parks, swimming pools, beaches, and bike paths.

Continued progress is being made to understand the environmental and policy factors that affect physical activity and identify promising multilevel, broad-spectrum interventions to address the nation's obesity epidemic. The CDC's Community Preventive Services Task Force reviewed research on interventions and found evidence for recommendations spanning the full McKinlay model. These include the following:

- Downstream health behavior change programs that increase social supports for physical activity and exercise (e.g., health care provider reminder systems plus provider education)
- Midstream requirements for school physical education classes that increase the time students spend in moderate or vigorous physical activity and "point of decision" prompts on elevators and escalators that encourage people to use nearby stairs
- Upstream efforts to create, or increase, access to safe, attractive, and convenient places for physical activity, along with informational outreach to change knowledge and attitudes about the benefits of and opportunities for physical activity

Additionally, the IOM used a systems approach to analyze hundreds of strategies for obesity prevention and prioritize the most promising recommendations (Glickman et al., 2012). Together, these guidelines have provided a strong, science-based blueprint for multisector efforts by professionals in public health, urban planning, transportation, parks and recreation, architecture, landscape design, public safety, and the mass media to close the gaps between recommended and actual physical activity levels for U.S. children and adults.

Some upstream efforts come in the form of federal payments that can help communities create or improve access to healthy options. The Patient Protection and Affordable Care Act (ACA), passed in 2010, provided states and communities with a new stream of funds to promote healthy living by creating and improving multiple factors—such as housing, education, child care, and food outlets—in ways that address health disparities, improve access to behavioral health services, and reduce and control behavioral risk factors.

Other federal and state health-related policy changes have been influential in reducing childhood obesity, particularly among children from low-income families who participate in the Special Supplemental Nutrition Program for Women, Infants, and Children (better known as WIC). A 2008 overhaul of the WIC food package changed the mix of foods covered by the program, making more fruits and vegetables, skim and low-fat milk, and whole grain breads and cereals available to participants. Grocery stores and schools serving WIC children changed their inventories to meet the new standards, which benefited not only WIC families but also entire communities. In 2013, evidence pointed to declining obesity rates among children from low-income communities in 18 states and one U.S. territory (CDC, 2013c).

Among U.S. cities, Philadelphia set itself apart by reporting a significant decrease in obesity between 2006 and 2010, particularly among school children in grades K through 12 and adolescents of color. These decreases emerged after the city instituted a decade-long, multipronged effort to combat obesity and influence health behavior. Over those 10 years, Philadelphia implemented the following:

- Nutrition education to public school students whose families are eligible for the federal Supplemental Nutrition Assistance Program

- Financial incentives to attract grocers to open stores in underserved areas
- A school districtwide wellness policy
- Improved nutritional offerings in schools, which included the removal of deep-fried foods, sodas, and sugar-sweetened beverages
- Improved in-store food marketing practices in local grocery and locally owned corner stores
- Required calorie postings at chain restaurants

With respect to high-risk populations and environments, systematic surveillance can increasingly monitor the prevalence of behavioral risk factors and related health-promoting programs, resources, and policies. Such surveillance systems, which already exist for tobacco control and are rapidly developing for physical activity, establish a national baseline that makes it possible to assess the effects of specific interventions and to evaluate important local, state, and national intervention efforts (Sallis et al., 2011). Although some events and political changes may create opportunities for rapid change, as did the Tobacco Master Settlement Agreement, a long-term view is essential. Most successful health promotion and social change efforts have required decades of hard work.

As we learned from the success of tobacco control, highly credible scientific evidence can persuade policy makers and withstand the attacks of those whose interests are threatened. Collaboration among public health researchers, advocates, communicators, strategists, and health care providers is needed to ensure that high-quality evidence reaches policy decision makers at the right times.

The difficulty of implementing effective broad-spectrum approaches should not be underestimated. Powerful political opponents benefit from the sale, promotion, and marketing of unhealthy products. Other barriers include industry lobbying, chronically limited public support for healthy public policies, and inadequate funding for and enforcement of effective policies and programs. Creating a favorable political climate requires advocacy in order to instigate broad public pressure and support for change, clear and well-communicated evidence of public demand and support for change, and evidence of the beneficial health and economic effects of proposed programs and policies.

CHANGING PROVIDER BEHAVIOR: CLOSING THE GAP BETWEEN BEST PRACTICE AND USUAL CARE

One of the most basic measures of national health care quality is the extent to which patients receive recommended, evidence-based care. Evidence-based guidelines exist for prevention-oriented primary care interventions related to behavioral risks, and putting these guidelines into practice has become an important objective for national health care **quality improvement** efforts.

The IOM's (2001) transformative report, *Crossing the Quality Chasm*, set forth a bold national agenda for improving health care quality across the full spectrum of care, from prevention to acute and chronic illness and palliative care, including health behavior change. A follow-up IOM report (Adams & Corrigan, 2003) selected health behavior change interventions for tobacco and obesity as two of the top 20 priorities for national action.

These reports and the reviews and recommendations issued over the past decade by the USPSTF and CDC's Community Preventive Services Task Force have had a significant influence on the prevention and public health provisions of the ACA, enacted in 2010. They helped researchers, health professionals, and policy makers understand the need for a multisystemic approach to obesity prevention—one that involved a range of recommendations to build sustainably healthy communities that offer opportunities for everyone to make healthy, productive choices. This strategy was outlined in the IOM's 2012 report, *Accelerating Progress in Obesity Prevention: Solving the Weight of the Nation* (Glickman et al., 2012), which emphasized the need for targeted health interventions to reduce the inequitable distribution of health promotion and health care resources and risk factors that contribute to health disparities among members of low-income, low-resource communities.

> The Institute of Medicine's 2012 Report, *Accelerating Progress in Obesity Prevention*, presents an ambitious vision of "a society of healthy children, healthy families, and healthy communities in which all people realize their full potential" made possible through "large-scale transformative changes focused on multi-level environmental and policy changes" (p. 19).

Despite strong evidence for behavioral prevention in primary care, significant gaps persist between recommended and actual care. One of the landmark studies of the quality of outpatient health care found that U.S. adults, on average, receive about *half* the services recommended for people with their specific health problems and even less—only 18%—of the recommended lifestyle screening and counseling services (McGlynn et al., 2003). It is safe to say that most patients who could benefit from health behavior change counseling—particularly those from lower-income and economically disadvantaged racial/ethnic populations, communities, and neighborhoods—are not receiving it. In most studies, patients receive only the first two of the 5 A's—*assessment* and *advice*.

- *Tobacco use:* According to national data in 2010, 68% and 19% of visits to office-based ambulatory care settings involved tobacco use screening and tobacco cessation counseling, respectively (DHHS, 2011). These percentages, though higher than those in the baseline year of 2007, are below the *Healthy People 2020* target.
- *Alcohol use:* A 2005 study found that less than one-third of individuals who saw a general medical provider were screened for alcohol or drug use (D'Amico, Paddock, Burnam, & Kung, 2005). The probability of problem drinkers in the study's sample being screened for alcohol use was less than 50%.
- *Physical inactivity and unhealthy diet:* National surveys indicate that in 2010, 9% of physician visits by children and adults included counseling about exercise (DHHS, 2011). Among patients diagnosed with diabetes, cardiovascular disease, or

hyperlipidemia, the percentage of their physician visits that included counseling or education related to exercise was 12%. Survey data also found that in 2010, 14% of physician visits by children and adults included counseling about nutrition or diet. This percentage increases to 19% for patients diagnosed with diabetes, cardiovascular disease, or hyperlipidemia.

- **Obesity:** In 2008, just under half of primary care physicians regularly assessed BMI for their child, adolescent, and adult patients (DHHS, 2011). Similarly, multiple surveys of family practitioners (Sesselberg, Klein, O'Connor, & Johnson, 2010) and pediatricians (Klein et al., 2010) found that only about half of these primary care providers (45% and 52%, respectively) routinely assess BMI in children over age 2. Among adult patients diagnosed with obesity, the percentage of physician visits that include counseling or education regarding weight reduction, physical activity, or nutrition was 28% (DHHS, 2011).

Systematic evidence reviews beginning in the 1990s have found that most educational approaches, including traditional continuing medical education (CME), had limited effect. More interactive and skills-based educational efforts that used principles of adult learning and social-learning theory (including modeling by respected peer "opinion leaders") were somewhat more effective. Multicomponent interventions that addressed the multiple intrapersonal and environmental barriers to provider adherence, especially system barriers, were most effective.

The limited success of "if you tell them, they will change" provider education strategies drew critical attention to the many system-level barriers to adherence to evidence-based guidelines and recommendations, including the pressure of time (in the face of more urgent medical issues), inadequate office supports, a lack of provider and patient resources, and missing financial incentives.

Follow-up studies confirmed that clinician training was most effective when combined with efforts to create office supports to prompt, facilitate, and reward the delivery of preventive interventions, especially behavioral counseling, and that the most successful interventions were not one-size-fits-all, but tailored to the unique circumstances present in any particular office practice.

Multilevel Models for Improving Delivery of Effective Health Behavior Change Interventions

Collectively, these findings led to a shift in understanding what the targets of interventions to change *provider* health care practices needed to be. Crabtree and colleagues (1998) introduced a **practice ecology model**, emphasizing the need to address not just the behavior of individual providers, but also the powerful effects of the health care systems and environments in which providers practice.

They and other proponents of a broader view of health care improvement emphasized the need for broad-spectrum strategies addressing multiple levels of influence: downstream intrapersonal/individual provider-level factors; midstream interpersonal/practice team, office microsystems and health plan

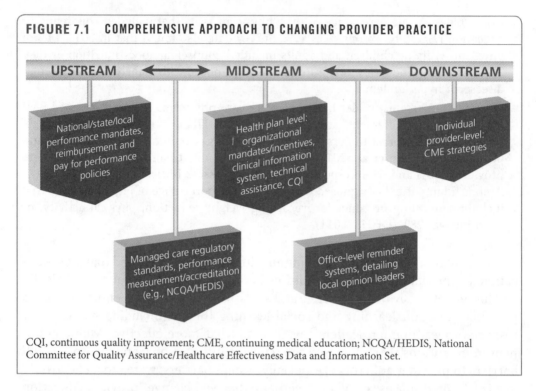

FIGURE 7.1   COMPREHENSIVE APPROACH TO CHANGING PROVIDER PRACTICE

UPSTREAM ⟵⟶ MIDSTREAM ⟵⟶ DOWNSTREAM

National/state/local performance mandates, reimbursement and pay for performance policies

Health plan level: organizational mandates/incentives, clinical information system, technical assistance, CQI

Individual provider-level: CME strategies

Managed care regulatory standards, performance measurement/accreditation (e.g., NCQA/HEDIS)

Office-level reminder systems, detailing local opinion leaders

CQI, continuous quality improvement; CME, continuing medical education; NCQA/HEDIS, National Committee for Quality Assurance/Healthcare Effectiveness Data and Information Set.

influences; and upstream macro-level health care systems and policies (Goodwin et al., 2001; see Figure 7.1).

Responding to the same evidence, the IOM's (2001) *Crossing the Quality Chasm* report recommended a fundamental reengineering of the nation's health care system—moving from a system designed primarily to support and pay for the delivery of reactive acute and remedial illness care to one that would support and pay for the proactive, preventive, and behavioral care needed to prevent and manage chronic disease.

It has been said that "an ounce of prevention takes a ton of office system change." Until recently, we lacked a coherent model for what this "ton of change" involved. Filling this void, Wagner, Austin, and Von Korff (1996) reviewed the research on effective chronic illness care and prevention and devised a model for the multiple interlocking systems supports required for effective planned, proactive chronic illness care—the **chronic care model**.

This model applies equally to the *prevention* and to the *treatment* of chronic disease, both of which require helping patients to change the behavioral risk factors that cause or complicate their illnesses. The chronic care model helped to pave the way for the concept of the "medical home" as a means for reorganizing primary care practices to improve health outcomes and reduce health care costs and disparities.

The six key elements of the chronic care model can be implemented at the level of the office practice or larger health care delivery system. Each element includes interventions that are planned rather than reactive, are patient-centered and informed by individually relevant patient data, are proactive, involve scheduled outreach and follow-up, and are population-based—that is, focused on an entire panel of patients with a specific behavioral risk factor, disease, or condition and not just on individuals who seek care. Both prevention and treatment of chronic conditions require regular (nonsymptom-driven) screening and counseling for health behavior change, involve ongoing planned care with proactive follow-up, depend on active patient involvement in decision making and adherence, and require links to supportive community resources and services.

As an example, the chronic care model proved a helpful heuristic for describing an organizationwide initiative at Group Health Cooperative of Puget Sound that integrates screening and treatment for tobacco use with routine primary care. This successful plan applied all six model elements as follows:

- *Health care organization:* Health plan leaders made reducing tobacco use their top prevention priority, provided financial and other incentives to providers (including hiring dedicated clinic counselors), and eliminated patient copayments for counseling.
- *Clinical information systems* were used to create a registry of the tobacco users enrolled in the health plan, track their use of treatment resources and programs, and generate proactive telephone quitline calls for patients and feedback reports for providers.
- *Decision support tools* included extensive provider training, ongoing consultation, automated patient assessment and guideline algorithms, and reminder tools.
- *Practice redesign* and *self-management support* included self-help materials and a telephone quitline to deliver counseling and pharmacotherapy without burdening the provider.
- *Community resources and policies* included referral to community and worksite quit-smoking clinics and related healthy lifestyle change programs and focused on stress management, exercise, and weight loss, as well as support for worksite smoking cessation. Their efforts also involved campaigns and smoking restrictions and expanded state funding for tobacco prevention and control programs.

The chronic care model has provided a unifying approach to health care quality improvement that cuts across different types of health behavior and chronic conditions with the promise of a more efficient, sustainable, and cost-effective approach to health care quality improvement. This is especially the case given the development of several successful continuous quality improvement (CQI) techniques for putting chronic care model–based system changes into place. Promising midstream CQI techniques have been used to design and test office system changes to find ways to eliminate barriers and strengthen the supports for recommended care, often through a series of "rapid cycle" (plan-do-study-act) improvement efforts.

Successful preventive CQI interventions have been delivered through learning collaboratives involving multiple health care teams from different organizations that meet and work over a 12- to 18-month period with faculty experts in CQI techniques and in the type of care targeted for improvement (e.g., tobacco dependence, obesity, diabetes management). Individual practice-level, chronic care model–based improvements involve planning, implementing, evaluating, and refining changes in individual practices. These efforts have substantially increased the proportion of patients—including the most disadvantaged patients—who receive evidence-based preventive care and for whom individual behavior change plans were developed and implemented.

Effective individual practice consultation models for CQI with a focus on multiple risk behavior change were pioneered in the STEP-UP (Study to Enhance Prevention by Understanding Practice) trial conducted by Goodwin and colleagues (2001). This randomized, controlled trial tested a brief practice-tailored approach to improving preventive service delivery, emphasizing improving rates of health habit counseling and the usage of effective community-based programs and supports for health behavior change.

Intervention practices received a 1-day practice assessment, an initial practicewide consultation, and several brief follow-up visits to assess and address practice-specific barriers. All interventions were delivered by a specially trained nurse facilitator who helped practices to identify promising changes and presented a menu of tools for implementing them (e.g., reminder systems, flow sheets, patient education materials, clinical information systems), including a practice improvement manual. This brief CQI intervention resulted in significant improvements at 6 and 12 months, which were maintained at a 24-month follow-up.

Improvements in behavioral counseling services were especially dramatic. The investigators attributed these lasting results to the maintenance of the practice and system changes that were made—changes that may have been easier to institutionalize because they were tailored to the unique characteristics of each practice.

The success of the STEP-UP trial and similar chronic care model–based primary care practice redesign approaches inspired the Robert Wood Johnson Foundation's Prescription for Health national program. This program funded 27 studies in primary care practice–based research networks to discover and test innovative ways of delivering 5 A's interventions for two or more health behaviors: tobacco use, sedentary lifestyle, unhealthy diet, and/or risky drinking.

Projects in round 1 of the program demonstrated that practices could identify at-risk patients and motivate them to make changes. Round 2 projects built linkages between clinical practices and community resources to reduce provider burden and help patients sustain behavior changes. Each project required policy and environmental changes in the practice (e.g., reminder systems, patient registries, performance incentives) to facilitate delivery of evidence-based counseling and related treatments and to facilitate use of needed follow-up support from community resources, such as telephone quitlines. Results showed that primary care providers were able to deliver effective health behavior change interventions when working in supportive health care systems and practices.

In the long run, just as upstream macro-level societal and policy change is needed to sustain individual behavior change, upstream macro-level health system and policy change is needed to improve care in office practices and health plans. Such changes include quality performance measurement and public reporting, "pay-for-performance" initiatives that reward providers based on the quality of care they offer, and improved information technology to drive and support care improvement.

Some research has found that providers were more likely to offer health behavior change counseling when a portion of their capitation payment depended on their doing so. Providers in physician organizations were found to be more likely to offer proven health promotion services if their performance measures were publicly reported or they received public recognition or economic benefit, and they had greater clinical information technology capacity (McMenamin et al., 2004).

> Just as upstream macro-level societal and policy change is needed to sustain individual behavior change, upstream macro-level health system and policy change are needed to support and improve care in office practices and health plans.

CONCLUSION

Changing health-related behavior represents a prime target for improving national health and health care. Never have we known more about the importance of addressing the lifestyle factors that pose the most serious threats to Americans' health, produce the greatest demands on our health system, and contribute most to health care costs. The growing burden of chronic disease, a national epidemic of obesity, and escalating health care costs—at a time when health care spending already is growing faster than the U.S. gross domestic product—makes establishing a stronger preventive orientation in the nation's health care and public health systems an urgent priority.

Never have we known as much about how to motivate, support, and assist individuals to make lasting lifestyle changes or how to support and assist health care professionals to deliver evidence-based preventive care aimed at behavior change. The tremendous parallel gains made in what we have learned about how to achieve effective health promotion for individuals and health care quality improvement for providers have created unprecedented potential.

The landmark ACA represents one promising strategy that places prevention at the heart of the efforts needed to improve the nation's health and health care. Its prevention-oriented provisions include (a) full Medicaid and Medicare coverage for all preventive health services recommended by USPSTF, including those focused on health behavior change; (b) funding for community-based prevention grants to implement programs and policy; (c) environmental changes to improve nutrition, increase physical activity, reduce tobacco use and substance abuse, and reduce health risk disparities; (d) funding for childhood obesity community demonstration projects; and (e) the establishment of a National Prevention, Health Promotion, and Public Health Council to set and track goals and objectives for improving health through federally supported prevention, health promotion, and public health programs.

The law also requires funding for the continuation and greater coordination of the USPSTF and CDC's Community Preventive Services Task Force. Combined, these efforts hold unprecedented potential to capitalize and build on the strong evidence for health-related behavior change created over the past three decades.

▶ CASE EXERCISE—COMPREHENSIVE PLAN FOR ADDRESSING RISK FACTORS

You have just been hired as the director of strategic planning for a health plan that insures 30% of the residents in a metropolitan area of 500,000. Most of those insured by this health plan are employed by large companies in the metropolitan area, and these companies pay for their employees' health insurance. The health plan leaders and the employers both recognize that their business model depends on their success in addressing behavioral risk factors that play a critical role in the prevention and management of chronic diseases, the containment of health care costs, and the enhancement of employee productivity.

In your new role, you are asked to create a comprehensive plan for addressing these behavioral risk factors—by improving both the clinical care provided and the plan's community-based efforts. Specifically, you want to develop strategies to reduce the levels of tobacco use, unhealthy diet, and physical inactivity. In constructing your plan, consider the following questions:

1. What mix of interventions would you need to consider that might change enrollee behavior, provider behavior, and community policies and environments and maximize the cost-effectiveness of this plan?

2. What is the evidence that these interventions would work?

3. What would be the implementation challenges of the plan?

DISCUSSION QUESTIONS

1. Briefly describe the effects of personal health behavior (e.g., tobacco use, risky drinking, diet, and physical activity) on individual and population health status and health care costs in the United States.

2. How have health behavior change programs and interventions evolved over the past 40 years?

3. In order to achieve effective behavioral interventions, most physicians use clinical practice guidelines that are based on the 5A's model. Briefly describe this model, using tobacco cessation counseling as an example.

4. Describe the parallel shifts that have taken place during the past 30 years in understanding what the essential targets must be for successful interventions (a) to increase patients' adherence to recommended prevention-oriented health behavior and (b) to increase providers' use of recommended clinical preventive behavior change interventions.

5. With reference to McKinlay's population-based intervention model, outline possible coordinated *downstream, midstream,* and *upstream* strategies that can be used to achieve one of the following: (a) curb binge drinking on a college campus; (b) increase smoking cessation, especially among pregnant smokers enrolled in a Medicaid managed care plan; or (c) increase physical activity and healthy eating among middle school students in an urban center. Be sure to mention the different sectors that would need to be involved (public health, law enforcement, local business, school officials, policy makers, community planning, transportation, health plan leaders/providers, and so on).

REFERENCES

Adams, K., & Corrigan, J. M. (Eds.). (2003). *Priority areas for national action: Transforming health care quality. Quality chasm series.* Washington, DC: National Academies Press.

Adler, N., Bachrach, C., Daley, D., & Frisco, M. (2013). *Building the science for a population health movement* [Discussion paper]. Washington, DC: Institute of Medicine.

American Cancer Society. (2012). Health risks of smokeless tobacco. Retrieved from http://www.cancer.org/cancer/cancercauses/tobaccocancer/smokeless-tobacco

Berke, E. M., Tanksi, S. E., Demidenko, E., Alford-Teaster, J., Shi, X., & Sargent, J. D. (2010). Alcohol retail density and demographic predictors of health disparities: A geographic analysis. *American Journal of Public Health, 100,* 1967–1971. doi:10.2105/AJPH.2009.170464

Centers for Disease Control and Prevention. (n.d.). Alcohol-related disease impact (ARDI) application. Retrieved from https://nccd.cdc.gov/DPH_ARDI/default/default.aspx

Centers for Disease Control and Prevention. (1964). Surgeon General's Report on Smoking and Tobacco Use. Retrieved from https://www.cdc.gov/tobacco/data_statistics/sgr/index.htm

Centers for Disease Control and Prevention. (2013). Community Preventive Services Task Force: Annual Report to Congress, 2013. Retrieved from https://www.thecommunityguide.org/sites/default/files/assets/2013-congress-report-full_0.pdf

Centers for Disease Control and Prevention. (2013b). Tobacco: Guide to community preventive services. Reducing tobacco use and secondhand smoke exposure. Retrieved from https://www.thecommunityguide.org/topic/tobacco

Centers for Disease Control and Prevention. (2013c). Vital signs: Obesity among low-income, preschool-aged children—United States, 2008–2011. *Morbidity and Mortality Weekly Report, 62*(31), 629–634. Retrieved from https://www.cdc.gov/mmwr/preview/mmwrhtml/mm6231a4.htm

Centers for Disease Control and Prevention. (2013d). Youth and tobacco use fact sheet. Retrieved from http://www.cdc.gov/tobacco/data_statistics/fact_sheets/youth_data/tobacco_use/#estimates

Centers for Disease Control and Prevention. (2016). The cost of excessive alcohol use. Retrieved from https://www.cdc.gov/alcohol/onlinemedia/infographics/cost-excessive-alcohol-use.html

Centers for Disease Control and Prevention. (2017). CDC social media tools, guidelines, and best practices. Retrieved from https://www.cdc.gov/socialmedia/tools/guidelines/index.html

Centers for Disease Control and Prevention. (2017). Tobacco use and pregnancy. Retrieved from https://www.cdc.gov/reproductivehealth/maternalinfanthealth/tobaccousepregnancy/index.htm

Centers for Disease Control and Prevention. (2018). Smoking is down, but almost 38 million American adults still smoke [Press release]. Retrieved from https://www.cdc.gov/media/releases/2018/p0118-smoking-rates-declining.html

Coups, E. J., Gaba, A., & Orleans, C. T. (2004). Physician screening for multiple behavioral health risk factors. *American Journal of Preventive Medicine, 27*(2 Suppl.), 34–41. doi:10.1016/j.amepre.2004.04.021

Crabtree, B. F., Miller, W. L., Aita, V. A., Flocke, S. A., & Stange, K. C. (1998). Primary care practice organization and preventive services delivery: A qualitative analysis. *Journal of Family Practice, 46,* 403–409.

D'Amico, E. J., Paddock, S. M., Burnam, A., & Kung, F. Y. (2005). Identification of and guidance for problem drinking by general medical providers: Results from a national survey. *Medical Care, 43*(3), 229–236. Retrieved from https://www.jstor.org/stable/3768221

Emmons, K. M., & Rollnick, S. (2001). Motivational interviewing in health care settings: Opportunities and limitations. *American Journal of Preventive Medicine, 20,* 68–74. doi:10.1016/S0749-3797(00)00254-3

Giovino, G. A., Chaloupka, F. J., Hartman, A. M., Joyce, K. G., Chriqui, J., Orleans, C. T., … Larkin, M. (2009). *Cigarette smoking prevalence and policies in the 50 states: An era of change—The Robert Wood Johnson Foundation impact teen tobacco chart book.* Buffalo: State University of New York at Buffalo.

Goodwin, M. A., Zyzanski, S. J., Zronek, S., Ruhe, M., Weyer, S. M., Konrad, N., & Stange, K. C. (2001). A clinical trial of tailored office systems for preventive service delivery: The Study to Enhance Prevention by Understanding Practice (STEP-UP). *American Journal of Preventive Medicine, 21,* 20–28. doi:10.1016/S0749-3797(01)00310-5

Glickman, D., Parker, L., Sim, L., Del Valle Cook, H., & Miller, E. A. (Eds.). (2012). *Accelerating progress in obesity prevention: Solving the weight of the nation.* Washington, DC: National Academies Press.

Glickman, D., Parker, L., Sim, L., Del Valle Cook, H., & Miller, E. A. (Eds.). (2013). *Creating equal opportunities for a healthy weight: Workshop summary.* Washington, DC: National Academies Press.

Hamilton, M. T., Hamilton, D. G., & Zedric, T. W. (2007). Role of low energy expenditure and sitting in obesity, metabolic syndrome, type 2 diabetes, and cardiovascular disease. *Diabetes, 56,* 2655–2667. doi:10.2337/db07-0882

Institute of Medicine. (1982). *Health and behavior.* Washington, DC: National Academies Press.

Institute of Medicine. (2001). *Crossing the quality chasm: A new health system for the 21st century.* Washington, DC: National Academies Press.

Institute of Medicine. (2013). *Creating equal opportunities for a healthy weight: Workshop summary.* Washington, DC: National Academies Press.

Jamal, A., Phillips E., Gentzke A. S., Homa, D. M., Babb, S. D., King, B. A., Neff, L. J. (2018). Current cigarette smoking among adults—United States, 2016. *Morbidity and Mortality Weekly Report, 67,* 53–59. doi:10.15585/mmwr.mm6702a1

Johnston, L. D., O'Malley, P. M., Bachman, J. G., & Schulenberg, J. E. (2013a). *Monitoring the future: National results on drug use, 1975–2012* (Vol. 2, College students and adults ages 19–50). Ann Arbor: University of Michigan, Institute for Social Research.

Klein, J. D., Sesselberg, T. S., Johnson, M. S., O'Connor, K. G., Cook, S., Coon, M., … Washington, R. (2010). Adoption of body mass index guidelines for screening and counseling in pediatric practice. *Pediatrics, 25,* 265–272. doi:10.1542/peds.2008-2985

Koh, H. K. (2010). A 2020 vision for healthy people. *New England Journal of Medicine, 362,* 1653–1656. doi: 10.1056/NEJMp1001601

Kumanyika, S. K., Parker, L., & Sim, L. J. (Eds.). (2010). *Bridging the evidence gap in obesity prevention: A framework to inform decision making.* Washington, DC: National Academies Press.

Maciosek, M. V., Edwards, N. M., Coffield, A. B., Flottemesch, T. J., Nelson, W. W., Goodman, M. J., & Solberg, L. I. (2006). Priorities among effective clinical preventive services: Methods. *American Journal of Preventive Medicine, 31,* 90–96. doi:10.1016/j.amepre.2006.03.011

McGinnis, J. M., & Foege, W. H. (1993). Actual causes of death in the United States. *Journal of the American Medical Association, 270,* 2207–2212. doi:10.1001/jama.1993.03510180077038

McGlynn, E. A., Asch, S. M., Adams, J., Keesey, J., Hicks, J., DeCristofaro, A., & Kerr, E. A. (2003). The quality of health care delivered to adults in the United States. *New England Journal of Medicine, 348,* 2635–2645. doi:10.1056/NEJMsa022615

McKinlay, J. B. (1995). The new public health approach to improving physical activity and autonomy in older populations. In E. Heikkinen, J. Kuusinen, & I. Ruoppila (Eds.), *Preparation for aging* (pp. 87–102). New York, NY: Plenum.

McMenamin, S. B., Schmittdiel, J., Halpin, H., Gillies, R., Rundall, T. G., & Shortell, S. M. (2004). Health promotion in physician organizations: Results from a national study. *American Journal of Preventive Medicine, 26,* 259–264. doi:10.1016/j.amepre.2003.12.012

Micha, R., Penalvo, J. L., Cudhea, F., Imamura, F., Rehm, C. D., Mozaffarian, D. (2017). Association between dietary factors and mortality from heart disease, stroke, and type 2 diabetes in the United States. *Journal of the American Medical Association, 317*(9), 912–924. doi:10.1001/jama.2017.0947

Miech, R. A., Johnston, L. D., O'Malley, P. M., Bachman, J. G., Schulenberg, J. E., & Patrick, M. E. (2018). *Monitoring the future: National survey results on drug use, 1975–2017: Volume I, Secondary school students.* Ann Arbor: Institute for Social Research, The University of Michigan. Retrieved from http://monitoringthefuture.org/pubs/monographs/mtf-vol1_2017.pdf

Mokdad, A. H., Ballestros, K., Echko, M., Glenn, S. Olsen, H. E., Mullany, E., . . . Murray, C. J. L. (2018). The state of U.S. health, 1990–2016: Burden of diseases, injuries, and risk factors among U.S. states. *Journal of the American Medical Association, 319*(14), 1444–1472. https://jamanetwork.com/journals/jama/fullarticle/2678018

Orleans, C. T., Ulmer, C. C., & Gruman, J. C. (2004). The role of behavioral factors in achieving national health outcomes. In T. J. Boll, R. G. Frank, & A. Baum (Eds.), *Handbook of clinical health psychology: Models and perspectives in health psychology* (Vol. 3, pp. 465–499). Washington, DC: American Psychological Association.

Powell, L. M., Han, E., & Chaloupka, F. J. (2010). Economic contextual factors, food consumption, and obesity among U.S. adolescents. *Journal of Nutrition, 140,* 1175–1180. doi:10.3945/jn.109.111526

Prochaska, J. O., & DiClemente, C. C. (1983). Stages and processes of self-change of smoking: Toward an integrative model of change. *Journal of Consulting and Clinical Psychology, 51,* 390–395. doi:10.1037/0022-006X.51.3.390

Richtel, M. (2013, October 26). The e-cigarette industry, waiting to exhale. *The New York Times.* Retrieved from http://www.nytimes.com/2013/10/27/business/the-e-cigarette-industry-waiting-to-exhale.html?adxnnl = 1&adxnnlx = 1388415666-ONxkwS17kyrjnWucGjHSGg

Rideout, V. J., Foehr, U. G., & Roberts, D. F. (2010). *Generation M2: Media in the lives of 8- to 18-year-olds.* Menlo Park, CA: Kaiser Family Foundation.

Robert Wood Johnson Foundation's Commission to Build a Healthier America. (2013). *Overcoming obstacles to health in 2013 and beyond.* Princeton, NJ: Robert Wood Johnson Foundation. Retrieved from http://www.rwjf.org/content/dam/farm/reports/reports/2013/rwjf406474

Sacks, J. J., Gonzales, K. R., Bouchery, E. E., Tomedi, L. E., & Brewer, R. D. (2015). 2010 National and state costs of excessive alcohol consumption. *American Journal of Preventive Medicine, 49*(5), e73–e79. doi:10.1016/j.amepre.2015.05.031

Sallis, J. F., Slymen, D. J., Conway, T. L., Frank, L. D., Saelens, B. E., Cain, K., & Chapman, J. E. (2011). Income disparities in perceived neighborhood built and social environment attributes. *Health & Place, 17,* 1274–1283. doi:10.1016/j.healthplace.2011.02.006

Saloner, B., & Lê Cook, B. (2013). Blacks and Hispanics are less likely than Whites to complete addiction treatment, largely due to socioeconomic factors. *Health Affairs, 32,* 135–145. doi:10.1377/hlthaff.2011.0983

Schlam, T. R., & Baker, T. B. (2013). Interventions for tobacco smoking. *Annual Review of Clinical Psychology, 9,* 675–702. doi:10.1146/annurev-clinpsy-050212-185602

Sesselberg, T. S., Klein, J. D., O'Connor, K. G., & Johnson, M. S. (2010). Screening and counseling for childhood obesity: Results from a national survey. *American Board of Family Medicine, 23,* 334–342. doi:10.3122/jabfm.2010.03.090070

Smedley, B. D., & Syme, S. L. (Eds.). (2000). *Promoting health: Intervention strategies from social and behavioral research.* Washington, DC: National Academies Press.

Smedley, B. D., & Syme, S. L. (Eds.). (2001). *Crossing the quality chasm: A new health system for the 21st century.* Washington, DC: National Academies Press.

Taylor, W. C., & Lou, D. (2012). *Do all children have places to be active? Disparities in access to physical activity environments in racial and ethnic minority and lower-income communities. A research synthesis.* Princeton, NJ: Active Living Research.

Treuhaft, S., & Karpyn, A. (2010). *The grocery gap: Who has access to healthy food and why it matters.* Oakland, CA: PolicyLink.

Troiano, R. P., Berrigan, D., Dodd, K. W., Mâsse, L. C., Tilert, T., & McDowell, M. (2008). Physical activity in the United States measured by accelerometer. *Medicine & Science in Sports & Exercise, 40,* 181–188. doi:10.1249/mss.0b013e31815a51b3

U.S. Department of Health and Human Services. (2000). *Healthy people 2010.* Washington, DC: Author.

U.S. Department of Health and Human Services. (2011). *Healthy people 2020.* Washington, DC: Author.

U.S. Department of Health and Human Services. (2014). *The health consequences of smoking—50 years of progress: A report of the Surgeon General.* Atlanta, GA: U.S. Department of Health and Human Services, Centers for Disease Control and Prevention, National Center for Chronic Disease Prevention and Health Promotion, Office on Smoking and Health.

U.S. Preventive Services Task Force. (1996). *Guide to clinical preventive services* (2nd ed.). Baltimore, MD: Williams & Wilkins.

Volpp, K. G., & Mohta, N. S. (2017). Patient engagement survey: Social networks to improve patient health. *NEJM Catalyst: Insights Report.* Retrieved from https://catalyst.nejm .org/survey-social-networks-patient-health

Wagner, E. H., Austin, B. T., & Von Korff, M. (1996). Organizing care for patients with chronic illness. *Milbank Quarterly, 74,* 511–544. doi:10.2307/3350391

Ward, B. W., Barnes, P. M., Freeman, G., & Schiller, J. S. (2012, March 21). *Early release of selected estimates based on data from the January–September 2011 National Health Interview Survey* [Online]. Retrieved from http://www.cdc.gov/nchs/data/nhis/early release/earlyrelease201203.pdf

White House Task Force on Childhood Obesity. (2010). *Report to the President: Solving the problem of childhood obesity within a generation.* Retrieved from https://letsmove.obama whitehouse.archives.gov/sites/letsmove.gov/files/TaskForce_on_Childhood_Obesity_ May2010_FullReport.pdf

Xu, X., Bishop, E. E., Kennedy, S. M., Simpson, S. A., Pechacek, T. F. (2014). Annual health-care spending attributable to cigarette smoking. *American Journal of Preventive Medicine, 48*(3), 326–333. doi:10.1016/j.amepre.2014.10.012

Yu, E., Rimm, E., Qi, L., Rexrode, K., Albert, C. M., Sun, Q., … F. B., & Manson, J. E. (2016). Diet, lifestyle, biomarkers, genetic factors, and rick of cardiovascular disease in the nurses' health studies. *American Journal of Public Health, 106*(9), 1616–1623. doi:10.2105/AJPH.2016.303316

8

Vulnerable Populations: Meeting the Health Needs of Populations Facing Health Inequities

Monique J. Vasquez, Jacqueline Martinez Garcel,
Elizabeth A. Ward, and Lourdes J. Rodríguez

LEARNING OBJECTIVES

▶ Understand the predisposing and enabling factors that increase the vulnerability of people disproportionately affected by health inequities

▶ Identify the growing number of health inequities

▶ Describe how the Great Recession has led to a strained social service sector

▶ Explain how the U.S. health care system provides and pays for services to vulnerable populations

▶ Discuss social needs of populations affected by health inequities and the safety net currently provided by the social service sector

▶ Identify challenges and opportunities to reduce health care costs and improve health outcomes of people disproportionately affected by health inequities

KEY TERMS

▶ behavioral health services

▶ cash assistance programs

▶ chronic illnesses

▶ Disproportionate Share Hospitals (DSH) program

▶ dual eligibles

▶ enabling factor

- ▶ fragmentation
- ▶ health need factor
- ▶ Medicaid
- ▶ Medicare
- ▶ patient engagement
- ▶ predisposing factor
- ▶ safety-net providers

TOPICAL OUTLINE

- ▶ Understanding factors and systems that affect people disproportionately affected by health inequities
- ▶ The growing number of health inequities
- ▶ Uneven footing after the Great Recession and a strained social service sector
- ▶ Organization and financing of health care, population/public health/ prevention, and other services for populations experiencing health inequities
- ▶ Social service needs
- ▶ Federal and state financing of care for vulnerable populations
- ▶ Challenges for service delivery and payment
- ▶ Emerging and tested ideas for better health delivery
- ▶ Opportunities in the ACA to meet health care needs of vulnerable populations
- ▶ Challenges of health care reform and threats to the ACA

INTRODUCTION

In order to better understand health, we must understand the way in which life experiences affect the health and well-being of different groups. When power and oppression result in groups being treated differently because of race, ethnicity, income, gender, sexual orientation, immigration status, ability level, or other factors, people in groups that have less power or social status are more vulnerable to health inequities. This vulnerability makes it harder for people to be healthy, to stay healthy, to prevent illness, and to have better outcomes when they become sick or ill. Throughout the 20th century, the United States—one of the wealthiest nations in the world—has made strides toward increasing access to health care for vulnerable populations. The advent of employer-based health insurance, passage of **Medicare**

> With the nation's population growing both older and more diverse in terms of demographics and income, policymakers face increasing challenges in ensuring that health care is provided to vulnerable populations, and at affordable costs.*

*To hear the podcast, go to https://bcove.video/2zGiJte or access the ebook on Springer Publishing Connect™.

and **Medicaid** in the 1960s, the establishment of community health centers in the 1970s, and the creation of the Children's Health Insurance Program in the 1990s all worked together to connect medically and socioeconomically disadvantaged populations to the U.S. health care system. The passage of the landmark Patient Protection and Affordable Care Act (ACA) in the 21st century was yet another major victory in narrowing the gap between those who have access to health care services and those who have been historically marginalized from them. Progress thus far, however, has barely scratched the surface of a mounting problem—the health and well-being of people living in the United States who are disproportionately affected by health inequities. There remain millions of people living in the United States who have not benefited from these improvements. Moreover, the solutions developed to address the needs of people disproportionately impacted by health inequities have been fragmented and categorical. Populations disproportionately affected by health inequities are strong. They have weathered and fought against generations of oppression, but our current system provides little support for the growing number of people disproportionately affected by health inequities. As demographics shift in the United States, the population is becoming older, the number of people of color is increasing, and a growing number of people are living with chronic disease(s). Income gaps have been increasing since the 1970s, and wealth gaps have increased dramatically, with the top 1% owning almost half (49%) of the wealth in 2016 (Stone, Trisi, Sherman, & Debot, 2015). At the same time, there is a strained social sector that provides support for vulnerable populations.

Current solutions come with growing price tags. As a result, they are at heightened risk of funding cuts. This is the case with the ACA, at threat of being repealed, undermining access to health care services for those who are already vulnerable to health inequities. Developing solutions that will contain health care expenditures *and* meet the health needs of vulnerable populations is one of the leading challenges facing policy makers in the United States.

In order to meet these shifting needs and address health inequities, our health care system must utilize innovative approaches to increase access to care and rethink the ways in which health care is delivered.

> Developing solutions that will contain health care expenditures and meet the needs of populations disproportionately affected by health inequities is one of the leading challenges facing policy makers in the United States.

This chapter examines the factors affecting populations disproportionately impacted by health inequities. The first section provides an overview of the segments of the population that fall under this category as well as a framework for understanding enablers of vulnerability. In subsequent sections, we explore the organization and financing of health care for vulnerable populations, examine limitations, and explore the importance of social services to achieve and maintain health. Finally, we discuss the role of the ACA in addressing the health needs of people experiencing disproportionate health inequities.

UNDERSTANDING FACTORS AND SYSTEMS THAT IMPACT PEOPLE DISPROPORTIONATELY AFFECTED BY HEALTH INEQUITIES

Whether we identify as part of this population ourselves or whether they are our friends, loved ones, or neighbors, the lives of people who are disproportionately affected by health inequities are interwoven into our communities and neighborhoods. People affected by inequities are everywhere, regardless of whether we live in a thriving metropolis, a gated suburban community, or a small town in rural America. In order to better understand how groups of people are impacted by health inequities, we must first distinguish between inequalities and inequities. Figure 8.1 illustrates the difference between the two terms.

The illustration shows three people confronted with a barrier, the fence, that prevents them from watching a ball game. The first panel shows what happens when an intervention seeks to be equal; although each individual has been provided with the same resources, one person is excluded from being able to see the game, even though they have equal access to the resource (the box). In the second panel, the same amount of resources (boxes) are distributed, but this time resources are distributed in an intentional way that takes into account the needs of each person relative to the barriers (the fence). Rather than seeking equality, health equity seeks to address the systemic barriers that groups of people face that result in disproportionate poor health outcomes. It can be tempting to view the individual on the right from a deficit lens or simply label them as "in need."

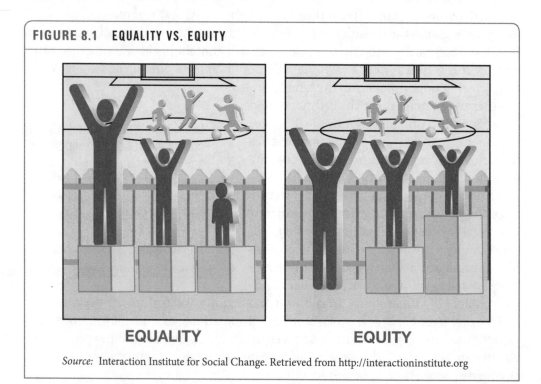

FIGURE 8.1 EQUALITY VS. EQUITY

EQUALITY   EQUITY

Source: Interaction Institute for Social Change. Retrieved from http://interactioninstitute.org

It is more useful, however, to recognize that there are a variety of factors that, when ignored, make it difficult for individuals and groups to overcome systemic barriers. The World Health Organization (WHO) defines health inequities as systematic differences in health that occur between and within countries and are avoidable and unfair (Commission on Social Determinants of Health, 2008). In their 2008 study, the WHO discusses the need to embrace a holistic view toward the social determinants of health in order to understand how "circumstances in which people grow, live, work and age, and the systems put in place to deal with illness" affect health inequities (Commission on Social Determinants of Health, 2008).

The United States has a long history of oppression, discrimination, social exclusion, and marginalization of groups that are non-European; that are poor, or not male; and who, because of these factors, are not part of an advantaged social or economic group. This history began with the colonists' violence, exploitation, and decimation of Native American peoples and the forced migration and enslavement of people from Africa. Despite improvements, mainly at the impetus of marginalized peoples pushing for change, many policies, systems, and institutions in the United States continue to oppress people of color; people who are poor; people living with physical disabilities; people with mental health issues; people practicing nondominant faiths; and people who identify as lesbian, gay, bisexual, transgender, or queer (LGBTQ). Factors such as poverty, discrimination, unbalanced power dynamics, and lack of equal and fair access to opportunities further contribute to poor health outcomes (Braveman, Arkin, Orleans, Proctor, & Plough, 2017). Braveman et al. (2011) discussed that these health inequities serve to further marginalize oppressed groups, noting that "Health differences adversely affecting socially disadvantaged groups are particularly unacceptable because ill health can be an obstacle to overcoming social disadvantage." The obstacles that people from historically marginalized populations face make them vulnerable to poor health status, poor health outcomes, and health care access.

Vulnerability can be influenced by a variety of factors, including disease status (such as chronic conditions, mental illness, HIV-positive status), demographics (such as socioeconomic status [SES], educational attainment, housing situation, racial/ethnic background, immigration or refugee status), age group (such as children or the elderly), or the ability to access health services (uninsured, those who live in a remote rural area, those who lack a regular source of care) (Aday, 2001). For instance, children, senior citizens, refugees, immigrants, non-native English speakers, formerly incarcerated individuals, people who experience homelessness, and many other groups are more vulnerable to health inequities due to risk of discrimination, oppression, and diminished agency or power.

Our humanity and the range of life experiences we face put us all at risk of being vulnerable at different points in our lives. We are all susceptible to a host of negative or stressful events such as sudden or chronic or acute illness, unemployment, homelessness, or divorce. There are, however, individual and community factors that mediate this risk. For instance, according to the Conservation of Resources theory, the effect of a stressful life event on a person who lives in a poor neighborhood with limited access to resources is much more adverse than that on a person who lives in a wealthy neighborhood with access to a variety of options to ameliorate the problem (Hobfoll, 2001).

The Conservation of Resources theory states that people are motivated to obtain, keep, and protect resources they value, which can range from a house or vehicle to marriage, employment, self-esteem, credit, knowledge, or money (Hobfoll, 2012). Resource loss, which can be caused by an adverse event or disaster, has a stronger impact on an individual than if they had gained resources. An individual will need to invest resources in order to recover or protect against resource loss, but those who already have limited resources prior to a disaster will have less capacity to manage stress and leverage resources when resources are lost (Hobfoll, 2012). As an example, over the last few decades, a series of natural disasters has caused many Americans to lose their loved ones, their homes, and their possessions and to be at risk for significant medical and/or mental health issues. Since 2005, extreme weather conditions caused by hurricanes Katrina, Rita, Harvey, Irma, and Maria devastated parts of Texas, Louisiana, Florida, and Puerto Rico. Everyone affected by a hurricane will experience resource loss, but the people with fewer resources—such as people living in poverty, renters, people with low-quality housing, people with low-levels of social support or social capital, people who have a disability or chronic medical condition, or people who are elderly—may find themselves with increased vulnerability because of their circumstances prior to the disaster. Vulnerability can be two fold as people who are disproportionately affected by inequities are also likely to live in high-risk areas, including flood zones and in substandard housing (Cutter & Emrich, 2006).

A Framework for Understanding Vulnerability

Shi and colleagues (2008) introduced a general model of vulnerability, which was adapted from a model from Andersen and Aday that categorized risks as predisposing, enabling, and need (Andersen, 1995). The general model of vulnerability can be used to understand the convergence of individual, social, community, and access-to-care risks (Shi & Stevens, 2010). In this model, individual risk factors, such as demographics (age, gender, race/ethnicity, SES), health status, health insurance, and individual belief systems associated with health behaviors, are studied in light of the larger context of a person's life. Environmental (or ecological) risk factors include the geographical location (rural versus urban), SES of an entire community (neighborhood income level and unemployment rates), resource inequalities, and the social capital (or social cohesion) of the neighborhood.

Vulnerability to poor health, as posited by this model, is determined by a convergence of predisposing, enabling, and need characteristics at the individual and ecological levels.

For example, a man who has hypertension (**health need factor**), is African American (**predisposing factor**), and is uninsured (**enabling factor**) would be

FIGURE 8.2 GENERAL MODEL OF VULNERABILITY

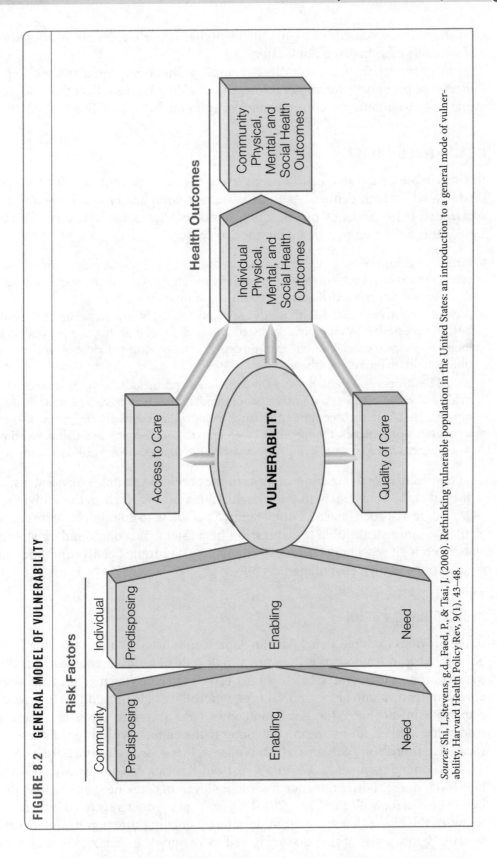

Source: Shi, L,Stevens, g.d., Faed, P., & Tsai, J. (2008). Rethinking vulnerable population in the United States: an introduction to a general mode of vulner-ability. Harvard Health Policy Rev, 9(1), 43–48.

considered more vulnerable than a man who has hypertension but is not part of a historically marginalized population.

In this model, *health needs* directly imply vulnerability, *predisposing factors* indicate the propensity for vulnerability, and *enabling factors* reflect the resources available to overcome the consequences of vulnerability (Shi & Stevens, 2010).

Health Need Factor

In this chapter, we frame *health needs* using the definition of *health* developed by the WHO, which defines health as a "state of complete *physical, mental,* and *social* well-being and not merely the absence of disease or infirmity" (WHO, 1948). This definition may be understood as follows:

- *Physical* health needs are characterized according to the physiological and physical status of the body. Problems affecting physical health include specific acute or chronic diseases (such as HIV/AIDS, diabetes, asthma) or disabilities.
- *Mental* (or *psychological*) health needs are characterized by emotional and behavioral health—in essence, by an individual's state of mind. Problems affecting mental health include specific mental illnesses, chronic dependence on drugs or alcohol, or a susceptibility to harm oneself or others.
- *Social* health needs extend beyond the individual and include both the quantity and quality of social contacts with other people. Individuals who have been marginalized or ostracized from their communities (such as individuals experiencing homelessness, immigrants or refugees, the formerly incarcerated, people living in an abusive home) would be characterized as having unmet social health needs (Aday, 2001).

Poor health along one dimension, as in the previous example's physical health, is very likely to converge with poor health along others, such as the individual's psychological or social needs. For instance, a person who does not have insurance would be more susceptible to depression because of the compounding stresses associated with receiving a diagnosis, managing a chronic health condition, and confronting the high cost of medical bills.

Predisposing Factor

In the previous example, being African American is listed as a predisposing factor because African Americans experience a multitude of health inequities, including higher chronic disease rates, barriers and obstacles to receiving medical care, worse disease outcomes, and higher mortality and morbidity rates; in addition to systemic disparities in income, educational outcomes, and access to resources, multiple studies have linked adverse health outcomes to the cumulative burden of stress and racial discrimination (Williams, 2012; Williams, Priest, & Anderson, 2016).

In a longitudinal study, 17- to 19-year-old African Americans who reported high levels of racial discrimination had higher levels of cytokine at age 22 than their peers (Brody, Yu, Miller, & Chen, 2015). Cyokine are proteins secreted by cells and found in the blood that serve an important modulating function in the immune system. Higher levels of cytokine are linked to low-grade inflammation, which can cause increased risk of chronic disease and problems associated with aging such as hypertension, obesity, insulin resistance, diabetes risk, and stroke. Researchers also found that youth who showed positive racial identity did not show the same association between discrimination and cytokine (Brody et al., 2015). Studies focused on adults show an association between hypertension risk, control of hypertension symptoms, and elevated blood pressure with perceived discrimination (Cuffee, Hargraves, & Allison, 2012). A survey conducted in 2017 of African Americans, Asian Americans, Latinos, Native Americans, White Americans, and LGBTQ adults asked about experiences with discrimination. African Americans reported experiencing high levels of discrimination when being considered for a promotion or receiving equal pay at work (57%), during job applications (56%), and being unfairly stopped or unfairly treated by police due to their race (National Public Radio, 2017). The American Psychological Association (APA) found that people who experienced discrimination reported worse health and higher levels of stress (APA, 2016).

Predisposing factors include not only individual risk but also community risk. Community risk includes issues that affect groups of individuals such as less access to parks and places to exercise, less access to affordable and accessible healthy foods, and increased stress levels from low-wage jobs (Shi, Stevens, Faed & Tsai, 2008). Socioeconomic determinants of health are structural determinants and conditions that influence health; they include a variety of factors such as economic stability, neighborhood and physical environment, education, food, community and social context, and certain characteristics of the health care systems (Heiman & Artiga, 2015). Health experts believe these factors have a much larger influence than health care itself (Heiman & Artiga, 2015), and the WHO places a high priority on addressing the social determinants of health and training a workforce that both understands and can raise public awareness about the social determinants (Commission on Social Determinants of Health, 2008).

FIGURE 8.3   SOCIAL DETERMINANTS OF HEALTH

Economic Stability	Neighborhood and Physical Environment	Education	Food	Community and Social Context	Health Care System
Employment	Housing	Literacy	Hunger	Social integration	Health coverage
Income	Transportation	Language	Access to healthy options	Support systems	Provider availability
Expenses	Safety	Early childhood education		Community engagement	Provider linguistic and cultural competency
Debt	Parks	Vocational training		Discrimination	
Medical bills	Playgrounds				
Support	Walkability	Higher education			Quality of care

Health Outcomes
Mortality, Morbidity, Life Expectancy, Health Care Expenditures, Health Status, Functional Limitations

Enabling Factors

Previously, we described that enabling factors mediate our access to resources necessary to overcome the consequences of vulnerability. One example is social capital. Social capital is measured by the quantity and quality of interpersonal ties among people and groups sharing a community, which can be defined geographically or by a common characteristic. It is critical for mitigating or minimizing the effect of negative life events on health. Family structure, friendship ties, religious organizations, and neighborhood connections provide social capital to members in the form of social support and associated feelings of belonging, psychological well-being, and self-esteem (Aday, 2001).

> A strong social support system is key to making a significant difference in the likelihood of starting—and sticking with—lifestyle changes.

Building on the example of an uninsured African American man who has hypertension and symptoms of depression: If, in addition, he is also socially isolated, with little or no social network in his community, it is unlikely that he will succeed in long-term efforts to improve his health, such as establishing healthier eating habits or adhering to a strict medication regimen. A strong social support system is key to making a significant difference in the likelihood of starting—and sticking with—lifestyle changes.

The general model of vulnerability is used throughout this chapter to illustrate best practices, including an examination of predisposing factors, enabling factors, and need; later in the chapter are recommendations for programs and policies that can improve the health outcomes of this population. Before we describe the network of existing services and programs—and their financing mechanisms—that care for the needs of vulnerable populations, we focus in the next section on why the number of vulnerable groups is increasing in the United States. This increase is one of the critical reasons health care leaders and policy makers must find more effective and efficient ways to address the needs of vulnerable populations than are currently available.

THE GROWING NUMBER OF HEALTH INEQUITIES

Three leading and concurrent factors have contributed to the growing number of populations who are currently at risk of disproportionally experiencing health inequities:

- The differential rise in prevalence of chronic conditions such as diabetes, cancer, and cardiovascular disease
- Shifting demographics of the overall U.S. population, especially the growing income inequality between rich and poor, the shift to a majority of people of color population, and the graying of the baby boomer generation
- An uneven footing after the Great Recession for already vulnerable communities and a strained social service sector

Prevalence of Chronic Conditions

Chronic illnesses, such as heart disease, diabetes, cancer, respiratory diseases, and arthritis, are ongoing medical conditions that can be treated but not cured. These conditions require constant management, and they significantly alter the daily life of those who suffer from them. The 2012 National Health Interview Survey estimated that 49.8% of civilians who are not institutionalized, or 117 million adults, had at least one chronic physical health condition. In the United States, the rise in chronic conditions has been unprecedented, and these conditions have exacted an enormous human and financial toll.

While everyone is at risk for developing a chronic illness, vulnerable groups are more likely to have a chronic illnesses because of disparities in resources and tools to prevent illness and maintain health and well-being. Lifestyle behaviors that can often be associated with the socioeconomic determinants of health—such as tobacco use; lack of regular physical activity; and consumption of diets rich in saturated fats, sugars, and salt—have greatly contributed to the increase in chronic conditions in the United States (Bauer, Briss, Goodman, & Bowman, 2014). Studies have shown that people who live in areas of more socioeconomic disadvantage are more likely to take part in these risky health behaviors (Diez-Roux, 2003; Do, 2009; Lang et al., 2009). In order to truly address health inequities, particularly as they pertain to socioeconomic determinants of health, we must explicitly focus on health equity throughout intervention design and implementation; otherwise, we run the risk of inadvertently increasing disparities in populations. For instance, public smoking campaigns in the past have been more effective with affluent educated populations, not because they are the ones who care more about their health, but because the interventions did not have marginalized populations and lower socioeconomic populations in mind during their implementation (Braveman et al., 2017).

Although having a chronic physical or mental health condition does not mean that an individual will not have a good quality of life, for many, one or more of these conditions can be disabling, thereby reducing the quality of life and leading to isolation and depression. Vulnerable groups are more likely to feel the impacts of chronic disease in a different way than populations with more resources or socieconocomic status. Groups with fewer resources may struggle to find and access care to monitor and treat their condition, to pay for treatment, and to have adequate social support. Additionally, vulnerable populations may struggle to change the very lifestyle behaviors that put them at risk for a chronic illness in the first place, because a diagnosis rarely has the ability to alter the socioeconomic determinants of health. Thus, it is difficult for already vulnerable populations to seek care and manage their illness. Chronic illness also impacts an individual's ability to maintain employment and care for themselves and family members, which in turn can increase their vulnerability. The prevalence of *multiple* chronic conditions—comorbidity of any combination of the previously mentioned conditions—makes it even harder to coordinate efforts and address the problems at hand. More than 25% of adults had two or three chronic conditions (Ward,

Schiller, & Goodman, 2014). These estimates look worse for specific segments of the population, especially people of color and the poor. If these trends continue unchanged, we can expect the number of adults with at least one chronic disease to reach more than 171 million by 2030 (Figure 8.4) (Wu & Green, 2000). Not only is the toll on life high—with 7 out of 10 deaths each year attributed to chronic conditions—but so is the toll on the health care system because people with chronic conditions account for more than 80% of hospital admissions (Partnership for Solutions, 2004).

Shifting Demographics in the United States

Growing Income Inequalities

In 2014, the United States marked the 50th anniversary of President Lyndon B. Johnson's War on Poverty. As a nation, however, the United States has fallen short of the commitment made in 1964 that American citizens would have a fair opportunity to pursue a productive future, earn a decent living wage, and live in a safe community with access to good schools. In 2016, more than 40.6 million Americans—approximately 12.5% of the population—were living at or below the federal poverty threshold ($24,600 for a family of four) (U.S. Census Bureau, 2017). In 2016, more than one-third of the poor—5.8% of the overall U.S. population—lived in deep poverty, earning less than $6,000 a year. While poverty rates have fluctuated with the economy, the number of people in deep poverty has increased over time from 3.7% of the population in 1975. The rate of deep poverty increased

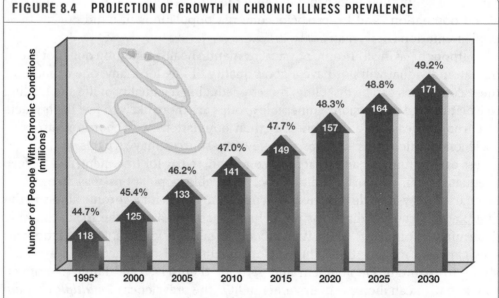

FIGURE 8.4   PROJECTION OF GROWTH IN CHRONIC ILLNESS PREVALENCE

Source: Wu, S.-Y., & Green, A. (2000). *Projection of chronic illness prevalence and cost inflation.* Santa Monica, CA: RAND Corporation. Retrieved from http://www.fightchronicdisease.org/ sites/ fightchronicdisease.org/files/docs/GrowingCrisisofChronicDiseaseintheUSfactsheet_81009.pdf

in the early 1980s, reaching 5.9% in 1983. It lowered again until 1993 where it peaked at 6.2% before going back to a range of 4.5% to 5.7%. The rate of deep poverty rose to its highest level in 2010 at 6.7% and has remained high since the recession, with 2016 as the first time it has dropped below 6% since that time (U.S. Census Bureau, 2017).

Poverty has persistently affected certain segments of the population more than others. Children under the age of 18 are more likely to live in poverty. In 2012, nearly 22% of children—one out of every five—were living in poverty. Certain racial and ethnic groups are more likely to be poor than others. Poverty rates for African Americans (27%) and Latinos (25%), as well as their children (38% and 33%, respectively), are significantly higher than for White Americans (10%) and their children (20%). To put this in perspective, one out of every three African American children and one out of every four Latino children lives in poverty. Single-parent families are also more likely to live in poverty. Thirty-one percent of female-headed households, for instance, live in poverty, compared with 6% of married-couple households. People with disabilities (28%) are more than twice as likely to live in poverty as their counterparts without a disability (12%).

Although poverty has been concentrated in cities and in rural communities throughout U.S. history, there has been a steady increase in the number of people living in poverty in suburban neighborhoods. In 2008, the number of suburban poor exceeded the urban poor in central cities by 1.5 million. Although the rates of poverty continue to be higher in urban areas than in suburbs (18% versus 9.5%), poverty rates are increasing at a faster pace in suburban areas (Allard & Roth, 2010). This is an especially troubling trend, since suburban communities tend to be mostly residential (with little or no access to commercial services), disconnected from public amenities (i.e., mass transit), and lacking in public spaces for social interaction.

Income—or lack thereof—is one of the key enablers of vulnerability. People with financial resources not only have the ability to obtain access to the highest-quality health services, but also have access to other material goods that benefit health and greater opportunities to build the social capital that can serve as a buffer for adverse life events. Income also has a more substantive and complex effect on health when it is considered in the context of a neighborhood. Concentrated wealth has a larger effect on the environment (neighborhood) that shapes a person's position along the socioeconomic gradient, which includes an individual's education level and employment opportunities. In the United States, where you live determines the quality of the education system your children have access to because the local tax base determines funding for public schools. In communities with concentrated poverty, students have lower average test scores, fewer qualified teachers, fewer interactions with colleges and potential employers, higher levels of teen pregnancy, and higher high school dropout rates than public schools in neighborhoods with more resources (Willms, 1999).

Thus far, we have explored the effect of absolute income and SES status on health and the role of SES as an enabling factor of vulnerability. However, distribution of income is also an important factor in determining the health of a

> People living in neighborhoods with many resources are more likely to engage in healthy behaviors, whether these behaviors are due to the wider availability of primary care services, stores offering healthy food, or environments for safe physical activities.

population. Income inequalities are on the rise in the United States; in fact, in 2012 the gap between the richest 1% and the remaining 99% was the largest it has been since the 1920s. According to recent analysis, the 400 richest people in the United States have more combined wealth than the bottom 150 million put together. The relationship between income inequality and health has broader implications in determining health outcomes beyond personal income. Concentrated wealth leads to concentrated poverty, which in turn leads to poor neighborhoods and communities.

Myriad studies have shown the correlation between disadvantaged communities and poor health outcomes (Diez-Roux, 2003; Do, 2009; Lang et al., 2009). The widening gap between rich and poor leads to a greater separation between the institutions, organizations, and services that promote and protect health. People living in neighborhoods with many resources are more likely to engage in healthy behaviors, whether these behaviors are due to the wider availability of primary care services, stores offering healthy food, or environments for safe physical activities. An entire population is at greater risk of poor health outcomes when they are persistently exposed to poverty, have limited access to high-quality health organizations, and have major stressors impeding their daily life activities.

Growing Numbers of People of Color

The U.S. Census Bureau predicts that by 2044, the United States will be made up by a majority of people of color as opposed to a nation with a majority White population. (Pastor, Scoggins, & Treuhaft, 2017). Our nation has not effectively addressed racial and ethnic inequities, which means that while the number of people of color increase, it is accompanied by the problematic and disproportionate burden created by systemic inequities that negatively impact people of color. There is a growing need to address these inequities, especially for the subset of people of color who are most vulnerable to health challenges due to low incomes and frequent challenges related to the social determinants of health. While it is the case that most people with low incomes face health challenges, being a person of color intersects with SES; thus, a person of color living in poverty will experience worsened health impacts than a person living in poverty without this identity. Inequities in health associated with race, for example, do not simply put patients of color at risk of receiving less effective care, they also appear to be often at risk of receiving more ineffective care (Schpero et al., 2017) when they receive care. Inequities are also associated with system related factors such as ambulance diversion (Hsia, Sarkar, & Shen, 2017), organ allocation protocols (Mathur, Ashby, Sands, & Wolfe, 2010; Patzer & McClellan, 2012), and implementation of care delivery models such as the patient-centered medical home (Washington et al., 2017).

The Graying of America

On January 1, 2011, the first baby boomers turned 65 years old. Over the next 5 years, 8,000 people will turn 65 each day, qualifying many for Medicare. The population aged 65 and over increased from 35 million in 2000 to 41 million in 2011 (an 18% increase). As of 2013, people over 65 represented 13% of the U.S. population, about one in every eight Americans. In 2030, when the entire baby boom generation will have turned 65, seniors will make up one-fourth of the population. The segment of the population 85 years and older is projected to increase from 5 million in 2011 to 9 million in 2030 (Knickman & Snell, 2002).

Baby boomers will live longer than previous generations because of improvements in health care, technology, and lifestyles. The elderly of 2030 will also be better educated than the current elderly population, with rates of college graduation two times higher and high school dropout rates one-third less than the current elderly generation (Knickman & Snell, 2002). This is good news for the future health of baby boomers because there is a strong association between education and disability. College graduates have a disability rate about half that of high school dropouts (Knickman & Snell, 2002). However, with the aging of America and longer average life spans, the rates of chronic conditions associated with an older population will also grow.

According to the Centers for Disease Control and Prevention (CDC), the average American over the age of 65 has multiple chronic conditions such as hypertension (72%), arthritis (51%), heart disease (31%), cancer (24%), and diabetes (20%). In 2010, about 13.6 million persons aged 65 or older were discharged from short-stay hospitals. Their rate of discharge is three times the comparable rate for persons of all ages. The average length of stay in a hospital is longer for older people. The average length of stay for persons aged 65 to 74 was 5.4 days; for those aged 75 to 84, it was 5.7 days; and for those aged 85 and over, it was 5.6 days. The comparable rate for persons of all ages was 4.8 days.

Health expenditures are a greater financial burden for older people, in particular for those with lower SES. The majority of Medicare recipients (83%) are over 65 (Centers for Medicare & Medicaid Services [CMS], 2016). In 2013, the average out-of-pocket health care expenditures for all Medicare recipients was $5,503. Average costs increased with age with people aged 65–74 with expenses at $4,676, people aged 75–84 at $5,745, and out of pocket costs rising to $10,208 for people 85 and over (Cubanski, Neuman, Damico, & Smith, 2018). This is an especially large amount given that half of all people enrolled in Medicare live on less than $26,000 a year, and the average Social Security income (SSI) in 2013 was $13,375. For elderly populations on Medicare with no other income other than SSI, out-of-pocket health care spending in 2013 averaged a large portion of their income at nearly a third (34%) for ages 65–74, 40% for those aged 75–84, and 74% for ages 85 and older. (Cubanski et al., 2018). These numbers are expected to increase by 2030 at 44%, 48%, and 87%, respectively. Out-of-pocket health care expenses made up a larger proportion of costs for women, even though they had slightly higher SSIs, their cost of care was higher, particularly for women over 75 (Cubanski et al., 2018).

Their age (a predisposing factor of vulnerability), coupled with the risk of financial hardship (an enabling factor) and the increased possibility of chronic conditions (another enabling factor), places older Americans—especially those living in impoverished neighborhoods—at highest risk of vulnerability.

UNEVEN FOOTING AFTER THE GREAT RECESSION AND A STRAINED SOCIAL SERVICE SECTOR

Between December 2007 and June 2009, the United States experienced an economic recession that was one of the longest and, by most measures, the worst since the Great Depression (Grusky, Western, & Wimer, 2011). This Great Recession began with the bursting of an $8 trillion housing bubble, which was then followed by massive job loss. A decade later, as a country, we find ourselves in a good news/bad news moment. The good news is that the Great Recession is behind us. While most economic markers experienced low points through 2009–2010, they began to recover by 2012–2014. For example, the annual Median Household Income in the United States recovered from the Great Recession low of $54,569 in 2012 to an record high of $60,309 by 2016 (Federal Reserve Economic Data [FRED], 2018). In December 2014, President Obama declared the Great Recession over and bailout measures instituted during the Bush and Obama administrations as mostly effective (Weisman, 2014).

The bad news is that, despite more fully employed people, wage increases have been sluggish and, since the Great Recession disproportionally affected already vulnerable populations, imposing a larger burden and negative impact—recovery has not been equitable. An analysis of the National Asset Scorecard and Communities of Color found that while during the Great Recession White families typically saw 16% of their wealth taken, African American families had more than half (53%) of their already proportionally lower wealth stripped away. Before the Great Recession, African American families had less than a dime of wealth for every dollar of wealth held by White families. After the recession, African American families had, on average, about 6 cents for every dollar compared to their White counterparts (Hamilton, Darity, Price Sridharan, & Tippett, 2015).

While the U.S. government passed a tax reduction plan aimed at alleviating the negative impact of the Great Recession, the benefits favored the wealthy more than low- to middle-income persons (Saez & Zucman, 2016). To offset the resulting budget deficits, policy makers reduced funding to the social service sector that aids vulnerable populations and keeps those at the edge from becoming vulnerable (Stern & Axinn, 2018). In sum, the positive direction of the overall economy has not been equitably distributed, and the tax cut is highly likely to exacerbate economic and hence health and other inequities.

The very same agencies that help to alleviate the economic and social effects on families and communities are being stretched to the limit while experiencing cuts to their own budgets. One of such agencies is the U.S. Department of Agriculture (USDA), which has experienced cuts to their Supplemental Nutrition

Assistance Program (SNAP). In 2018, SNAP benefits averaged close to $1.40 per person per meal (Center on Budget and Policy Priorities, 2018). These cuts affect some of the most vulnerable populations that participate in SNAP—including 22 million children (10 million of whom live in "deep poverty," with family incomes below 50% of the poverty line) and 9 million people who are elderly or have a serious disability. Furthermore, while SNAP caseload declined as the economy improved and the country recovered from the Great Recession, some of the decline (at least 500,000 people) is the result of a provision that limits SNAP benefits for unemployed adults aged 18–49 who are not disabled or raising children. The 3-month limit, while contributing to falling caseloads, threatens to put individuals over the vulnerability edge.

ORGANIZATION AND FINANCING OF HEALTH CARE, POPULATION/PUBLIC HEALTH/PREVENTION, AND OTHER SERVICES FOR POPULATIONS EXPERIENCING HEALTH INEQUITIES

We have defined vulnerable populations and described the pathways through which predisposing and enabling factors lead to vulnerability. We have also described three main reasons why the number of vulnerable groups is projected to grow. In this section, we provide an inventory of the existing resources and strategies set in place to care for the vulnerable. First, we offer a brief description of institutions and structures within the health care system that deliver services for vulnerable populations. Then, we describe financing mechanisms at the federal, state, and private levels that support health care and social services for vulnerable groups. More thorough and general treatments (not specific to vulnerable populations) of some of the topics presented here are offered in other chapters of this book.

Public Hospitals

Public hospitals make up a large part of the safety net, providing services to large portions of people who are uninsured, the underinsured, and those on Medicaid and often serve some of the sickest, poorest, and most vulnerable populations. The mission of a public hospital within the safety net system is, quite simply, to be the guarantor of health for the public (Gourevitch, Malaspina, Weitzman, & Goldfrank, 2008). Public hospitals focus on providing care to the most vulnerable groups within a community: the homeless, the disabled, documented and undocumented immigrants, high-risk mothers and infants, and those with limited proficiency in speaking and reading English. Public hospitals also provide services to the incarcerated, respond to disasters within communities, provide trauma care, and administer behavioral health and substance abuse treatment when necessary (Gourevitch et al., 2008).

Most patients who receive health care services from public hospitals are low income and uninsured; they also suffer disproportionately from preventable chronic health conditions. Many of these patients visit the emergency department (EDs) of public hospitals to receive primary care because they lack a primary care provider. Patients who use the ED for most of their health care, regardless of urgency, are referred to as high utilizers (see case exercise 2).

Federally Qualified Health Centers

Federally qualified health centers (FQHCs) are systems of **safety-net providers** that serve predominantly vulnerable groups living in underserved communities. These centers are overseen by the Health Resources and Services Administration (HRSA) of the U.S. Department of Health and Human Services (DHHS).

The FQHC program allocates special Medicare and Medicaid cost-based reimbursement payments to health centers for legislatively specified services. To qualify as an FQHC, a safety-net provider must meet the following criteria:

- Provide services in communities identified as "predominantly medically underserved areas" or provide services to a target population documented to be underserved
- Offer the required primary and preventive health services, meet specific staffing requirements, and offer a sliding-fee payment scale for services rendered
- Participate in an ongoing quality assurance program
- Have a governing board of directors that includes representatives from the populations served

FQHCs include these facilities:

- Community health centers (CHCs)
- Migrant health centers (MHCs)
- Health care for the homeless centers (HCHs)
- Public housing primary care centers (PHPCCs)

Community Health Centers

Riding on the successful passage of the 1964 Civil Rights Act and President Johnson's War on Poverty efforts, Tufts University physicians H. Jack Geiger and Count Gibson submitted proposals to the federal Office of Economic Opportunity (OEO) for funding to establish what they called "neighborhood health centers" in inner-city, underserved areas across the United States (Hawkins & Groves, 2011). The Economic Opportunity Act of 1964 provided federal funds for two such centers; both were built in Boston, Massachusetts, in 1965 (National Center for Farmworker Health, n.d.). Building on a community-based health care model already thriving in South Africa, these two CHCs offered comprehensive primary health care that focused on outreach, disease prevention, social support services, and patient education activities, including nutritional education and counseling and sanitation education. Dr. Geiger and Dr. Gibson believed that treating patients with dignity and respect, regardless of age, race, health status, or income level, and engaging them in their own health and health care were of critical importance and promoted these beliefs as central tenets of CHC care (Adashi, Geiger, & Fine, 2010). These numbers have increased over the last few years. In 2010, there were more than 8,000 CHCs, which served about 20 million people in the United States, or 5% of the population (Adashi et al., 2010); in 2015 more than 9,750 CHCs served more than 24.3 million individuals, or about nearly 8.3% of U.S. residents. More than half the population served (55%) lived in rural areas. This number of CHCs has increased in the past few years, in part due to the increase in federal funding, and the ACA's provisions, which increased the number of people eligible for in individuals eligible to receive care. A trust fund specifically for health centers was also created through the ACA (Paradise et al., 2017).

Migrant Health Centers

MHCs serve the migrant and seasonal farm workers who come to the United States each year to harvest, plant, and tend to agricultural crops. Patients pay for care on a sliding scale (an average visit costs $30). Currently, 156 MHCs operate within the CHC system in the United States. In 2011, the federal government spent $166 million to help pay for the care of close to 1 million migrant and seasonal farmworkers (Galewitz, 2012).

Health Care for the Homeless Centers

Although eligible for federally funded health care, approximately 70% of homeless health center patients lack health insurance and face significant barriers to care elsewhere in their communities (National Health Care for the Homeless Council, 2008). The Health Care for the Homeless program was initially authorized under the Stewart B. McKinney Homeless Assistance Act of 1987. HCHs provide comprehensive medical services to the homeless, including pediatric and adult primary care, screening, health education, referrals for specialty medical care, transportation services, social service outreach, and both long- and short-term rehabilitative care. By statute, the HCH program receives 8.7% of the total health center appropriations for all FQHCs.

Public Housing Primary Care Centers

PHPCCs are health centers that provide comprehensive medical care and social support services to individuals who live in public and assisted housing. Currently there are 63 PHPCCs in 25 states and Puerto Rico, and these centers provided services to nearly 171,731 public and assisted housing residents in 2012 (National Center for Health in Public Housing, 2012).

RURAL HEALTH CLINICS AND RURAL HEALTH NETWORKS

Rural health clinics (RHCs) were created as a result of the Rural Health Clinic Services Act of 1977. This federal legislation provided reimbursement not just for services provided by full-time doctors but also for preventive and primary care services done by health professionals called mid-level providers (MLPs), such as nurse practitioners (NPs) and physician assistants (PAs) at clinics in underserved rural areas across the United States. This legislation was established both to alleviate the burden on the limited number of full-time doctors and specialists and to cut down on emergency care spending (DHHS, Office of Rural Health Policy, 2006).

Rural health networks (RHNs)—also known as rural health alliances, cooperatives, or affiliations—are systems of care in rural areas that include at least one rural hospital and two other separate community health organizations, such as a nursing home or a public health unit. These networks operate by pooling resources in ways such as developing continuing education programs, investing money in electronic medical record systems for easier care coordination between providers, and supporting advocacy activities within the communities served by the RHN (DHHS, Office of Rural Health Policy, 2006). These networks were created out of necessity to foster collaboration and discourage reduction in services due to unwarranted competition (Moscovice, Gregg, & Lewerenz, 2003).

Indian Health Services

Because of the history of oppression and enduring health inequities Native Americans are considered a special group and have continued to face disproportionate health inequities. The relationship between the U.S. federal government and North American native peoples (Indian tribes) began in 1787 and has evolved ever since with various laws, treaties, and executive orders to protect their status (DHHS, Indian Health Services [IHS], 2014).

The IHS has an annual budget of about $4.8 billion and is the primary federal health care provider for approximately 2.2 million of the estimated 3.7 million American Indians and Alaska Natives who belong to the more than 567 federally recognized tribes in 37 states (DHHS, IHS, 2017).

Through a network of 45 hospitals and more than 293 clinics, IHS programs provide Native Americans with preventive, primary, dental, and emergency medical care; mental health and substance abuse prevention and treatment; nutrition education; access to referrals and resources; and social service support, including (but not limited to) assistance in applying for federally designated public housing for Native Americans and other need-based benefit programs such as SNAP, Women, Infants, and Children (WIC), and Temporary Assistance for Needy Families (TANF).

Mental Health and Chemical Dependency Services

In 1963, Congress passed the Mental Retardation Facilities and Community Health Centers Construction Act, which provided federal funding for the development and implementation of community-based mental health centers (CMHCs). With the exception of the most severely mentally ill, most previously institutionalized patients were released into their communities and encouraged to seek care at these new CMHCs and other, similar facilities (Unite for Sight, n.d.).

Unfortunately, CMHCs are underfunded and understaffed; as a result, many people living with mental illness or chemical dependence are not receiving the proper comprehensive care they need. Many ultimately end up homeless or in prison. According to the *Journal of Community Mental Health*, the combination of deinstitutionalization and inadequate and underfunded community care has led to transinstitutionalization, a phenomenon in which prisons, instead of psychiatric or detoxification facilities, become the main providers of highly structured, controlled living environments for the severely mentally ill and chemically dependent (Prins, 2011).

Not only are mentally ill individuals more likely to be incarcerated or homeless, they also contribute significantly to the cost of ED care in hospitals across the country. By one federal estimate, spending by general hospitals to care for these patients will nearly double in 1 year—from $20.3 billion in 2013 to $38.5 billion in 2014 (Creswell, 2013).

Special Populations: HIV/AIDS Programs

Legislation to address the AIDS epidemic was first enacted in 1990 as the Ryan White Comprehensive AIDS Resources Emergency (CARE) Act. Since then, the legislation has been amended and reauthorized four times to accommodate new and emerging medical and social needs; it is now called the Ryan White HIV/AIDS Program (Henry J. Kaiser Family Foundation, 2013). HRSA estimates that more than 500,000 individuals receive at least one medical, health, or related support service through a Ryan White program each year (Henry J. Kaiser Family Foundation, 2013). The multiple parts of the Ryan White Program all emphasize risk reduction and prevention through interventions at both individual and community levels. For those affected, intensive case management in a community-based health care setting is critical to a long life (Aday, 2001).

Despite the delayed response to the HIV/AIDS epidemic in the United States, the wraparound services provided through the Ryan White Program serve as a model for responding to health needs with a whole person approach. No other vulnerable population has been able to advocate as effectively for that level of support.

SOCIAL SERVICE NEEDS

Spanish philosopher José Ortega y Gasset posited, "*Yo soy yo y mi circunstancia, y si no la salvo a ella no me salvo yo*", which loosely translates as "I am myself and my circumstance; if I do not help it, I cannot help myself." In that same spirit, social needs are the *circunstancia* that enables the events that lead people with predisposing characteristics to become vulnerable. Toward the end of the 19th century and sporadically throughout the 20th century, the United States made attempts to advance social change. Examples include President Franklin D. Roosevelt's New Deal in response to the Great Depression; the previously mentioned War on Poverty waged by President Johnson; President John F. Kennedy's work in support of progressive taxation, affordable housing, and extension of social welfare, and President Barack Obama's passage of the Patient Protection and Affordable Care Act (ACA). The existing safety net of social services is an amalgam of programs that, though not completely infallible, provides some support for vulnerable populations, potentially making the difference between maintaining good health outcomes and succumbing to illness.

In this section, we highlight three types of social service programs: (a) food assistance, (b) monetary assistance, and (c) housing assistance.

Food Assistance

All food assistance programs listed in this section are administered and funded through the USDA Food and Nutrition Service Agency.

Supplemental Nutrition Assistance Program

The first food assistance program was implemented in May 1939 but was shut down in 1943 because "unmarketable food surpluses and widespread unemployment no longer existed" (USDA, Food and Nutrition Service, n.d.). It wasn't until President Kennedy came along 18 years later that a second food assistance program was implemented. Kennedy's program eliminated the concept of different stamps for different foods and encouraged beneficiaries to use their stamps to buy healthy food (USDA, Food and Nutrition Service, n.d.). In September 2007, the Food Stamp Program was renamed SNAP (Supplemental Nutrition Assistance Program) to decrease the stigma associated with the term "food stamps" and to encourage those who need benefits to apply for them. SNAP enrollment has generally increased over time and was at its highest point in 2013, when more than 47 million individuals received SNAP benefits. Since 2013, this number of SNAP enrollees has declined annually to mid-2010 levels with more than 42 million receiving SNAP benefits in 2017 (U.S. Department of Agriculture, 2018).

Women, Infants, and Children

The Special Supplemental Nutrition Program for Women, Infants, and Children was authorized by the Child Nutrition Act of 1966 and officially launched in 1974. WIC state agencies receive federal funding to pay for WIC foods, nutrition-related services, and administrative costs (Association of State and Territorial Health Officials, 2010). Pregnant, breastfeeding, or postpartum women, as well as infants and children up to age 5, are eligible for benefits if (a) they meet a predetermined income standard; (b) they already receive SNAP, Medicaid, or TANF benefits; or (c) they have documentation from a medical professional explaining that the mother, her children, or both are at nutritional risk (Kent, 2006). Preliminary data for 2017 estimates that WIC had more than 7.2 million participants. The program costs an average of $41.22 per month per participant (USDA, Food and Nutrition Service, 2018).

Other Federal and Private Food Programs

The USDA Food and Nutrition Service administers 11 additional supplemental nutrition programs, ranging from reduced-price or free lunch programs for elementary school children (The National School Lunch Program [NSLP]) to emergency food assistance programs that organize and fund food banks, pantries, and soup kitchens to distribute food items to low-income people (USDA, Food and Nutrition Service, n.d.).

The rise in food insecurity since the 1980s has not kept up with federal food program availability. Thus, a network of private food assistance programs has emerged to try to fill the gap between need and federal support. This private food assistance network relies on food donations; at-cost bulk purchasing; and food rescue of perishable, nonperishable, and prepared foods (Daponte & Bade, 2006).

Monetary Assistance

Support for vulnerable individuals and families in the form of monetary assistance is aimed at offering both short-term and long-term financial relief to meet basic needs. Several federal agencies administer monetary assistance.

Temporary Assistance for Needy Families

TANF is a monthly **cash assistance program** for low-income families with children established under the Personal Responsibility and Work Opportunity Reconciliation Act of 1996 as a replacement to the Aid to Families with Dependent Children (AFDC) program. TANF is overseen by the Office of Family Assistance (part of the DHHS Administration for Children & Families), but control over implementation is given to states (Purtell, Gershoff, & Aber, 2012).

Supplemental Security Income

President Richard M. Nixon passed the federal Social Security Amendments of 1972 in an effort to centralize the administration of Social Security and reduce inequalities among the state-run adult assistance programs already in existence. Today, the federal Supplemental Security Income (SSI) program administers cash assistance each month to eligible individuals aged 65 and older, the blind, and mentally or physically disabled children and adults. A preset federal benefit rate determines benefit levels (U.S. Social Security Administration, n.d.).

Unemployment Insurance

Unemployment insurance (UI) is available to people who have lost their jobs through no fault of their own but as a result of circumstances such as employer cutbacks. Federal funds are distributed through the U.S. Department of Labor to each state; states then administer their UI programs according to state-determined criteria.

Housing Assistance

The first major investment in housing assistance in the United States took place in 1932, when—in the midst of widespread unemployment and homelessness resulting from the Great Depression—Congress passed the Emergency Relief and Construction Act (U.S. Department of Housing and Urban Development, n.d.). This act created the Reconstruction Finance Corporation (RFC), an agency whose responsibility it was to make loans to private corporations that were providing housing for low-income families. From 1932 to 1956, four housing acts were enacted; these continued through the 1960s and into the 1970s. Funding included federal investments in new housing construction; the preservation of existing housing resources; and the development of safer, better public housing communities.

The McKinney-Vento Homeless Assistance Act of 1987 established the Supportive Housing Program (SHP) especially for the homeless. The 2009 American Recovery and Reinvestment Act (ARRA) included new housing programs, most notably the Homelessness Prevention and Rapid Re-Housing Program (HPRP). This program allocated $1.9 billion in funding to homelessness housing. Funds allocated for HPRP helped with short-term or medium-term rental assistance and housing relocation and stabilization services, including such activities as mediation, credit counseling, security or utility deposits, utility payments, moving cost assistance, and case management.

This section has not presented an exhaustive list of federal and private social services available for vulnerable populations. For example, in terms of housing, there are services that offer long-term care for elderly and disabled people, such as nursing homes, and supportive at-home services that allow for aging in place, such as home health aides.

The next section offers a more detailed picture of the payment system that covers the health care of vulnerable populations.

FEDERAL AND STATE FINANCING OF CARE FOR VULNERABLE POPULATIONS

There are three main payers for health care for the vulnerable: (a) the federal government; (b) the states; and (c) private sources, including employers, insurers, and philanthropic organizations.

At the federal level, the primary health care payment programs are Medicare, Medicaid, and the Children's Health Insurance Plan (CHIP). These programs are managed by the CMS; however, each state has the power to administer its Medicaid program. Medicaid-eligible individuals typically include low-income individuals and families who fall below a certain federal poverty level (FPL) threshold and those receiving SSI. As we discuss toward the end of the chapter, the ACA has greatly increased the enrollment for both CHIP and Medicaid.

Medicaid provided health coverage for approximately 34.5 million children (including the 6.5 million receiving coverage through CHIP), 26.7 million adults, 5.7 million seniors, and 10.6 million persons with disabilities on average monthly in 2016 at a total cost of $565.5 billion (CMS, 2018a). CMS reports that under the current law, national health spending is expected to grow under in the period 2017–2026, at an average rate of 5.5% each year, resulting in an estimated $5.7 trillion in 2026 (Center for Medicare & Medicaid Services, 2018b).

Individuals eligible for Medicare include the elderly (ages 65 and older), some people under 65 with qualifying disabilities, and people with kidney failure requiring dialysis. The most recent estimate of Medicare expenses in 2016 reported a yearly program cost of $672.1 billion, with beneficiaries exceeding 57.1 million, including 8.8 million people who are disabled, and 48.1 million people aged 65 and older (CMS, 2018b).

Individuals who are **dual eligibles** qualify for both Medicare and Medicaid and are among the sickest and poorest in the United States; more than half have three or more chronic conditions, and more than 40% have a mental health diagnosis (CMS, 2018c). This population is three times more likely than the Medicare-only population to be disabled (Fontenot & Stubblefield, 2011). Although they represent a relatively small percentage of the overall Medicare and Medicaid populations, the cost for people who are dual eligible totals $306 billion (approximately 33%) of annual spending between the two programs (CMS, 2018c). Disproportionate levels of funding for state Medicaid programs means the resources available for people with dual eligibility vary from state to state. Part of the high cost can be reduced through better care coordination and treatment, as individuals who are dual eligible must also bear the burden of navigating both programs. The Medicare-Medicaid Coordination Office aims to increase effectiveness and coordination between the two programs; however, this is only a recent development as it was created by section 2602 of the ACA (CMS, 2011).

There is a segment of the vulnerable population that neither qualifies for subsidized care nor receives care through an employer or other private funder. To offset the burden of offering care for the uninsured, federal law offers a modified payment strategy called the Medicaid and Medicare **Disproportionate Share Hospital (DSH) program**. DSH payments are available to qualifying hospitals that have a high number of Medicaid and Medicare patients and uninsured individuals (Mitchell, 2013). Under the ACA federal payments through the DSH were scheduled to be reduced in 2014. This reduction of a total of $43 billion was delayed and will take place in 2018, starting with a $2 billion cut. The reduction is set to increase incrementally until it reaches a $8 billion cut by 2025. This will significantly reduce DSH funds, as federal spending for DSH allotments in 2014 was $11.7 billion (Cunningham, Rudowitz, Young, Garfield, & Foutz, 2016). Cuts to DSH pose risks to safety net hospitals and public hospitals that serve higher numbers of populations who are either without insurance, on Medicaid or Medicare and who rely more heavily on DSH funding (Cunningham et al., 2016).

CHALLENGES FOR SERVICE DELIVERY AND PAYMENT

The systems of care and financing mechanisms currently available in the United States, well intentioned as they are, fall short of their goal of taking care of vulnerable populations. At best, the programs and services are disjointed and, at worst, they offer temporary solutions that deal with isolated problems, and for very targeted populations. For instance, a person's drug or alcohol dependency may preclude him or her from eligibility for supportive housing. Yet, stable housing has been linked to recovery from addictions. The common response by policy makers—and common practice by researchers—is to focus on distinct populations when examining and addressing the needs of vulnerable populations. Disparate and disjointed programs are created to address the needs of children, the elderly, the physically disabled, the chronically ill, the mentally ill, substance abusers, persons with HIV/AIDS, the homeless, residents of rural areas, immigrants, individuals with limited or no English proficiency—the list goes on and on. Yet, the distinctions among many of these vulnerable groups are thin and artificial. Many of these groups share common traits and experience a convergence of multiple vulnerable characteristics. These subpopulations are more likely to live in poor communities; less likely to have access to high-quality health and education; and less likely to have the financial resources to secure adequate, stable, affordable housing.

The programs and services available are not very cost-effective; this puts them at the mercy of critics who would prefer less government involvement in the care of vulnerable individuals and their families. The current market-driven health care delivery and payment system is one that gives providers financial incentives for the volume, not the quality, of services delivered. Some areas for improvement related to delivery and payment are discussed later. In this section, we first point out how (and where) the current ways in which care is delivered and payment is structured fall short of their goal to take care of the vulnerable while containing cost. Second, we highlight emerging service delivery models and innovative payment strategies created to reach the Triple Aim—better care for individuals, better health for populations, and lower cost—as it pertains to vulnerable populations.

A Fragmented Delivery System

Health care initiatives to reduce the barriers created by vulnerability rarely recognize the common overlap of risk factors, and few studies have examined the combined influences of multiple risks on obtaining needed health care services (Shi & Stevens, 2005). The main issues that emerge in a review of delivery systems created to care for vulnerable populations include (a) fragmented and siloed structures and (b) a focus on health and psychological needs that does not always recognize the link between social needs and health.

> Health care initiatives to reduce the barriers created by vulnerability rarely recognize the common overlap of risk factors, and few studies have examined the combined influences of multiple risks on obtaining needed health care services.

Fragmentation refers to care that is delivered by different providers who are not co-located or within proximity of each other. Where fragmentation exists, patients must make and manage multiple appointments that may require, for example, more days off from work to attend appointments. Silo structures refer to care offered by multiple providers who do not consult with each other. An endocrinologist, for instance, may be unaware of the medications prescribed by a psychiatrist treating a patient's depression—which may have weight gain as a side effect, thus disrupting the patient's diabetes management.

Although there has been budding awareness of the importance of meeting social and other nonclinical needs in relationship to health, the U.S. delivery system has not made the necessary transformation to make this possible. For example, food insecurity would make it hard for a person managing cardiovascular disease to eat more fruits and vegetables because that person may depend on a local emergency food provider that is unequipped to receive and distribute produce.

Volume Versus Value

A major weakness of our current payment system is that it encourages a volume-driven health care system rather than a value-driven health care system. Under fee-for-service (FFS), providers (such as hospitals, physicians, and health centers) gain increased revenue and profit by delivering more services to people.

This payment model becomes an enormous barrier to delivering effective and efficient care to vulnerable populations. Providers have little or no incentive to spend the necessary time with an individual who has complex medical, behavioral, and social needs in order to determine a course of action that will address the underlying complexities of the patient's life. Providers are more likely to address the present health crisis affecting the individual—usually by delivering more diagnostic tests, prescribing more medication, or making more referrals to costly specialists. FFS payment systems also reinforce fragmentation of care by paying multiple providers for multiple services or tests for the same patient, regardless of whether the care is coordinated or duplicative.

Behavioral and social services operate in an entirely different realm than medical care; such a vast, complex web of disconnected services is available for vulnerable populations that the time and effort required to coordinate and manage transitions across necessary services are beyond any reimbursement rate set by public or private payer. Instead, there is a perverse payment system that rewards the provider for delivering more health care services, rather than addressing (by connecting patients to critical services) the pressing social and behavioral problems that negatively affect the patient's health outcomes.

Reactive Versus Preventive Care

Only a small fraction of health care spending is devoted to the promotion of healthier behavior, despite the fact that preventable chronic diseases are linked to smoking, obesity, lack of exercise, and drug and alcohol use (DeVol et al., 2007). There are very few incentives in the health care system to promote prevention and early intervention, especially in the case of chronic diseases. Only a small percentage of health care spending is devoted to promoting healthier behavior, despite the fact that preventable chronic diseases are linked to lifestyle behaviors, such as smoking, exercise, and drug and alcohol use, and to social determinants of health (McGinnis, Russo, & Knickman, 2002). This is explored more in Chapter 5 on population health.

EMERGING AND TESTED IDEAS FOR BETTER HEALTH DELIVERY

Health care leaders and policy makers are grappling with how to improve our health delivery system. In this section, we highlight emerging service delivery models created to improve health outcomes for vulnerable groups while containing the cost of care. Definitions and descriptions of these budding models are explained, along with case studies that have implemented these models.

Delivery Strategies That Work

Growing evidence shows that three distinct delivery strategies—care coordination, patient engagement and team-based care, and integration of care—help to meet the needs of vulnerable populations. We describe these strategies and discuss the *meaningful* use of data to drive them.

Care Coordination

Creating successful integrated delivery systems for vulnerable populations requires several factors: (a) an emphasis on primary care; (b) coordination of all care, including behavioral, social, and public health services; and (c) accountability for population health outcomes (Witgert & Hess, 2012). The Agency for Healthcare Research and Quality (AHRQ) defines care coordination as:

> [T]he deliberate organization of patient care activities between two or more participants (including the patient) involved in a patient's care to facilitate the appropriate delivery of health care services. Organizing care involves the marshaling of personnel and other resources needed to carry out all required patient care activities, and is often managed by the exchange of information among participants responsible for different aspects of care. (AHRQ, 2014)

According to a 2011 report published by the American Hospital Association, promising practices that will improve care coordination include (among other practices) conducting periodic home visits, facilitating and encouraging data sharing through the use of integrated health information systems (i.e., electronic medical records [EMRs]), providing non–health care services such as transportation to appointments, and employing and incorporating specially trained teams of providers that are aware of each patient's cultural and language backgrounds and can administer guidance and advice as they see fit (Fontenot & Stubblefield, 2011).

Patient Engagement and Team-Based Care

Patient engagement is generally defined as the process of involving individuals in their health care, disease management, or preventive behaviors. Providers can—and do—play an important role in the health outcomes of their patients; however, after a patient has left the doctor's office, the patient's health is largely in his or her own hands. Low income, lack of education, language barriers, and not having a regular source of care are some of the many risk factors that may create significant barriers to accessing necessary health care services (Shi & Stevens, 2005). Patients are expected to follow recommended care management plans, communicate regularly with their providers, and make positive lifestyle changes; however, patients—especially those within vulnerable populations—lack the energy, money, knowledge, and skills needed to navigate successfully their often complex health conditions, regardless of whether they are sick or well (Center for Advancing Health, 2010).

Patient engagement works best when it involves a team that not only possesses clinical expertise, but also considers patients' socioeconomic needs (such as the importance to clinical outcomes of stable housing) and provides coordination (e.g., across multiple providers or between community-based organizations and the health system). The ideal care team includes not only physicians and nurses directing decisions related to medical care, but also psychiatrists, psychologists, or other licensed clinical social workers who support behavioral and mental health, as well as social workers who can provide counseling and access to social services via referrals (Manahan, 2011; Volkmann & Castanares,

2011). More and more, such multidisciplinary teams include outreach specialists and community health workers, especially when addressing the needs of vulnerable populations (Martinez Garcel, 2012; Volkmann & Castanares, 2011). A 2014 report on Bronx Lebanon Hospital's utilization of community health workers (CHWs) showed that CHWs help to reduce the number of ED visits and hospitalizations, thus reducing health care costs and contributing to the management of chronic disease (Findley, Matos, Hicks, Chang, & Reich, 2014). Case Exercise 8.1 expands on the Bronx-Lebanon Hospital example (Findley et al., 2014).

CHWs play a critical role in patient engagement. They can explain reasons for their actions in layman's terms and provide a support system that allows patients to feel they have the power to navigate the system and take control of their condition. When care coordination includes the support of individuals such as CHWs, patients have the help they need to think through how to integrate self-management of their chronic conditions into their existing life circumstances and—in the best of cases—are directed to the auxiliary services they need to get a handle on their nonmedical problems, stabilize their routines, and have better health outcomes.

Bringing It All Together: An Integrated System

Populations that are vulnerable due to low income or poor health stand to benefit from the integration of care. Integrated health care delivery systems provide or arrange a coordinated continuum of health care services to a defined population, and these delivery systems hold themselves accountable for the outcomes and health status of their patients (Witgert & Hess, 2012). By ensuring appropriate care, avoiding duplication of services, and reducing fragmentation within a preventive framework, integrated delivery systems seek to promote health care equality while controlling costs.

Use of Data in Improving Care

EHRs (electronic health records) and advances in information technology (including geographic information systems) have created new opportunities to improve the effectiveness and efficiency of care—particularly for vulnerable populations. Such technological advances have facilitated the use of large data sets to inform health care delivery and to conduct comprehensive cost and utilization analysis by population type, geography, and more.

One of the most compelling examples of data-reliant integrated care is the work of New Jersey's Camden Coalition of Healthcare Providers (CCHP), which utilizes the Camden Health Information Exchange (HIE) to track, monitor, and target services for the highest-cost patients across health systems in Camden. Case Exercise 8.2 expands on the example of the Camden Coalition.

▶ CASE EXERCISE 8.1—PATIENT ENGAGEMENT: BRONX-LEBANON HOSPITAL DEPARTMENT OF FAMILY MEDICINE'S PATIENT-CENTERED MEDICAL HOME

The South Bronx is home to a vibrant community, albeit poor, young, and with high rates of every illness now reaching epidemic proportions in the United States: diabetes, asthma, HIV, drug use, and obesity, to name a few. It is also the home of the Bronx-Lebanon Hospital Department of Family Medicine's Patient-Centered Medical Home.

The hospital's chair of family medicine, Dr. Douglas Reich, was grappling with the department's goal of improving health outcomes for the patients with the most complex life contexts. Beyond completing the very important clinical tasks of diagnosis and treatment, Reich's clinicians lacked the time and the skills to conduct meaningful discussions that would help to provide a better context for patients' care: What were the barriers to following a treatment regimen? What was getting in the way of managing illness? Was there room for prevention? An even greater challenge was reaching the hundreds of people who were in need of health care but going without.

In 2007, the Community Health Worker (CHW) program was established. CHWs, supervised directly by the department chair, received extensive training to fulfill their role as care managers. Integration into the care team was achieved by creating opportunities for shared learning and cross-education about team roles, for CHWs and clinical members alike, through continuing education, rounds, staff meetings, and so on.

Achieving CHW program sustainability required additional infrastructure, and protocol changes were necessary, the following among them:

- Recognition of CHW team contributions, including assessments and feedback within the department and hospital administration
- Shared group visits with a CHW and a physician
- Elaboration of the care management process
- Focus of work on interactions with patients

The patients assigned to CHWs demonstrated improvements in medication compliance, increased self-management of chronic conditions, and showing up for follow-up primary care appointments. In several cases, there has been a reduction of ED use and inpatient hospitalization. The CHW program at Bronx-Lebanon Hospital Department of Family Medicine has yielded important lessons for other patient-centered medical homes interested in expanding their care teams to enhance patient engagement.

▶ CASE EXERCISE 8.2—INTEGRATED CARE: CAMDEN COALITION OF HEALTH CARE PROVIDERS

Founded in 1828, Camden, New Jersey, was once the center of a thriving manufacturing industry. As with many other U.S. cities, deindustrialization led to high poverty rates that, coupled with political corruption and consistently high rates of violent crime, earned the city the dubious title of poorest city in the country. In addition to high unemployment rates, Camden is home to many Medicaid and Medicare beneficiaries and to others who are uninsured.

Dr. Jeffrey Brenner, a family physician operating a solo practice in Camden, recognized patterns of overspending that did not result in better health outcomes for Camden residents. In 2002, he and a small group of other primary care providers began meeting over breakfast once a month to discuss the issues they faced in their practices. It quickly became evident that all of the providers experienced many of the same barriers. In 2003, Dr. Brenner and colleagues founded the Camden Coalition of Healthcare Providers and set out to convince local stakeholders that an integrated health delivery model, in which patient data were shared and care coordinated, would result in better care for Camden residents (Gawande, 2011).

The coalition showed how vulnerable populations, in absence of a well-integrated and supportive health care system, have higher numbers of ED visits, suffer from more chronic disease, have access to fewer preventive services, and seek more reactive care than their peers living less chaotic lives. The analysis looked at 480,000 records for 98,000 patients by pooling data from the major health care institutions serving Camden for the period between 2002 and 2009. They results showed that 50% of Camden residents used the ED or the hospital in one year. Those individuals with the highest number of ED visits and hospitalizations citywide ("super utilizers") accounted for 324 visits in five years and 113 visits in one year. Thirty percent of costs were incurred by 1% of patients, 80% of costs were incurred by 13% of patients, and 90% of costs were incurred by only 20% of patients. The most expensive patient incurred $3.5 million in health care costs.

For vulnerable populations, crisis is the baseline. At the heart of crisis is the confluence of economic, social, geographic, and demographic factors that create the conditions for poor health and make management of illness a difficult task. When conducting a spatial analysis of Camden hospital cost data, the coalition found areas of the city with high concentrations of utilizers. In fact, several buildings each year were responsible for between $1 and $3 million in hospital costs. Furthermore, 6% of city blocks accounted for 18% of patients and 37% of billable visits.

The Camden team created an integrated model of care in response to these findings. Members of the care team check in with individual patients to ask about issues including, but not limited to, their unfilled prescriptions, reasons for missing appointments, and any emerging health issues. All patients have access to the coalition's health care crisis hotline, always staffed by a health care provider who can offer advice in an emergency situation.

Since the coalition formed in 2003, analysis of the data from the first 36 super utilizers has shown a 40% reduction in hospital and ED visits per month, and a 56% reduction in their average combined hospital bills (from $1.2 million to $500,000; Gawande, 2011).

Opportunities in the ACA to Meet Health Care Needs of Vulnerable Populations

On March 23, 2010, President Obama signed the ACA into law and altered the landscape of U.S. health care policy, with the intention to increase and improve health care access and quality of care for vulnerable populations. In addition, the ACA provided major investments to expand FQHCs and initiated efforts to change how health care is delivered and paid for in the United States.

The sections below discuss the and the improvements and opportunities for increased access under the ACA as well as its gaps and current limitations.

Increased Insurance Coverage for Individuals

One of the most immediate effects of the ACA is that it has increased coverage for millions of people, particularly for low-income adults (Sommers, Blendon, Orav, & Epstein, 2016). The United States is currently at a historically low uninsured rate (Kantarjian, 2017); in 2010 an estimated 48.3 million people were uninsured, in 2015 that number dropped to 28.7 (National Health Interview Survey, 2015). The ACA has played a significant role in increasing coverage and has provided a variety of pathways that allow people to access coverage who might otherwise not be eligible (Kantarjian, 2017; Frean et al., 2016). This included a provision that allowed for extended coverage from a parent's insurance until a young adult was 26 years old and expanded Medicaid eligibility to adults with incomes up to 138% of the FPL. It also included tax credits and subsidies based on income for people within 100% and 400% of the FPL, which lowered the cost of insurance through the health care marketplace, and laws that prevented insurers from discrimination against individuals with preexisting health condition and an insurance mandate (Frean et al., 2016).

While researchers could not explain all of the increases in health insurance coverage through the ACA, they estimate that of the 60% they can link to specific provisions, 40% of the gains are due to price subsidies and 60% is from Medicaid expansion (Frean et al., 2016). As of January 2018, all but 18 states have adopted Medicaid expansion (Henry J. Kaiser Family Foundation, 2018). While the decision to not expand Medicaid has resulted in disproportionate rates of access to care among states, the expansion of Medicaid is linked to an increase in coverage, even in states where coverage was not expanded. In states where Medicaid was expanded, uninsured people who were previously ineligible enrolled in Medicaid for the first time. In non-Medicaid expansion states, scholars believed a "woodwork effect" took place in which individuals who were previously eligible for Medicaid but had not been enrolled seemingly came out of the woodwork (Frean et al., 2016).

Improving Access to Community Health Centers

The ACA included large investments to expand FQHCs. Through the expanded availability of health insurance, particularly Medicaid, to low-income people, the ACA also included large investments in expanding FQHCs to improve care to this population. For instance, the law appropriated $11 billion in mandatory funding increase for Section 330 grants from 2011 to 2015. The law also boosts funding for FQHCs through increased payment rates for primary care physicians serving Medicaid beneficiaries. As of 2014, Medicaid providers will be paid at 100% of the rate paid to Medicare providers. These provisions will lead to increased access to primary care for vulnerable populations, both by increasing the capacity of this safety net and by creating a financial incentive through increased reimbursement for physicians to accept more people covered by Medicaid.

Advancing Payment and Delivery Reform

The ACA called for several underlying themes to alter proposed models of care and payment structures: (a) a move toward value-based purchasing of health services; (b) increased coordination of health, social services, and prevention; and (c) better integration of physical and **behavioral health services**. The proposed models can potentially have a positive effect on the health outcomes of vulnerable populations while reducing the cost of services delivered to this population.

For example, the ACA encourages state Medicaid programs to develop medical homes, known as Health Homes, for Medicaid patients with two or more chronic conditions or patients who have one serious and persistent mental health condition. The CMS issued specific elements that need to be included as part of a Health Home. These elements include comprehensive care management; intensive care transition services for patients moving out of acute care services (such as hospitals, home-based care, and outpatient facilities); care coordination among physical health, behavioral health, and social and community services (such as supportive housing); and individual and family support to patients.

Through better coordination of services through primary care, specialty and hospital care, behavioral health, social service support, and stronger patient monitoring, Health Homes could improve health outcomes and reduce unnecessary care. One study estimated that the U.S. health system would save approximately $175 billion over 10 years if primary care providers shifted to this coordinated system of care (The Lewin Group, 2009).

The ACA has also prompted a move away from the traditional FFS model to payment models that would align reimbursement and incentives to the value of care provided and hold providers accountable for health outcomes. This move toward value-based purchasing of services is central to a major Medicare demonstration supported by the ACA: accountable care organizations (ACOs).

ACOs are groups of doctors, hospitals, and other health care providers who come together voluntarily to give coordinated, high-quality care to their Medicare patients (Bachrach, Bernstein, & Karl, 2012). As defined by the ACA, ACOs must manage the health care needs of a minimum of 5,000 Medicare beneficiaries for at least three years. The goal of an ACO is to ensure that patients, especially the chronically ill, get the right care at the right time, while avoiding unnecessary duplication of services and preventing medical errors. This approach to care should lead to reductions in the total cost of care for the assigned population of patients. Providers participating in an ACO will share accrued savings with Medicare. In the end, providers get paid more for keeping their patients healthy and out of the hospital—as opposed to getting paid more only for providing more services. If an ACO is unable to save money, it can potentially be at risk for losing money associated with the costs of investments made to improve care, or it may have to pay a penalty if it does not meet performance and savings benchmarks.

Additional payment reform efforts enacted by the ACA include bundled payment demonstration programs and reduced payments for potentially preventable readmissions and complications. The common goal of all of these efforts is to improve the quality of care and rein in cost of health care, with a special focus on vulnerable populations.

Limitations of the ACA

Through the ACA, it is up to each individual state to expand eligibility for Medicaid. As of January 16, 2018, 18 states have rejected the Medicaid expansion (Henry J. Kaiser Family Foundation, 2018). As a result, an estimated 4.8 million uninsured adults in 2016 were estimated to fall in a coverage gap, where they did not earn enough to qualify for Medicaid but did not make enough money to qualify for federal subsidies to help them buy into the health exchanges (Buettgens & Kenney, 2016). People of color are disproportionality affected by a lack of Medicaid expansion, as they make up more than half of those who are in the coverage gap, including an estimated 1.2 million African Americans (Buettgens & Kenney, 2016). This is in part because the states where Medicaid expansion was not passed are also states where there is a high proportion of people of color (Garfield, Damico, Stephens, & Rouhani, 2014). Texas, Florida, and Georgia account for more than 50% of people who would be eligible for Medicaid if it were expanded (Kantarjian, 2017). In addition to the gap in coverage, there are many low-income people who qualified for ACA subsidies but did not enroll in the Marketplace because of high premium costs.

The ACA specifically excludes undocumented immigrants and their families from its provisions, leaving out the approximately 11 million undocumented immigrants who reside in the United States. These same individuals and families are likely to live in poverty, experience language and cultural barriers to accessing health care services, and have higher risk factors for chronic conditions.

As a result of these ACA limitations, the safety-net hospitals that provide care to vulnerable populations will experience a significant burden. This is especially troubling in the states with high concentrations of undocumented immigrants and a higher proportion of people who remain ineligible for insurance. Under the ACA, a reduction is scheduled in payments to disproportionate share hospitals, which have helped to absorb the effects of providing uncompensated care. This reduction will add to the strain on the resources of these institutions (Davis, 2012).

Another important limitation of the ACA that will affect the health and well-being of vulnerable populations is its narrow focus on the traditional health care system. Although the law sets in motion delivery system and payment transformations that will help to bridge traditional health care institutions with agencies, programs, and services that address some of the key drivers of poor health (such as housing and behavioral health services), it falls short of making the necessary investments in the social service sector that will help vulnerable populations get on—and stay on—the path to a healthy life. The United States is one of only three industrialized countries to spend most of its health and social services budget on health care itself (Bradley & Taylor, 2013). For every dollar the United States spends on health care, an additional 90 cents is spent on social services. In peer countries, for every dollar spent on health care, an additional $2 is spent on social services. Researchers who looked at spending across health care relative to social services found that countries with high health care spending compared with social spending had lower life expectancy and higher infant mortality rate than countries that favored social spending. European countries that have made greater investments in social services relative to health have experienced leaps in life expectancy (well over 80 years) and infant mortality rates that are half those in the United States. Most medical providers concur with this logic. In a Robert Wood Johnson Foundation–funded national survey, four out of five physicians agreed that unmet social needs lead directly to worse health.

If the United States is to make a dent in improving the health outcomes of vulnerable populations, we must go beyond shifting dollars from one part of the health care system to another. Rather, we must make a transformative shift in where the investments are made—and accept that subpar social conditions have a direct consequence on health. As Bradley and Taylor state:

> Homelessness isn't typically thought of as a medical problem, but it often precludes good nutrition, personal hygiene, and basic first aid, and it increases the risks of frostbite, leg ulcers, upper respiratory infections, and trauma from muggings, beatings, and rape. (Bradley & Taylor, 2013)

A program in Boston that tracked the medical expenses of 119 chronically homeless people found that, in a five-year period, these individuals accounted for 18,834 emergency department visits estimated to cost more than $12 million.

Challenges of Health Care Reform and Threats to the ACA

At this time, health care reform is largely debated issue. There is heated political debate over whether health care is a right or is a privilege, which individuals should be eligible for care, and how health care can be improved. President Trump has used a series of executive orders to alter aspects of the ACA (Adamcyzk, 2017; Sanger-Katz, 2017). There have been several attempts in Congress to dismantle the ACA, including the American Health Care Act of 2017, which would put 23 million people at risk of losing their insurance, but so far these orders have not passed in Congress (Pearl, 2017). In October 2017, the DHHS announced it would no longer make payments after President Trump's decision to stop making payments to insurance companies that subsidize care for low-income members

(Alonso-Zaldivar, 2017; Sanger-Katz, 2017). This cut impacts insurers' decisions about future pricing and coverage, which further affects low-income members ability to afford insurance if cost goes up.

CONCLUSION

Populations adversely impacted by health inequities are at greatest risk of poor physical, behavioral, and social health. They have high rates of disease burden and mortality. When receiving care, people who are poor, people of color, and people who have faced historical oppression have the hardest time accessing timely, high-quality health care and, when receiving care, are more likely to have worse health outcomes than the general population. Despite an extensive body of literature and myriad federal efforts to eliminate these inequities in health and health care between vulnerable groups and the general population, the United States has barely made progress.

> The prevalence of vulnerable populations is increasing; if we fail to institute policies and programs to improve the health of vulnerable populations, little will be done to contain the cost of care in the United States.

To some extent, the topic of eliminating disparities has been diluted and overused. It is almost as though the topic of health disparities has become an accepted part of our health literary repertoire. But this issue contains an underlying, explosive problem: The prevalence of vulnerable populations is increasing; if we fail to institute policies and programs to improve the health of vulnerable populations, little will be done to contain the cost of care in the United States. We will continue to spend more on health but have significantly poorer health status compared with other industrialized countries.

In this chapter, we have offered an integrated framework that sets examines how health inequities disproportionately affect certain groups due to social and economic contexts. As opposed to examining the health of discrete subgroups of people disproportionately impacted by health inequities, which are not mutually exclusive, the chapter provided a general overview of the predisposing and enabling factors that lead to vulnerability. The approach reflects the co-occurrence of risk factors *and* helps to explain why existing approaches to meet the health needs of this population will continue to fall short. Though well intended, current policies and programs are a patchwork of categorical, fragmented, and uncoordinated attempts that cost a lot of money.

Health inequities are primarily a social issue created through social forces. It will be addressed adequately only through broader social, communitywide investments. A shift to community-oriented policies and programs that address the social origins of vulnerability can lead to greater improvements in health outcomes. These programs and policies should aim to produce networks of collaboration and integration—rather than wedges of bureaucratic division—across medical care, public health, social and economic solutions, and policies that permanently fix the risks and consequences of vulnerability. Investing time, energy, and resources in improving the health of vulnerable populations as a national priority is more than a social and moral imperative—it is an economic one. The human and financial costs of this problem weigh heavily on the future of the United States to continue as a beacon of justice and equality and a global financial leader. Who are considered vulnerable populations, and what does this tell us about the nature of the problems that predispose and enable vulnerability in the United States?

▶ CASE EXERCISE 8.3—PLAN FOR REFUGEES

The commissioner of health in a large, mostly urban county has secured your services as a consultant to identify strategies to meet the needs of the growing refugee population legally settling in her region. A refugee is a person who has fled from his or her home country and cannot return because of a well-founded fear of persecution based on religion, race, nationality, political opinion, or membership in a particular social group. The commissioner of health has at her disposal both federal and state resources and good relationships with colleagues from other county agencies, such as planning, transportation, education, aging, and so on.

As a consultant, you have been asked to propose a coordinated plan to use existing resources and relationships to better serve the needs of the growing refugee population. When considering your plan, be sure to address the following questions:

1. What type of information would you collect, and how would you use it?
2. Whom else would you engage in developing a plan?
3. How will you ensure that the refugee population has access to existing and new services?
4. Explain how your plan will meet the immediate and long-term needs of this group as part of an improved system of health care and social services.

DISCUSSION QUESTIONS

1. How have shifting demographics, the rise in prevalence of chronic conditions, and the strained social service sector contributed to the growing number of vulnerable populations?
2. A wide array of medical and social services exists to help meet the complex needs of vulnerable populations; however, the United States has been unable to curb health care costs or improve health outcomes for this segment of the population. What are some of the underlying problems with the current approach to services for vulnerable populations?
3. How does the current payment system fall short in meeting the needs of vulnerable populations?
4. Review the limitations for meeting the needs of vulnerable populations in the ACA provisions. Propose ways in which you would address these limitations using (a) new policies, (b) existing policies and structures, and (c) innovative ideas (such as public/private partnerships).

REFERENCES

Adamcyzk, A. (2017, January 21). What Trump's Obamacare executive order means. *Time*. Retrieved from http://time.com/money/4642125/trump-obamacare-executive-orde

Adashi, E. Y., Geiger, J. H., & Fine, M. D. (2010). Health care reform and primary care—The growing importance of the Community Health Center. *New England Journal of Medicine, 362*, 2047–2050. doi:10.1056/NEJMp1003729

Aday, L. (2001). *At risk in America: The health and health care needs of vulnerable populations in the United States* (2nd ed.). San Francisco, CA: Jossey-Bass.

Agency for Healthcare Research and Quality. (2014). *Care coordination, quality improvement* (structured abstract). Rockville, MD: Author.

Allard, S. W., & Roth, B. (2010). *Strained suburbs: The social service challenges of rising suburban poverty*. Metropolitan opportunity series (Vol. 7). Washington, DC: The Brookings Institution Metropolitan Policy Program. Retrieved from http://www.brookings.edu/research/reports/2010/10/07-suburban-poverty-allard-roth

Alonso-Zaldivar, R. (2017, October 12). Trump plans to "immediately" stop ACA payments to insurers. *Associated Press*. Retrieved from https://www.pbs.org/newshour/politics/trump-plans-stop-aca-payments-insurers

American Psychological Association. (2016). *Stress in America: The impact of discrimination*. Retrieved from https://www.apa.org/news/press/releases/stress/2015/impact-of-discrimination.pdf

Andersen, R. M. (1995). Revisiting the behavioral model and access to medical care: Does it matter? *Journal of Health and Social Behavior, 36*(1), 1–10.

Association of State and Territorial Health Officials. (2010). MCH technical assistance SNAP & WIC side-by-side comparison. Retrieved from http://www.astho.org/Programs/Access/Maternal-and-Child-Health/Technical-Assistance/Materials/SNAP-and-WIC-Side-by-Side-Comparison

Bachrach, D., Bernstein, W., & Karl, A. (2012). *High-performance health care for vulnerable populations: A policy framework for promoting accountable care in Medicaid* (M. Hostetter, Ed.). New York, NY: The Commonwealth Fund. Retrieved from https://www.commonwealthfund.org/sites/default/files/documents/___media_files_publications_fund_report_2012_nov_1646_bachrach_high_performance_hlt_care_vulnerable_populations_medicaid_aco_v2.pdf

Bauer, U. E., Briss, P. A., Goodman, R. A., & Bowman, B. A. (2014). Prevention of chronic disease in the 21st century: Elimination of the leading preventable causes of premature death and disability in the USA. *Lancet, 384*(9937), 45–52. doi:10.1016/S0140-6736(14)60648-6

Bradley, E. H., & Taylor, L. (2013). *The American health care paradox: Why spending more is getting us less*. New York, NY: PublicAffairs Books.

Braveman P., Arkin, E., Orleans, T., Proctor, D., & Plough, A. (2017). *What is health equity? And what difference does a definition make?* Princeton, NJ: Robert Wood Johnson Foundation.

Braveman, P., Kumanyika, S., Fielding, J., LaVeist, T., Borrell, L. N., Manderscheid, R., & Troutman, A. (2011). Health disparities and health equity: The issue is justice. *American Journal of Public Health, 101*(S1), S149–S155.

Brody, G. H., Yu, T., Miller, G. E., & Chen, E. (2015). Discrimination, racial identity, and cytokine levels among African-American adolescents. *Journal of Adolescent Health, 56*(5), 496–501.

Buettgens, M., & Kenney, G. (2016). What if more states expanded Medicaid in 2017? Changes in eligibility, enrollment, and the uninsured. Retrieved from http://www.rwjf.org/content/dam/farm/reports/issue_briefs/2016/rwjf430492

Center for Advancing Health. (2010). *A new definition of patient engagement: What is it, and why is it important?* Washington, DC: Author. Retrieved from http://www.cfah.org/file/CFAH_Engagement_Behavior_Framework_current.pdf

Center on Budget and Policy Priorities. (2018). Chart book: SNAP helps struggling families put food on the table. Retrieved from https://www.cbpp.org/research/food-assistance/chart-book-snap-helps-struggling-families-put-food-on-the-table.

Centers for Medicare and Medicaid Services. (2016). Medicare enrollment/trends. Retrieved from https://www.cms.gov/Research-Statistics-Data-and-Systems/Statistics-Trends-and-Reports/CMS-Statistics-Reference-Booklet/Downloads/2016_CMS_Stats.pdf

Centers for Medicare and Medicaid Services. (2018a). Fast facts. Retrieved from https://www.cms.gov/fastfacts

Centers for Medicare and Medicaid Services. (2018b). National Health Expenditure Projections 2017–2026. Retrieved from https://www.cms.gov/Research-Statistics-Data-and-Systems/Statistics-Trends-and-Reports/NationalHealthExpendData/Downloads/ForecastSummary.pdf

Centers for Medicare and Medicaid Services (2018c). People enrolled in Medicare and Medicaid. Medicare-Medicaid Coordination Office Fact Sheet. Retrieved from https://www.cms.gov/Medicare-Medicaid-Coordination/Medicare-and-Medicaid-Coordination/Medicare-Medicaid-Coordination-Office/Downloads/MMCO_Factsheet.pdf

Commission on Social Determinants of Health. (2008). Closing the gap in a generation: Health equity through action on the social determinants of health. *Final Report of the Commission on Social Determinants of Health*. Geneva, Switzerland: World Health Organization.

Creswell, J. (2013, December 25). ER costs for mentally ill soar, and hospitals seek better way. *New York Times*. Retrieved from http://www.nytimes.com/2013/12/26/health/er-costs-for-mentally-ill-soar-and-hospitals-seek-better-way.html?_r = 0

Cubanski, J., Neuman, T., Damico, A., & Smith, K. (2018). Medicare beneficiaries' out-of-pocket health care spending as a share of income now and projections for the future. Henry J. Kaiser Family Foundation. Retrieved from https://www.kff.org/medicare/report/medicare-beneficiaries-out-of-pocket-health-care-spending-as-a-share-of-income-now-and-projections-for-the-future

Cuffee, Y. L., Hargraves, J. L., & Allison, J. (2012). Exploring the association between reported discrimination and hypertension among African Americans: A systematic review. *Ethnicity & Disease, 22*(4), 422–431.

Cunningham, P., Rudowitz, R., Young, Y., Garfield, R., & Foutz, J. (2016). Understanding Medicaid hospital payments and the impact of recent policy changes. Henry J. Kaiser Family Foundation. Retrieved from https://www.kff.org/report-section/understanding-medicaid-hospital-payments-and-the-impact-of-recent-policy-changes-issue-brief

Cutter, S. L., & Emrich, C. T. (2006). Moral hazard, social catastrophe: The changing face of vulnerability along the hurricane coasts. *Annals of the American Academy of Political and Social Science, 604*(1), 102–112.

Daponte, B. O., & Bade, S. (2006). How the private food assistance network evolved: Interactions between public and private responses to hunger. *Nonprofit and Voluntary Sector Quarterly, 35*(4), 668–690.

Davis, C. (2012). *Q & A: Disproportionate share hospital payments and the Medicaid expansion*. Washington, DC: National Health Law Program. Retrieved from http://www.healthlaw.org/publications/qa-disproportionate-share-hospital-payments-and-the-medicaid-expansion#.VMEVw_nF8yQ

Dean, S., Rosenbaum, D., & Foley, A. (2013). SNAP benefits will be cut for nearly all participants in November 2013. Center on budget and policy priorities. Retrieved from http://www.cbpp.org/cms/?fa=view&id=3899

Devi, S. (2011). Native American health left out in the cold. *Lancet, 377*(9776), 1481–1482. doi:10.1016/S0140-6736(11)60586-2

DeVol, R., Bedroussian, A., Charuworn, A., Chatterjee, A., Kim, I. K., Kim, S., & Klowden, K. (2007). *An unhealthy America: The economic burden of chronic disease*. Santa

Monica, CA: Milken Institute. Retrieved from http://assets1b.milkeninstitute.org/assets/Publication/ResearchReport/PDF/chronic_disease_report.pdf

Diez-Roux, A. V. (2003). Residential environments and cardiovascular risk. *Journal of Urban Health, 80*(4), 569–589.

Do, D. P. (2009). The dynamics of income and neighborhood context for population health: Do long-term measures of socioeconomic status explain more of the Black/White health disparity than single-point-in-time measures? *Social Science and Medicine, 68*(8), 1368–1375.

Findley, S., Matos, S., Hicks, A., Chang, J., & Reich, D. (2014). Community health worker integration into the healthcare team accomplishes the Triple Aim in a patient-centered medical home: A Bronx tale. *Journal of Ambulatory Care, 37*(1), 82–91. Retrieved from http://chwcentral.org/sites/default/files/Community_Health_Worker_Integration_Into_the.10.pdf

FRED—Federal Reserve Economic Data. (2018). Retrieved from https://fred.stlouisfed.org

Fontenot, T., & Stubblefield, A. G. (2011). Caring for vulnerable populations. American Hospital Association 2011 Committee on Research. Retrieved from http://www.aha.org/research/cor/caring/index.shtml

Federal Reserve Bank of St. Louis and U.S. Office of Management and Budget. (2018). Real Median Household Income in the United States [MEHOINUSA672N]. Retrieved from FRED, https://fred.stlouisfed.org/series/MEHOINUSA672N

Galewitz, P. (2012, June 6). Migrant health clinics caught in crossfire of immigration debate. *Kaiser Health News*. Retrieved from http://www.kaiserhealthnews.org/stories/2012/june/07/migrant-health-clinics-immigration-debate.aspx

Garfield, R., Damico, A., Stephens, J., & Rouhani, S. (2014). The coverage gap: Uninsured poor adults in states that do not expand Medicaid—An update. Menlo Park, CA: Kaiser Family Foundation. Retrieved from http://www.nasuad.org/sites/nasuad/files/the-coverage-gap-uninsured-poor-adults-in-states-that-do-not-expand-medicaid-issue-brief.pdf

Garr, E. (2011). *The landscape of repression: Unemployment and safety net services across urban and suburban America*. Metropolitan opportunity series: Vol. 12. Retrieved from http://www.brookings.edu/research/papers/2011/03/31-recession-garr

Gawande, A. (2011, January 24). The hot spotters: Can we lower medical costs by giving the neediest patients better care? *The New Yorker*. Retrieved from http://www.newyorker.com/reporting/2011/01/24/110124fa_fact_gawande?currentPage = 3

Gourevitch, M. N., Malaspina, D., Weitzman, M., & Goldfrank, L. (2008). The public hospital in American medical education. *Journal of Urban Health, 85*(5), 779–786. doi:10.1007/s11524-008-9297-4

Grusky, D. B., Western, B., & Wimer, C. (Eds.). (2011). *The great recession*. New York, NY: Russell Sage Foundation.

Hamilton, D., Darity, S., Price, A., Sridharan, V. & Tippett, R. (2015). *Umbrellas don't make it rain: Why studying and working hard isn't enough for black Americans*. Chapel Hill, NC: Duke Center on Social Equity, Duke University. Retrieved from https://socialequity.duke.edu/research/wealth

Hawkins, D., & Groves, D. (2011). The future role of community health centers in a changing health care landscape. *Journal of Ambulatory Care Management, 34*(1), 90–99. Retrieved from http://www.nachc.org/client/documents/The_Future_Role_of_Community_Health_Centers_in_a.11.pdfhttp://www.nachc.org/client/documents/The_Future_Role_of_Community_Health_Centers_in_a.11.pdf

Heiman, H. J., & Artiga, S. (2015). Beyond health care: The role of social determinants in promoting health and health equity. *Health, 20*(10), 1–10.

Henry J. Kaiser Family Foundation. (2011). Affordable Care Act Provisions Relating to the Care of Dually Eligible Medicare and Medicaid Beneficiaries. Focus on Health Reform. Retrieved from https://kaiserfamilyfoundation.files.wordpress.com/2013/01/8192.pdf

Henry J. Kaiser Family Foundation. (2013). The Ryan White AIDS program. Retrieved from http://kff.org/hivaids/fact-sheet/the-ryan-white-program

Henry J. Kaiser Family Foundation. (2018). Status of state action on the Medicaid expansion decision. Retrieved from https://www.kff.org/health-reform/state-indicator/state-activity-around-expanding-medicaid-under-the-affordable-care-act/?currentTimeframe=0&sortModel=%7B%22colId%22:%22Location%22,%22sort%22:%22asc%22%7D

Henry J. Kaiser Family Foundation. (n.d.,-a) Total Medicaid spending: FY 2016. Retrieved from https://www.kff.org/medicaid/state-indicator/total-medicaid-spending/?currentTimeframe=0&sortModel=%7B%22colId%22:%22Location%22,%22sort%22:%22asc%22%7D#

Henry J. Kaiser Family Foundation. (n.d.,-c) Total number of Medicare beneficiaries. Retrieved from https://www.kff.org/medicare/state-indicator/total-medicare-beneficiaries/?currentTimeframe=0&sortModel=%7B%22colId%22:%22Location%22,%22sort%22:%22asc%22%7D

Hobfoll, S. E. (2001). The influence of culture, community, and the nested-self in the stress process: Advancing conservation of resources theory. *Applied Psychology: An International Review, 50*(3), 337–421.

Hobfoll, S. E. (2012). Conservation applied psychology: An international review, of resources and disaster in cultural context: The caravans and passageways for resources. *Psychiatry, 75*(3), 227–232.

Hsia, R. Y., Sarkar, N., & Shen, Y. (2017). Impact of ambulance diversion: Black patients with acute myocardial infarction had higher mortality than whites. *Health Affairs, 36*(6), 1070–1077.

Kantarjian, H. M. (2017). The Affordable Care Act, or Obamacare, 3 years later: A reality check. *Cancer, 123*(1), 25–28.

Kent, G. (2006). WIC's promotion of infant formula in the United States. *International Breastfeeding Journal, 1*(8). doi:10.1186/1746-4358-1-8

Kiel, P. & Nguyen, D. (2018). [Insert article title.] *ProPublica*. Retrieved from http://projects.propublica.org/bailout

Knickman, J. K., & Snell, E. K. (2002). The 2030 problem: Caring for aging baby boomers. *Health Services Research, 37*(4), 849–884. doi:10.1034/j.1600-0560.2002.56.x

Lang, I. A., Hubbard, R., Andrew, M. K., Llewellyn, D. J., Melzer, D., & Rockwood, K. (2009). Neighborhood deprivation, individual socioeconomic status, and frailty in older adults. *Journal of the American Geriatrics Society, 57*(10), 1776–1780. doi:10.1111/j.1532-5415.2009.02480.x

The Lewin Group. (2009). *The path to a high performance U.S. health system: Technical documentation*. Washington, DC: Author.

Manahan, B. (2011). The whole systems medicine of tomorrow: A half-century perspective. *Explore: The Journal of Science and Healing, 7*(4), 212–214.

Martinez Garcel, J. (2012). Casting an A-team to deliver results: Embedding and sustaining the role of community health workers in medical homes. *Medical Home News, 4*(2), 6–7.

Mathur, A. K., Ashby, V. B., Sands, R. L., & Wolfe, R. A. (2010). Geographic variation in end-stage renal disease incidence and access to deceased donor kidney transplantation. *American Journal of Transplantation, 10*(4 Pt 2), 1069–1080.

McGinnis, J., Russo, P. W., & Knickman, J. K. (2002). The case for more active policy attention to health promotion. *Health Affairs, 21*(2), 78–93. doi:10.1377/hlthaff.21.2.78

McLeod, J. D., & Kessler, R. C. (1990). Socioeconomic status and differences in vulnerability to undesirable life events. *Journal of Health and Social Behavior, 31*, 162–172. Retrieved from http://www.ncbi.nlm.nih.gov/pubmed/2102495

McMorrow, S., Kenney, G. M., Long, S. K., & Anderson, N. (2015). Uninsurance among young adults continues to decline, particularly in Medicaid expansion states. *Health Affairs, 34*(4), 616.

Mitchell, A. (2013). *Medicaid disproportionate hospital share payments.* Congressional Research Service report. Washington, DC: Government Printing Office. Retrieved from https://www.fas.org/sgp/crs/misc/R42865.pdf

Moscovice, I., Gregg, W., & Lewerenz, E. (2003). *Rural health networks: Evolving organizational forms and functions.* Minneapolis, MN: University of Minnesota School of Public Health Rural Health Research Center. Retrieved from http://rhrc.umn.edu/wp-content/files_mf/formsandfunctions2.pdf

National Center for Farmworker Health. (n.d.). Migrant health center legislation. Retrieved from http://www.ncfh.org/?pid = 186

National Center for Health in Public Housing. (2012). Public housing primary care program. Retrieved from http://www.nchph.org/wp-content/uploads/2013/11/NCHPH-PHPC1.pdf

National Health Care for the Homeless Council. (2008). The basics of homelessness. Retrieved from http://www.nhchc.org/resources/general-information/fact-sheets

National Health Interview Survey. (2015). Long-term trends in health insurance coverage. Retrieved from https://www.cdc.gov/nchs/data/nhis/earlyrelease/trendshealthinsurance1968_2015.pdf

National Public Radio/Robert Wood Johnson Foundation/Harvard T. H. Chan School of Public Health. (2017). Discrimination in America: Experiences and views of African Americans. Retrieved from https://cdn1.sph.harvard.edu/wp-content/uploads/sites/21/2017/10/NPR-RWJF-HSPH-Discrimination-African-Americans-Final-Report.pdf

Paradise, J., Rosenbaum, S., Markus, A., Sharac, J., Tran, C., Reynolds, D., & Shin, P. (2017). Community Health Centers: Recent role of the ACA. The Henry J. Kaiser Family Foundation. Retrieved from https://www.kff.org/report-section/community-health-centers-recent-growth-and-the-role-of-the-aca-issue-brief

Partnership for Solutions. (2004). *Chronic conditions: Making the case for ongoing care, September 2004 update.* Baltimore, MD: Johns Hopkins University. Retrieved from http://www.partnershipforsolutions.org/DMS/files/chronicbook2004.pdf

Pastor, M., Scoggins, J., & Treuhaft, S. (2017). Bridging the racial generation gap is key to America's economic future. Retrieved from http://nationalequityatlas.org/sites/default/files/RacialGenGap_%20final.pdf

Patzer, R. E., & McClellan, W. M. (2012). Influence of race, ethnicity, and socioeconomic status on kidney disease. *Nature Reviews Nephrology, 8*(9), 533–541.

Pearl, R. (2017, December 18). The 3 biggest healthcare stories of 2017. *Forbes.* Retrieved from https://www.forbes.com/sites/robertpearl/2017/12/18/the-3-biggest-healthcare-stories-of-2017/#323ba15653e4

Prins, S. J. (2011). Does transinstitutionalization explain the overrepresentation of people with serious mental illnesses in the criminal justice system? *Community Mental Health Journal, 47*(6), 716–722. doi:10.1007/s10597-011-9420-y

Purtell, K. M., Gershoff, E. T., & Aber, J. L. (2012). Low income families' utilization of the federal "safety net": Individual and state-level predictors of TANF and food stamp receipt. *Children in Youth Services Review, 34*(4), 713–724. doi:10.1016/j.childyouth.2011.12.016

Robertson, B., & Ramiah, K. (2017). Essential data: Our hospitals, our patients—Results of America's essential hospitals 2015 annual member characteristics survey. *Essential Hospitals.* Retrieved from https://essentialhospitals.org/wp-content/uploads/2017/06/AEH_VitalData_2017_Spreads_NoBleedCropMarks.pdf

Saez, E., & Zucman, G. (2016). Wealth inequality in the United States since 1913: Evidence from capitalized income tax data. *Quarterly Journal of Economics, 131*(2), 519–578. doi:10.1093/qje/qjw004

Sanger-Katz, M. (2017, October 12). What we know about Trump's twin blows to Obamacare. *The New York Times.* Retrieved from https://www.nytimes.com/2017/10/12/upshot/

what-did-trumps-health-care-executive-order-do.htmlhttps://www.nytimes
.com/2017/10/12/upshot/what-did-trumps-health-care-executive-order-do.html

Schpero, W. L., Morden, N. E., Sequist, T. D., Rosenthal, M. B., Gottlieb, D. J., & Colla, C. H. (2017). For selected services, blacks and Hispanics more likely to receive low-value care than whites. *Health Affairs, 36*(6), 1065–1069.

Shi, L., & Stevens, G.D. (2005). Vulnerability and unmet health needs: The influence of multiple risk factors. *Journal of General Internal Medicine, 20*(2), 148–154. doi:10.1111/j.1525-1497.2005.40136.x

Shi, L., & Stevens, G. (2010). *Vulnerable populations in the United States* (2nd ed.). San Francisco, CA: Jossey-Bass Rethinking vulnerable populations in the United States: An introduction to a general model of vulnerability.

Shi, L., Stevens, G. D., Faed, P., & Tsai, J. (2008). Rethinking vulnerable populations in the United States: An introduction to a general model of vulnerability. *Harvard Health Policy Review, 9*(1), 43–48.

Sommers, B. D., Blendon, R. J., Orav, E. J., & Epstein, A. M. (2016). Changes in utilization and health among low-income adults after Medicaid expansion or expanded private insurance. *Journal of the American Medical Association Internal Medicine, 176*(10), 1501–1509. doi:10.1001/jamainternmed.2016.4419

Stern, M. J., & Axinn, J. (2018). *Social welfare: A history of the American response to need* (9th ed.). Merrill Social Work and Human Services Series. New York, NY: Pearson.

Stone, C., Trisi, D., Sherman, A., & Debot, B. (2015). A guide to statistics on historical trends in income inequality. *Center on Budget and Policy Priorities*, 26. Retrieved from https://www.cbpp.org/research/poverty-and-inequality/a-guide-to-statistics-on-historical-trends-on-income-inequality

Unite for Sight. (n.d.). Module 2: A brief history of mental illness and the U.S. mental health care system. Retrieved from http://www.uniteforsight.org/mental-health/module2

U.S. Census Bureau. (2017). Historical poverty tables: People and families—1959 to 2016. Data. Retrieved from https://www.census.gov/data/tables/time-series/demo/income-poverty/historical-poverty-people.html

U.S. Department of Agriculture, Food and Nutrition Service. (n.d.). Food and Nutrition Service (FNS) programs and services. Retrieved from http://www.fns.usda.gov/programs-and-services

U.S. Department of Agriculture, Food and Nutrition Service. (2018). Supplemental Nutrition Assistance Program participation and costs, 1969–2017. Retrieved from https://www.fns.usda. gov/pd/supplemental-nutrition-assistance-program-snap

U.S. Department of Health and Human Services, Health Resources and Services Administration. (n.d.). HIV/AIDS programs: Legislation. Retrieved from http://hab.hrsa.gov/abouthab/legislation.html

U.S. Department of Health and Human Services, Indian Health Services. (2018). Indian Health Services Profile. Retrieved from https://www.ihs.gov/newsroom/factsheets/ihsprofile/

U.S. Department of Health and Human Services, Office of Rural Health Policy. (2006). *Comparison of the rural health clinic and federally qualified health center programs*. Washington, DC: U.S. Government Printing Office. Retrieved from http://www.hrsa.gov/ruralhealth/policy/confcall/comparisonguide.pdf

U.S. Department of Housing and Urban Development. (n.d.). HUD historical background. Retrieved from http://www.hud.gov/offices/adm/about/admguide/history.cfm

U.S. Social Security Administration. (n.d.). SSI federal payment amounts for 2014. Retrieved from http://www.ssa.gov/OACT/cola/SSI.html

Volkmann, K., & Castanares, T. (2011). Clinical community health workers: Linchpin of the medical home. *Journal of Ambulatory Care Management, 34*(3), 221–233.

"Vulnerable". (n.d.). *Merriam-Webster online*. Retrieved from http://www.merriam-webster .com/dictionary/vulnerable

Ward, B. W., Schiller, J. S., & Goodman, R. A. (2014). Peer reviewed: Multiple chronic conditions among U.S. adults: A 2012 update. *Preventing Chronic Disease, 11,* E62. doi:10.5888/pcd11.130389

Washington, D. L., Steers, W. N., Huynh, A. K., Frayne, S. M., Uchendu, U. S., Riopelle, D., . . . & Hoggatt, K. J. (2017). Racial and ethnic disparities persist at Veterans Health Administration patient-centered medical homes. *Health Affairs, 36*(6), 1086–1094.

Weisman, J. (2014, December 19). U.S. declares bank and auto bailouts over, and profitable. *New York Times*. Retrieved from https://www.nytimes.com/2014/12/20/business/us-signals-end-of-bailouts-of-automakers-and-wall-street.html?_r=0

Williams, D. R. (2012). Miles to go before we sleep: Racial inequities in health. *Journal of Health and Social Behavior, 53*(3), 279–295.

Williams, D. R., Priest, N., & Anderson, N. B. (2016). Understanding associations among race, socioeconomic status, and health: Patterns and prospects. *Health Psychology, 35*(4), 407–411. doi:10.1037/hea0000242

Willms, D. (1999). *Inequalities in literacy skills among youth in Canada and the United States*. Ottawa, ON, Canada: Minister of Industry.

Witgert, K., & Hess, C. (2012). *Including safety-net providers in integrated delivery systems: Issues and options for policymakers*. National Academy of Health Policy. New York, NY: The Commonwealth Fund. Retrieved from http://www.nashp.org/sites/default/files/Including.SN_.Providers.in_.IDS_.pdf

World Health Organization. (1948). *Constitution of the World Health Organization*. Geneva, Switzerland: Author.

Wu, S. Y., & Green, A. (2000). *Projection of chronic illness prevalence and cost inflation*. Santa Monica, CA: RAND corporation. Retrieved from http://www.fightchronicdisease.org/sites/fightchronicdisease.org/files/docs/GrowingCrisisofChronicDiseaseintheUSfactsheet_81009.pdf

MEDICAL CARE: TREATING AMERICANS' MEDICAL PROBLEMS

Chapter 9

The Health Workforce

Joanne Spetz and Susan A. Chapman

LEARNING OBJECTIVES

▶ Identify who is part of the health workforce

▶ Understand the importance of the entire health workforce in delivering health care services

▶ Describe the different education paths for the health workforce

▶ Critically assess the reasons for shortages of health care providers

▶ Review new models and new roles of deploying health workers

▶ Assess the effects of health reform on the health workforce

KEY TERMS

▶ health professionals

▶ interprofessional education

▶ labor market

▶ licensure

▶ on-the-job training

▶ scope of practice

TOPICAL OUTLINE

▶ Who is part of the health workforce?

▶ Traditional approaches to health workforce planning

▶ Health workforce education

▶ Critical issues for the health workforce

▶ Building the future health care workforce

INTRODUCTION

The health care workforce is essential to the delivery of health care; essentially all types of health services require the contributions of individual workers. The health care workforce includes well-known professionals such as nurses, pharmacists, and dentists; it also includes many other, less obvious professions that encompass a wide variety of technicians, therapists, assistants, administrative personnel, and managers. In 2016, there were approximately 16.4 million jobs in the health care industry in the United States, and compensation for these jobs accounted for nearly half of total health care spending—$1.03 billion of the $2.1 billion spent on health care (U.S. Bureau of Economic Analysis, 2017; U.S. Bureau of Labor Statistics, 2017). The health workforce's central role in all aspects of health care and its significant contribution to total health care costs guarantee that any policies intended to change how health care is financed or delivered will be fundamentally shaped by their interactions with the workforce. This fact becomes more complex when one recognizes that the health workforce plays an important role in economic development and income distribution. Health care jobs often pay well and are stable, and they are frequently filled by people living where the health care is provided (Gitterman, Spetz, & Fellowes, 2004; Zacker, 2011). As health reform reshapes the system of health care in the United States, we will continue to see major changes in the size, composition, and practice of health professionals. Such changes will be complicated by the broader role of health care employment in our economy and society.

> By about 2025, the nation's health care sector is expected to be facing a shortfall of *2.3 million* new workers.*

WHO IS PART OF THE HEALTH WORKFORCE?

The health workforce includes all **health professionals** and workers who contribute to the delivery of health care. The determination of who falls into this definition can involve some debate. Many occupations are consistently classified as within the health workforce, such as physicians, radiation technologists, dental assistants, and nurses. Health occupations also include people who do not work in health care delivery settings but instead provide health services in homes, educational institutions, and other places, such as home care aides, personal care assistants, and school nurses (Bipartisan Policy Center, 2011; Matherlee, 2003). In 2016, these and related health care occupations included more than 13.1 million people, accounting for nearly 1 in 12 workers in the United States (U.S. Bureau of Labor Statistics, 2017).

The largest health care occupation is registered nurses (RNs), of whom about 2.9 million were employed in 2016 (U.S. Bureau of Labor Statistics, 2017). RNs work in nearly all health care settings; about 54.4% work in hospitals (Budden, Moulton, Harper, Brunell, & Smiley, 2016). Personal care aides, of whom there are about 1.5 million, are the second-largest occupation in health care and primarily

---

*To hear the podcast, go to https://bcove.video/2zI5NTt or access the ebook on Springer Publishing Connect™.

provide services and support in the home. Unlicensed nursing assistants are the third-largest health care occupation, with about 1.4 million workers employed. Unlicensed nursing assistants usually work in hospitals and long-term care facilities. About 603,000 certified nursing assistants and 702,400 licensed practical/vocational nurses work in skilled nursing facilities (U.S. Bureau of Labor Statistics, 2017). About 649,850 physicians were employed in the United States in 2016.

Other large occupations in health care include home health aides, medical assistants, dental assistants, pharmacy technicians, and emergency medical technicians/paramedics. The health care occupations also include licensed alternative and complementary providers, such as chiropractors and acupuncturists. Table 9.1 presents data on the wide variety of health care practitioner and support occupations in the United States with jobs in hospitals, outpatient settings, and long-term care.

The broadest definition of the health workforce includes anyone who works in a health care occupation or the health care industry, even if that worker is not directly involved in providing health care services—for example, insurance billing specialists, facilities managers, accountants, and other occupations. Within the health care industry, about 3.3 million people are employed in office, administrative, and support occupations, such as secretaries and administrative assistants,

TABLE 9.1 HEALTH CARE OCCUPATIONS IN THE UNITED STATES: 2016

OCCUPATION	NUMBER OF WORKERS
Registered nurse	2,857,180
Nursing assistant	1,443,150
Personal care aide	1,492,250
Home health aide	814,300
Licensed practical nurse/vocational nurse	702,400
Physician/surgeon	649,850
Medical assistant	623,560
Pharmacy technician	398,390
Dental assistant	327,290
Pharmacist	305,510
Emergency medical technician/paramedic	244,960
Radiological technologist	200,650
Physical therapist	216,920
Dental hygienist	204,990
Medical records and health information technician	200,140
Medical and clinical laboratory technologist	166,730

information and records clerks, food preparation and food service workers, custodial services, security, and education and training.

This chapter focuses on the workforce of more than 16 million people dedicated to delivering medical care services broadly defined. In addition, many other American workers focus on efforts to promote health among the population. Workers in public health departments across the country deliver essential social services that impact people's health and well-being and other practitioners deliver alternative health care services. Researchers, advocates, innovators, and others focus on developing new approaches to delivering health care and keeping people healthy. All these workforce resources are dedicated to the American health enterprise. Approximately 450,000 people work in public health agencies that focus on a broad range of activities that prevent poor health at the community level (Sumaya, 2012). It is more difficult to assess the scope of health promotion work done in other sectors, but it is clear that many people spend time on activities that affect the health of Americans throughout the private, public, and nonprofit sectors.

TRADITIONAL APPROACHES TO HEALTH WORKFORCE PLANNING

Approaches to health workforce planning vary across countries. Countries with national health care systems often closely manage the employment of health professionals, as well as the pipeline of new graduates from education programs. Many countries, including the United States, do not have a highly centralized health care system and engage in limited national health workforce planning efforts. Planning is left primarily to the private sector and local government agencies.

The traditional supply-and-demand approach to workforce planning compares the number of working health professionals to estimates of the demand for health workers. Projections of supply are typically built from data about the current number of workers, the number of new entrants per year, the number leaving the profession per year, and the share that is employed. In some cases, supply estimates account for other factors that may affect supply, such as the loss of health professionals to international migration. However, supply estimates rarely can estimate changes in overall supply that might arise due to the development of new health care occupations.

Projections of demand are usually based on current approaches to providing health care services. Some demand projections attempt to establish a targeted number of providers in order to deliver a desired level of services to the population. However, this "ideal" need-based demand may not align with budgetary realities and thus not match the demand we actually see in the **labor market**. For example, during economic recessions, demand for health workers usually drops even though demand for health services may remain stable because employers have less money for hiring. If the amount of money available in the health system is not sufficient to recruit workers and pay salaries, need-based demand and economic demand will diverge.

Two fundamental shortcomings of workforce planning are that (a) it is usually tied to current care delivery models and (b) it treats each health professional independently. Innovative approaches to care delivery and team-based care could address many reported shortages of health professionals. For example, a growing body of research argues that new, integrated primary care delivery models, effective use of information technology, and expanded roles for nonphysician health professionals could solve shortages of primary care physicians (Auerbach et al., 2013; Bodenheimer & Smith, 2013; Green, Savin, & Lu, 2013;

> A growing body of research argues that new, integrated primary care delivery models, effective use of information technology, and expanded roles for nonphysician health professionals could solve shortages of primary care physicians.

Rosenthal, 2014; U.S. Health Resources and Services Administration [HRSA], 2016; Willard & Bodenheimer, 2012). For example, the patient-centered medical home (PCMH) model of care (described in more detail below) brings together teams of physicians, advanced practice clinicians such as nurse practitioners (NPs), licensed nurses, medical assistants, health coaches, community health workers, and other professionals. Each worker plays a unique and expanded role, and this team-based approach can improve patient outcomes and satisfaction while reducing the demand for physician time (Alexander et al., 2015). But health workforce planning models are not designed to account for the variety of ways in which such teams might be structured and how they can shift demand for each type of professional.

HEALTH WORKFORCE EDUCATION

Educational and training requirements vary significantly across health care occupations: Some health workers enter the field without a high school diploma, whereas others complete many years of postgraduate education. Many occupations, such as personal care aides and medical secretaries, require little or no formal preparation, and training occurs on the job. In other occupations, such as medical assistants and pharmacy technicians, there is variation in employers' preferences for formal education programs versus longer-term, **on-the-job training**.

Most technical health care occupations require some formal postsecondary education but not a degree; such occupations include surgical technicians, licensed practical/vocational nurses, and emergency medical technicians. A large share of education in these occupations occurs in private vocational schools; for example, about 82% of medical assistants are trained in private and for-profit schools (U.S. National Center for Education Statistics, 2015). These schools often lack program-specific accreditation and standardized curricula. Some technical professions, such as dental hygienist, respiratory therapist, clinical laboratory technician, and radiology technician, require at least an associate degree. Registered nursing requires a minimum of an associate degree in most states, but many RNs complete baccalaureate education before becoming licensed. Finally, professions such as medicine, pharmacy, physical therapy, and optometry require postgraduate education, typically at the doctoral level.

Postsecondary education is available from many institutions: private vocational schools, public adult school programs, community colleges, and public and private colleges and universities. The costs of educational programs vary significantly. Private education is generally much more expensive than public education; in the 2014–2015 academic year, annual costs for public postsecondary education institutions averaged $16,188, whereas these costs averaged $37,424 for private institutions (U.S. National Center for Education Statistics, 2016). Although prospective students might prefer to attend public institutions, these often have many fewer admission spaces than applicants. Health worker education is relatively expensive to deliver because it often requires the use of laboratories and clinical sites and involves closely supervised clinical training. Many public colleges and universities receive a fixed amount of funding per student, regardless of the major field of study. Thus, these schools face a financial loss if they expand their health professions programs rather than expanding less-costly programs. Moreover, because most health care jobs have relatively high pay, it can be difficult for colleges to recruit faculty.

> Differences in the costs of educational programs affect choices made by students, especially when cost is compared with expected earnings.

Differences in the costs of educational programs affect choices made by students, especially when cost is compared with expected earnings. For example, the education of a primary care physician requires 4 years of postgraduate medical school education, followed by 3 or more years of residency. Preparation for a specialized field of medicine requires more time; for example, a cardiologist must complete 2 or 3 years of postresidency fellowship after his or her residency. Some research has demonstrated that medical students' choice of specialty is influenced by potential earnings compared with education debt and that the lower earnings of primary care physicians do not compare favorably, even though other fields of medicine require more years of residency and fellowship training (Bodenheimer, Berenson, & Rudolf, 2007; Grayson, Newton, & Thompson, 2012; Hauer et al., 2008). Similar patterns have been reported for dentistry (Nicholson, Vujicic, Wanchek, Ziebert, & Menezes, 2015). There also are mismatches between the cost of education and expected earnings for many lower-skill health occupations. For example, medical assistant wages averaged $15.17 per hour in 2016 (U.S. Bureau of Labor Statistics, 2017), yet some medical assistants attend private training programs that charge tuition and fees of more than $10,000 for a program of less than 1 year (U.S. Department of Education, 2018).

Interprofessional Education

Health workforce education is traditionally focused on single professions. Physicians attend medical schools, nurses study in nursing schools, and dentists attend dental schools. These siloed education programs rarely offer opportunities to learn together either in the classroom or through clinical experience. Alternative health care professionals, such as chiropractors, are rarely educated alongside physicians or other professionals. However, a growing body of evidence finds that **interprofessional education** (IPE) and subsequent interprofessional practice, can improve the ability of health care professionals to provide high-quality patient-centered care (Barr, Koppel, Reeves, Hammick, & Freeth, 2005), including mental health care (Richards et al., 2013). Although the rapid emergence of initiatives to promulgate IPE seems recent, their roots date back to more than 40 years ago, when the Institute of Medicine (IOM) published "Educating for the Health Team" (1972). The IOM's second report on this subject, "Health Professions Education: A Bridge to Quality" (Greiner & Knebel, 2003), brought more attention to the imperative to revamp health workforce training. The report's authors argued that the silo approach to educating health professionals contributes to continuing problems in the health care system.

Many private foundations, advocacy groups, and educational institutions are now actively developing and implementing IPE programs to address future health care needs. The Interprofessional Education Collaborative—a consortium that includes national organizations representing educators in allopathic and osteopathic medicine, dentistry, nursing, public health, and pharmacy—has made specific recommendations regarding the competencies required for successful interprofessional collaborative practice (Interprofessional Education Collaborative, 2011). The competencies fall under four domains: (a) values and ethics for interprofessional practice, (b) roles and responsibilities for collaborative practice, (c) interprofessional communication, and (d) interprofessional teamwork and team-based care. The National Center for Interprofessional Practice and Education, established through a cooperative agreement between the federal government and four private foundations, is leading, coordinating, and studying the advancement of interprofessional collaboration, with a particular focus on the effect of IPE on quality, patient outcomes, and costs.

Innovative Models for Health Workforce Education

Traditionally, health professional students receive didactic instruction in the classroom setting and develop clinical skills in health care delivery settings such as hospitals, dental offices, and primary care clinics. As health professions programs have expanded, there has been increasing competition for clinical education sites, and some sites have reduced the number of students allowed to train due to concerns about patient safety, demands for longer orientation periods, and restrictions on access to electronic health records (Hayden, Smiley, Alexander, Kandong-Edgren, & Jeffries, 2014; Ironside & McNelis, 2009). The development of increasingly sophisticated patient simulators, including high-fidelity mannequins, has facilitated growing use of simulation-based clinical education (Hayden et al., 2014) as has recognition that simulation can be used to develop clinical skills without risk to patients (Ziv, Wolpe, Small, & Glick, 2006). In 2002, only 66 nursing programs were known to use patient simulators (Nehring & Lashley, 2004), but by 2010 at least 917 programs were using this technology (Hayden, 2010). Reviews of simulation in prelicensure education for multiple health professions, including medicine, nursing, and rehabilitation therapy, find that use of simulation is associated with high satisfaction and confidence as well as similar clinical performance between groups that have varying levels of simulation experience during their education (Alanazi, Nicholson, & Thomas, 2017; Cant & Cooper, 2017; Hayden et al., 2014; Laschinger et al., 2008). Simulation education also is playing an increasing role in supporting IPE and the development of skills to practice effectively in health care teams (Palaganas, Epps, & Raemer, 2014).

Technological development also has fostered the growth of online health professions education for both initial education and continuing postlicensure education. Prelicensure programs frequently use "flipped classroom" and "blended classroom" approaches, in which there is a combination of in-person and online learning modules (Wittich et al., 2017). Research on blended learning in health professions education indicates that it has positive effects on learning both didactic and clinical content (Liu et al., 2016; McCutcheon, Lohan, Traynor, & Martin, 2015). Postlicensure education, including both advanced degree programs and continuing education for license renewal, is increasingly offered online, in web-based formats, and via videoconferencing (Cook et al., 2008). These strategies are highly effective for licensed professionals (Chipps, Brysiewicz, & Mars, 2012; Cook et al., 2008; Du et al., 2013; Richmond, Copsey, Hall, Davies, & Lamb, 2017). These innovative education approaches can improve the accessibility of postlicensure degree programs and continuing education for those living in rural communities (Chipps et al., 2012) and with mobility limitations (Marcyjanik & Zorn, 2011).

In the face of rising costs and lengthy programs for health professions education, some U.S. schools have launched and expanded shorter training programs, most notably for medicine. Three-year medical education programs are not new; during the early 1970s, it was reported that 27% of schools of medicine offered 3-year programs (Beran, 1979). Additional schools offered 6-year combined B.S.-M.D. programs. However, these programs were largely abandoned owing to quality of life issues for students and faculty and the preference among residency directors for 4-year program graduates (Kettel, Dinham, Drach, & Barbee, 1979; Trzebiatowski & Peterson, 1979), even though there were no systematic reports of inadequacy of student preparation (Beran, 1979; Garrard & Weber, 1974; Hallock et al., 1977; Kettel et al., 1979). In the 2000s, interest in 3-year medical school programs was renewed in both allopathic and osteopathic medical schools, primarily as a strategy to increase interest in primary care (Bell, Ferretti, & Ortoski, 2007; Raymond, Kerschner, Hueston, & Maurana, 2015). Some of these programs combine a 3-year undergraduate medical program with a 3-year family or internal medicine residency. In 2012, it was reported that more than 60 medical schools offered combined B.S.-M.D. programs lasting 6 or 7 years, and a small but growing number of schools were offering 3-year medicine-only programs (Eaglen et al., 2012; Emanuel & Fuchs, 2012; Raymond et al., 2015). Accelerated education programs also are growing for nursing, including master's degree entry and second-bachelor's degree programs designed for students with bachelor's degrees in non-nursing fields (Aktan et al., 2009; Lindsey, 2009).

Increasing Educational Expectations

Concurrent with trends toward accelerated education and innovative education delivery modalities has been a push among some professions, including pharmacists, NPs, certified registered nurse anesthetists, and physical therapists, to increase educational standards. For example, to support expanded roles of pharmacists in direct patient care and collaborative practice, in 2004 the Accreditation Council for Pharmacy Education ended approval of 5-year bachelor's of pharmacy programs and made the Doctor of Pharmacy (PharmD) the only accredited pharmacy degree in the United States (Council on Credentialing in Pharmacy, 2010; Maine, Knapp, & Scheckelhoff, 2013; Schommer, Cline, & Larson, 2005). That same year, the American Association of Colleges of Nursing (AACN) approved a position statement that supported adoption of the doctor of nursing practice (DNP) degree by 2020 as the entry-level standard for advance practice RNs, which includes NPs, certified nurse midwives, clinical nurse specialists, and nurse anesthetists (Martsolf, Auerbach, Spetz, Pearson, & Muchow, 2015). Although the nurse anesthesia certification board has dictated that all new graduates must receive a DNP by 2025, only 25% of advance practice RN programs offered the option for baccalaureate-educated RNs to go directly to a DNP in 2015. For PAs, entry-level doctoral programs are now being launched, with the first one focused on emergency medicine at Baylor University. Physical therapy, occupational therapy, laboratory medicine, speech therapy, and audiology also have moved toward a clinical doctorate as the recommended or required entry-level education.

Many other health occupations are moving toward greater education requirements, including some that do not require bachelor's-level education. The IOM recommended in 2011 that 80% of RNs attain a bachelor's or higher degree by 2020 (IOM, 2011a), although this target will not be reached by that year. Similarly, the American Association for Respiratory Care issued a statement in 2015 that the share of respiratory therapists holding or working on a bachelor's degree should rise from 65% to 80% by 2020 (American Association for Respiratory Care, 2015).

Supporters of increasing education standards for health professionals focus on the additional time required to develop skills in patient care management as well as development and execution of quality improvement programs. Those who oppose these education changes argue there is no evidence that higher educational requirements lead to better patient care and that higher levels of education increase costs for students and the health care system (Dickerson & Trujillo, 2009; Martsolf et al., 2015; Siler & Randolph, 2007).

CRITICAL ISSUES FOR THE HEALTH WORKFORCE

The implementation of the Patient Protection and Affordable Care Act (ACA) and a growing focus on the affordability of health care have brought new urgency to the need to reform the delivery of health care in the United States.

> For nearly 20 years, it has been recognized that significant changes are needed to improve the quality of care, increase the health status of the U.S. population, and control health care costs.

For nearly 20 years, it has been recognized that significant changes are needed to improve the quality of care, increase the health status of the U.S. population, and control health care costs (IOM, 2001; Kohn, Corrigan, & Donaldson, 2000). These changes, however, may be difficult to implement in the face of ongoing and worsening shortages of health professionals. The most critical issues facing the health workforce now, in addition to the educational reforms described earlier, include ongoing shortages; changes in health care financing, which are rapidly spurring changes in the organization of care delivery; developing a workforce that can effectively coordinate the care of patients; integrating physical health care services with behavioral health and dental care; optimizing the use of information technologies in care delivery and quality improvement; the need to revamp regulations so that health professionals can meet health care needs more efficiently and effectively; and leveraging the potential of health care labor unions and labor–management partnerships.

Health Professional Shortages

The expansion of insurance coverage under the ACA led to a surge in the demand for health services (Wishner & Burton, 2017), which exacerbated preexisting shortages of primary care providers and other health professionals (Bodenheimer & Pham, 2010; Colwill, Cultice, & Kruse, 2008; IHS Inc., 2015; Institute of Medicine, 2014; Nicholson, 2009) and heightened concerns that there is not an adequate workforce to meet the health care needs of the population (Ormond & Bovbjerg, 2011). Even if the ACA were to be modified or repealed, population growth, the aging of the U.S. population, and increased rates of chronic illness are expected to increase the workloads of primary care providers over the next 15 years (Colwill et al., 2008; IOM, 2008). The proportion of the U.S. population over age 65 is rising rapidly, from 14.9% in 2015 to a projected 20.6% in 2030 (U.S. Census Bureau, 2014). This is important for the health care workforce for several reasons:

- Health care for older Americans costs more than for other age groups. Data from 2006 show average annual costs ranging from about $11,000, for those ages 65 to 74, to nearly $24,000 annually, for those over age 85 (Federal Interagency Forum on Aging-Related Statistics, 2010, p. 50). Those costs rise even more when one adds the cost of chronic conditions: Costs average $5,100 for those with no chronic conditions to more than $25,000 annually for those with more than five chronic conditions.

- Older adults use more services from health professionals. Those over age 65 account for about 26% of all physician visits, 35% of all hospital stays, 34% of prescriptions, and 90% of nursing home use (IOM, 2008).

- Many health professions' curricula do not contain significant content in caring for older adults. At a time when we will most need generalists and specialists in geriatric care, the U.S. workforce is ill-prepared for these challenges (Kottek, Bates, & Spetz, 2017).

- Members of the workforce that provide the bulk of long-term care in the home, community, and nursing homes are poorly paid, lack recognition for their work, and have high rates of job dissatisfaction and turnover (IOM, 2008).

Shortages exist when demand is greater than supply. The economic response to a shortage is an increase in wages, which leads to greater supply (because compensation is more lucrative) and lower demand (because labor costs employers more). However, this normal economic response does not always occur in the labor markets for health professionals. First, wages may not change. The historical fee-for-service (FFS) reimbursement system favors specialized, complex, and procedurally oriented services. Because standard office visits receive lower payment, total compensation for primary care providers is lower. Significant changes in payment methods will be needed to rectify this differential; accountable care organizations (ACOs), PCMHs, and other such innovations may have some impact, but the degree to which they will support growth of the primary care workforce is yet unknown.

The second reason health care labor markets might not follow standard economic behavior is that their supply is constrained by **licensure** and educational requirements. The time required to prepare a new health care professional for entry into the workforce can be many years. For example, the education of a primary care physician requires 4 years of medical school education, followed by 3 or more years of residency. Interest in primary care among medical school students has been dropping for years, with particularly little interest in family medicine (Council on Graduate Medical Education, 2010; McGaha, Schmittling, DeVilbiss Bieck, Crosley, & Pugno, 2010). Registered nurses, who must have a license recognized by the state in which they practice, must complete at least 2 years of postsecondary education before they are qualified to take a licensing examination (Buerhaus, Staiger, & Auerbach, 2009). Many other health professions, including physical therapists, medical technologists, and respiratory therapists, face similar licensing and education requirements.

Further constraining the supply of health professionals are limits on educational capacity. Allied health educational programs exemplify some of the challenges in producing an adequate number of health professionals. Educational programs can be expensive to operate, with small class sizes and the cost of supplies for clinical practicums. This is true for many occupations, including radiologic technicians, imaging specialties, and medical laboratory technologists. Many allied health professions education programs are taught in community college settings, where financial resources may be more limited than in universities and private colleges (IOM, 2011b).

In addition to the challenge of educating enough health professionals, there is often a problem with the geographic distribution of those workers. In the United States, it has historically been difficult to recruit professionals into rural and poorer urban areas, particularly when jobs are plentiful elsewhere (Bourgueil, Mouseques, & Tajahmadi, 2006). Despite direct government interventions in the form of academic stipends and loan forgiveness programs, access to primary care in particular remains a problem in many states and in specific regions of some states. Several analyses of health workforce needs for the ACA have reported that the maldistribution of professionals is a critical problem across professions (e.g., Bates, Blash, Chapman, Dower, & O'Neil, 2011). These and other studies have reported that training and retaining allied health workers in rural areas is also a challenge (California Hospital Association, 2011). For this reason, many rural health care programs use a "grow your own" approach recruiting and training students from rural areas to increase the likelihood they will stay to work in the area (IOM, 2011b).

Health worker shortages, and the rising wages that accompany them, have led many health policy experts to advocate for increasing the roles of nonphysicians and allied health workers in care delivery. As discussed above, greater use of team-based care and nonphysician health professionals could address physician shortages, at least to some degree (Auerbach et al., 2013; Bodenheimer & Smith, 2013; HRSA, 2016). Similarly, licensed vocational nurses, who have a certificate or associate degree, can perform many tasks reserved for RNs (Seago, Spetz, Chapman, Dyer, & Grumbach, 2004). The degree to which health care delivery systems engage in the substitution of health professionals depends both on their relative wages and regulations that designate the **scope of practice** of each professional.

Changes in Health Care Financing and the Organization of Care

Some provisions of the ACA are intended to increase the efficiency of health care delivery and are likely to affect the mix of health workers demanded. Performance-based payment programs, for example, give health care organizations a financial incentive to focus on implementing models of care that can increase the quality of care at a reasonable cost (Davis & Guterman, 2007). For example, many studies have found that higher RN staffing levels in hospitals are linked to better patient outcomes (e.g., Aiken, Clarke, Sloane, Sochalski, & Silber, 2002; Kane, Shamliyan, Mueller, Duval, & Wilt, 2007; Lang, Hodge, Olson, Romano, & Kravitz, 2004; Needleman, Buerhaus, Mattke, Stewart, & Zelevinsky, 2002). Historically, however, hospitals have had little financial incentive to increase nurse staffing because higher-quality nursing care is not rewarded and nursing wages are expensive. Performance-based payment may lead hospitals to reconsider the value of increasing nurse staffing because there could be a financial gain in improving quality (Kurtzman & Buerhaus, 2008).

Two other innovations in health care financing are Medicare's bundled payment and ACO programs, both of which create financial incentives for health care providers to take full responsibility for an episode of care. This is a significant change from the FFS approach by allowing health care organizations to retain financial savings from delivering care efficiently, as long as quality is improved or maintained. The potential for financial gain gives health care providers an incentive to reassess their processes for providing care. ACOs have increased their use of interprofessional health care teams, particularly for patients with high costs and complex illness (Sandberg, Erikson, & Yunker, 2017). Bundled payments, which provide a single payment for hospital services during both initial hospitalization and any subsequent hospitalization for a fixed period of time, also lead hospitals to invest in services to prevent rehospitalizations.

> Bundled payments, which provide a single payment for hospital services during both initial hospitalization and any subsequent hospitalization for a fixed period of time, also lead hospitals to invest in services to prevent rehospitalizations.

Care Coordination

The diffusion of payment systems that provide incentives to increase the efficiency of care delivery has given hospitals incentives to reduce the length of hospital stay and ambulatory care providers incentives to reduce unnecessary ambulatory care and emergency department visits. This places increased importance on coordinating the continuation of care and communication with the health care team in the home. Care coordination and the employment of care managers are associated with reduced hospitalizations and avoidable emergency department visits (Conway, O'Donnell, & Yates, 2017; Erikson, Pittman, LaFrance, & Chapman, 2017; Sandberg et al., 2017). Research has shown that health systems are making greater investments in hiring and training nurses, social workers, medical assistants, and other workers for care coordination (Ladden et al., 2013). These workers hold a variety of job titles, including care coordinator, care manager, case manager, and care navigator (Erikson et al., 2017). Erikson and colleagues (2017) found that health systems often hire RNs for patients requiring clinical management and social workers for patients needing social services; however, these roles are often blended. As care coordination jobs become more prevalent in the future, a challenge will be preparing the workforce for the skills needed in these new roles: team communication, use of remote monitoring technology, telehealth, and working with family caregivers.

The ACA also includes provisions to support the PCMH model of care. A PCMH engages a team of providers in the delivery of care, typically including physicians, NPs, RNs, medical assistants, health educators, and pharmacists. Ideally, behavioral and mental health services are integrated into the PCMH (Bates et al., 2011). Medical assistants might conduct expanded health assessments and review patient records to identify those who need contact to ensure follow-up appointments and prescription refills occur (Chapman & Blash, 2017). RNs often engage in care coordination and management, linking patients to specialists and other services. Health coaches support patients in adopting care plans including diet and exercise, and community health workers engage patients with community and social support services. Evaluations of the PCMH model finds it has positive impacts on quality of care and use of preventive services as well as lower overall costs of care (Alexander et al., 2015). This and similar team-based approaches to providing primary care services may help to address anticipated shortages of primary care providers by increasing the roles of other health care professionals (Auerbach et al., 2013; Bates et al., 2011). In order for these models of care to be fully successful, however, educational programs need to be realigned to focus on interprofessional teams.

Integration of Physical Health, Behavioral Health, and Dental Care

Behavioral health care includes services for mental health and substance use disorders. The demand for behavioral health care services has increased for two primary reasons. The Mental Health Parity and Addiction Equity Act of 2008, along with the ACA, ensured that mental health and substance abuse benefits be no more restrictive than those for medical and surgical care (Frank, Beronio, & Glied, 2014). The ACA included mental health care as one of 10 essential benefits in all health care plans offered in the state insurance exchanges (Beronio, Po, Scopec, & Glied, 2013). Even prior to these changes, there were national shortages of behavioral health providers. HRSA identifies approximately 4,000 mental health professional shortage areas in the United States (U.S. Health Resources and Services Administration, 2016). Behavioral health providers include a wide range of professionals and levels of preparation, including psychiatrists, psychologists, psychiatric mental health nurse practitioners (PMHNPs), social workers, substance abuse counselors, and persons with lived experience called peer providers who support persons in the recovery process. Some of the challenges in assuring access to behavioral health care workers include a lack of growth in the number of psychiatry trainees for more than a decade (National Resident Matching Program, 2017), PMHNP scope of practice limitations (Phoenix, Hurd, & Chapman, 2016), maldistribution of the available workforce geographically and between public and private practice, and the stigma of working in behavioral health. Behavioral health is generally not well integrated with primary care services because services are often provided at separate locations and have different payment systems and electronic health records, and care coordination among the team members is difficult. There are promising efforts in integrating primary and behavioral health care, but much more needs to be done (Skillman, Snyder, Frogner, & Patterson, 2016).

Oral health care also has traditionally been separated from medical care, even though dental disease has impacts on respiratory disease, cardiovascular disease, and diabetes (IOM, 2011c). Dental pain accounts for more than

1.3 million emergency department visits each year and up to 5% of adult primary care visits (Allareddy et al., 2014; IOM, 2011c). Increasing awareness of the importance of oral health, along with requirements in the ACA that state Medicaid plans insure oral health services for children, has prompted integration of dental and medical services by some providers. Some federally qualified health centers and private medical groups have trained pediatricians to provide enhanced dental screening and apply fluoride varnish to children's teeth (Braun et al., 2017; Pahel, Rozier, Stearns, & Quiñonez, 2011). NPs and physician assistants employed in primary care settings also are delivering similar services (Mertz, Spetz, & Moore, 2017).

Information Technologies and the Workforce

The continuing evolution of information technology in health care is changing the work of health professionals as well as the way they communicate with each other and with family members. Electronic health records enable health workers to exchange information rapidly and to engage patients more actively in care. Electronic health records that facilitate greater use of telephone communication with patients have been associated with a decrease in primary care visits (Chen, Garrido, Chock, Okawa, & Liang, 2009) as well as fewer avoidable hospitalizations (Lammers, McLaughlin, & Barna, 2016). Even though the expanded use of electronic health records is improving efficiency, enhancing quality, and increasing patient engagement in health care, the implementation of such technologies has demanded notable changes in skills and workflow. Electronic health records organize information differently than traditional paper charts, and health professionals need to navigate through structured menus to enter information rather than rely on simple templates and free text. Many organizations have found that in the short term these systems—and changes to the systems—disrupt workflow, and workers with poor typing and computer skills are challenged to use them (Spetz, Phibbs, & Burgess, 2012). To make the best use of these systems, health workers need enhanced computer skills, and health care organizations must carefully redesign workflow to take best advantage of what electronic health records offer.

Telemedicine also is rapidly changing the capacity of the health care workforce, particularly in rural areas. Early use of telemedicine was limited largely to telephone communication, but high-resolution digital imaging, real-time two-way video communication, and rapid transmission of electronic health records make it possible for remote clinicians to access enough information to engage in complex consultations remotely. Rural communities are increasingly using electronic consultations to give patients access to specialists without traveling. Widespread adoption of these technologies in both urban and rural settings could greatly expand the capacity of the current workforce to meet health care needs (Courneya, Palattao, & Gallagher, 2013; Green et al., 2013; Weiner, Yeh, & Blumenthal, 2013).

The Need for Regulatory Reform

The growth of team-based models of care, such as the PCMH, and continuing concerns about shortages of physicians have led many researchers and policy analysts to argue that nonphysician providers can and should play a larger role in the delivery of primary care. For example, about half of NPs focus on the provision of primary care services (Spetz, Fraher, Li, & Bates, 2015). Many studies demonstrate that the quality of care delivered by NPs is at least equivalent to that of physicians, and some research has found that NPs have stronger patient communication skills (Horrocks, Anderson, & Salisbury, 2002; Lenz, Mundinger, & Kane, 2004; Newhouse et al., 2011). However, NPs face scope-of-practice laws that require them to work under physician supervision and limit their ability to prescribe medications (Sekscenski, Sansom, Bazell, Salmon, & Mullan, 1994; Wing, O'Grady, & Langelier, 2005). Removal of these barriers would enable NPs to practice to their fullest potential to meet health care needs (IOM, 2011a). Regulations also limit the work of other health professionals, such as licensed practical nurses (LPNs) and medical assistants (Seago et al., 2004).

More than three-fourths of health workers are employed in licensed occupations. These occupations practice in the context of regulations regarding their scope of practice which, for some states, stipulate whether they must be supervised or collaborate with other professionals and whether they can be reimbursed directly by insurance companies (Kleiner & Park, 2010). The often-stated purpose of scope-of-practice regulation across the professions is consumer protection: safeguarding consumers who cannot independently evaluate the skills or competence of health practitioners. State regulations, including licensure requirements, are meant to outline the basic education, skills, and competency of a health care professional. Sometimes these regulations outline what practitioners of a particular profession can do safely, and in some cases the regulations focus on what members of the profession are not allowed to do. Both the breadth of work permitted and prohibitions can be found in some state regulations. When there is overlap in the potential roles of health professionals, scope of practice regulations are more controversial and vary more across states (Kleiner, Marier, Park, & Wing, 2014). Health care organizations also control the practice of health professionals by establishing their own rules about what each provider can and cannot do. For example, some hospitals do not permit NPs and PAs to oversee patient care, and pharmacists are restricted from managing medications in some organizations.

The effect of NP scope-of-practice regulations has been studied more than those of other professions. There is substantial variation in the scope of practice permitted across states (Christian, Dower, & O'Neil, 2007). In 23 states and the District of Columbia, NPs are permitted to provide care independently, but in other states NPs are not permitted to practice without physician collaboration or supervision, often requiring written practice protocols and sometimes including restrictions on the number of NPs with whom a physician may collaborate (American Association of Nurse Practitioners, 2017). Even when NPs can practice

independently, they may be required to have a collaborative or supervisory relationship with a physician to prescribe medications. Restrictive scope-of-practice
regulations for NPs have been linked to lower utilization of primary care services (Stange, 2013) and higher costs in retail health care clinics (Spetz & Parente,
2013). At the same time, several systematic reviews have concluded that primary
care services provided by NPs are of similar quality as physician care (Horrocks
et al., 2002; Lenz et al., 2004; Newhouse et al., 2011). In order to fully leverage the
capacity of the health workforce and align care processes to emerging financial
incentives, scope-of-practice regulations may need to be reconsidered.

Since 2000, there has been a trend toward regulatory changes that allow many
NPs and PAs greater practice independence (Gadbois, Miller, Tyler, & Intrator,
2014). Other professions also have seen expansions in their scope of practice.
Dental hygienists are now practicing more autonomously in many states than in
the past, particularly in public health settings such as schools, nursing homes,
and correctional facilities (Mertz et al., 2017). In addition, new categories of
licensed health professionals have been added, such as dental therapists, who
are authorized to diagnose dental disease, treat caries, and perform extractions
in Minnesota, Maine, and Vermont as well as within the Alaskan Native Tribal
Health Consortium (Nash, 2009; Pew Charitable Trusts Dental Campaign, 2016).

Health Care Unions and Labor–Management Partnerships

Growing numbers of health care workers are represented by unions; this trend
dates to the 1970s when regulations permitted employees of nonprofit organizations to become unionized and eased the unionization of public-sector workers.
About 14% of health practitioner and technical workers are represented by unions,
as are 10% of health care support occupations (U.S. Bureau of Labor Statistics,
2014). Unionized health workers tend to receive higher wages than those not represented by unions. Unions also have sought other concessions from employers,
particularly hospitals, such as establishment of fixed nurse-to-patient ratios, preferred shifts based on employment tenure, and improved health and retirement
benefits. Health care workers have engaged in highly visible strikes and labor
actions; they are politically active, supporting legislation and candidates.

Some employers have developed good working relationships with their
unions. For example, in 1997 the Service Employees International Union, which
represents multiple health occupations, and 10 other unions partnered with
Kaiser Permanente in a landmark agreement. The partnership focused on multiple
goals, including improving quality of care for members, making Kaiser Permanente more competitive in its markets, making Kaiser Permanente an "employer of
choice," and providing Kaiser Permanente employees with the "maximum possible
employment and income security" (Kochan, McKersie, Eaton, & Adler, 2009). Since
then, the unions and Kaiser Permanente have worked closely together to establish
internal training programs, scholarships and grants for pursuing advanced education, and job transition programs. When Kaiser Permanente established a systemwide health information technology system, it worked with the union to ensure

that employees received training and to find new roles for workers, such as clerks, whose jobs would be obviated by the electronic records. Although this partnership has not been without challenges, it has served as one model of a collaborative labor–management approach, rather than an adversarial relationship.

CONCLUSION: BUILDING THE FUTURE HEALTH CARE WORKFORCE

The health workforce is central to the health care system, and changes in its deployment and utilization will have significant effects on health care quality and costs. The ACA and rising concerns about the efficiency of health care delivery are bringing renewed attention to the importance of team-based care models, IPE, and scope-of-practice regulations. At the same time, concerns and ongoing and emerging shortages of health workers persist. The U.S. Bureau of Labor Statistics estimates that the number of people employed in health occupations will rise to more than 15 million by 2026, accounting for nearly 1 in 11 jobs. The importance of this workforce to both health care and the overall economy will keep the health professions in the policy spotlight for the foreseeable future.

▶ CASE EXERCISE—WORKFORCE RECRUITMENT PLAN

You are the newly hired director of human resources (HR) for a large inner-city health care organization. The CEO has asked you to develop a strategic response to numerous HR problems. The main problem has been the inability to recruit new physicians and RNs. This problem is compounded by a lack of teamwork among clinicians and between service departments and a high rate of turnover of some of the best workers while less able workers remain employed.

In writing your strategic response, consider the following questions:

1. What strategies could be undertaken in the short term to address these problems?

2. What approaches could be taken in the long term?

3. Which of these approaches can be undertaken by the HR department on its own, and which require collaboration with employee groups and/or HR directors at neighboring employers?

4. Choose three short-term priorities and defend them. How might they segue into a long-term strategy?

DISCUSSION QUESTIONS

1. What are advantages of need-based models of demand? What are disadvantages of this approach to estimating demand?

2. If changes to scope-of-practice regulations could help to abate health worker shortages and reduce the cost of health care, why are such changes not made?

3. What specific skills are needed for health care practitioners to coordinate care across hospital, outpatient, skilled nursing, and home care settings?

REFERENCES

Aiken, L., Clarke, S., Sloane, D., Sochalski, J., & Silber, J. (2002). Hospital nurse staffing and patient mortality, nurse burnout, and job dissatisfaction. *Journal of the American Medical Association, 288*, 1987–1993.

Aktan, N. M., Bareford, C. G., Bliss, J. B., Connolly, K., DeYoung, S., Lancellotti Sullivan, K., & Tracy, J. (2009). Comparison of outcomes in a tailored versus accelerated nursing curriculum. *International Journal of Nursing Education Scholarship, 6*, Article 13.

Alanazi, A. A., Nicholson, N., & Thomas, S. (2017). The use of simulation training to improve knowledge, skills, and confidence among healthcare students: A systematic review. *Internet Journal of Allied Health Sciences and Practice, 15*(3), article 2.

Alexander, J. A., Markovitz, A. R., Paustian, M. L., Wise, C. G., El Reda, D. K., Green, L. A., & Fetters, M. D. (2015). Implementation of patient-centered medical homes in adult primary care practices. *Medical Care Research and Review, 72*(4), 438–467.

Allareddy V., Rampa, S., Lee, M. K., Allareddy, V., & Nalliah R. P. (2014). Hospital-based emergency department visits involving dental conditions: Profile and predictors of poor outcomes and resource utilization. *Journal of the American Dental Association, 145*(4), 331–337.

American Association for Respiratory Care. (2015). AARC BOD sets 80% bachelor degree goal by 2020. Retrieved from http://www.aarc.org/aarc-bod-sets-80-bachelor-degree-goal-by-2020

American Association of Nurse Practitioners. (2017). State practice environment. Retrieved from https://www.aanp.org/legislation-regulation/state-legislation/state-practice-environment

Auerbach, D. I., Chen, P. G., Friedberg, M. W., Reid, R., Lau, C., Buerhaus, P. I., & Mehrotra, A. (2013). Nurse-managed health centers and patient-centered medical homes could mitigate expected primary care physician shortage. *Health Affairs, 32*(11), 1933–1941.

Barr, H., Koppel, I., Reeves, S., Hammick, M., & Freeth, D. (2005). *Effective interprofessional education: Argument, assumption and evidence.* Oxford, UK: Blackwell Publishing.

Bates, T., Blash, L., Chapman, S., Dower, C., & O'Neil, E. (2011). *California's health care workforce: Readiness for the ACA era.* San Francisco: Center for the Health Professions at the University of California.

Bell, H. S., Ferretti, S. M., & Ortoski, R. A. (2007). A three-year accelerated medical school curriculum designed to encourage and facilitate primary care careers. *Academic Medicine, 82*(9), 895–899.

Beran, R. L. (1979). The rise and fall of three-year medical school programs. *Academic Medicine, 54*(3), 248–249.

Beronio, K., Po, R., Skopec, L., & Glied, S. (2013). Affordable Care Act will expand mental health and substance use disorder benefits and parity protections for 62 million Americans. ASPE Research Brief, Department of Health and Human Services, Office of the Assistant Secretary for Planning and Evaluation. Retrieved from https://aspe.hhs.gov/sites/default/files/pdf/76591/rb mental.pdf

Bipartisan Policy Center. (2011). The complexities of national health care workforce planning. Washington, DC: Bipartisan Policy Center. Retrieved from http://bipartisanpolicy.org/wp-content/uploads/sites/default/files/Workforce%20study_Public%20Release%20040912.pdf

Bodenheimer, T., Berenson, R. A., & Rudolf, P. (2007). The primary care-specialty income gap: Why it matters. *Annals of Internal Medicine, 146*(4), 301–306.

Bodenheimer, T., & Pham, H. H. (2010). Primary care: Current problems and proposed solutions. *Health Affairs, 29*(5), 799–805.

Bodenheimer, T. S., & Smith, M. D. (2013). Primary care: Proposed solutions to the physician shortage without training more physicians. *Health Affairs, 32*(11), 1881–1886.

Bourgueil, Y., Mouseques, J., & Tajahmadi, A. (2006). *Improving the geographical distribution of health professionals: What the literature tells us. Health economics letter*. Paris, France: Institute for Research and Information in Health Economics.

Braun, P. A., Widmer-Racich, K., Sevick, C., Starzyk, E. J., Mauritson, K., & Hambidge, S. J. (2017). Effectiveness on early childhood caries of an oral health promotion program for medical providers. *American Journal of Public Health, 107*(S1), S97–S103.

Budden, J. S., Moulton, P., Harper, K. J., Brunell, M. L., & Smiley, R. (2016). The 2015 National Nursing Workforce Survey. *Journal of Nursing Regulation, 7*(1), S4–S92.

Buerhaus, P. I., Staiger, D. O., & Auerbach, D. I. (2009). *The future of the nursing workforce in the United States: Data, trends, and implications*. Sudbury, MA: Jones & Bartlett.

California Hospital Association. (2011). Critical roles: California's allied health workforce follow-up report. Retrieved from http://www.calhospital.org/critical-roles

Cant, R. P., & Cooper, S. J. (2017). Use of simulation-based learning in undergraduate nurse education: An umbrella systematic review. *Nurse Education Today, 49*, 63–71.

Chapman, S. A. & Blash, L. (2017). New roles for medical assistants in innovative primary care practices. *Health Services Research, 52*(1), 383–406.

Chen, C., Garrido, T., Chock, D., Okawa, G., & Liang, L. (2009). The Kaiser Permanente electronic health record: Transforming and streamlining modalities of care. *Health Affairs, 28*(2), 323–333.

Chipps, J., Brysiewicz, P., & Mars, M. (2012). A systematic review of the effectiveness of videoconference-based tele-education for medical and nursing education. *Worldviews on Evidence-Based Nursing, 9*(2), 78–87.

Christian, S., Dower, C., & O'Neil, E. (2007).*Overview of nurse practitioner scopes of practice in the United States*. San Francisco: University of California Center for the Health Professions. Retrieved from http://futurehealth.ucsf.edu/Content/29/2007–12_Overview_of_Nurse_Practitioner_Scopes_of_Practice_In_the_United_States_Discussion.pdf

Colwill, J. M., Cultice, J. M., & Kruse, R. L. (2008). Will generalist physician supply meet demands of an increasing and aging population? *Health Affairs, 27*, w232–w241.

Conway, A., O'Donnell, C., & Yates, P. (2017). The effectiveness of the nurse care coordinator role on patient-reported and health service outcomes: A systematic review. *Evaluation and the Health Professions*, 1–34. E-pub ahead of print, retrieved from http://journals.sagepub.com/doi/abs/10.1177/0163278717734610

Cook, D. A., Levinson, A. J., Garside, S., Dupras, D. M., Erwin, P. J., & Montori, V. M. (2008). Internet-based learning in the health professions: A meta-analysis. *Journal of the American Medical Association, 300*(10), 1181–1196.

Council on Credentialing in Pharmacy. (2010). Scope of contemporary pharmacy practice: Roles, responsibilities, and functions of pharmacists and pharmacy technicians. *Journal of the American Pharmacist Association, 50*(2), e35–e69.

Council on Graduate Medical Education. (2010). *COGME 20th report: Advancing primary care*. Rockville, MD: Health Resources and Services Administration. Retrieved from http://www.hrsa.gov/advisorycommittees/bhpradvisory/cogme/Reports/index.html

Courneya, P. T., Palattao, K. J., & Gallagher, J. M. (2013). HealthPartners' online clinic for simple conditions delivers savings of $88 per episode and high patient approval. *Health Affairs, 32*(2), 385–392.

Davis, K., & Guterman, S. (2007). Rewarding excellence and efficiency in Medicare payments. *Milbank Quarterly, 85*, 449–468.

Dickerson, A. E., & Trujillo, L. (2009). Practitioners' perceptions of the occupational therapy clinical doctorate. *Journal of Allied Health, 18*(1), e47–e53.

Du, S., Liu, Z., Liu, S., Yin, H., Xu, G., Zhang, H., & Wang, A. (2013). Web-based distance learning for nurse education: A systematic review. *International Nursing Review, 60*(2), 167–177.

Eaglen, R. H., Arnold, L., Girotti, J. A., Cosgrove, E. M., Green, M. M., Kollisch, D. O., … Tracy, S. W. (2012). The scope and variety of combined baccalaureate-MD programs in the United States. *Academic Medicine, 87*(11), 1600–1608.

Emanuel, E. J., & Fuchs, V. R. (2012). Shortening medical training by 30%. *Journal of the American Medical Association, 307*(11), 1143–1144.

Erikson, C. E., Pittman, P., LaFrance, A., & Chapman, S. A. (2017). Alternative payment models lead to strategic care coordination workforce investments, *Nursing Outlook, 56,* 737–745.

Federal Interagency Forum on Aging-Related Statistics. (2010). *Older Americans 2010: Key indicators of well-being* [Forum]. Washington, DC: U.S. Government Printing Office.

Frank, R. G., Beronio, K., & Glied, S. A. (2014). Behavioral health parity and the Affordable Care Act. *Journal of Social Work in Disability and Rehabilitation, 13*(1–2), 31–43.

Gadbois, E. A., Miller, E. A., Tyler, D., & Intrator, O. (2014). Trends in state regulation of nurse practitioners and physician assistants, 2001 to 2010. *Medical Care Research and Review, 72*(2), 200–219.

Garrard, J., & Weber, R. G. (1974). Comparison of three- and four-year medical school graduates. *Academic Medicine, 49*(6), 547–553.

Gitterman, D., Spetz, J., & Fellowes, M. (2004). The other side of the ledger: Federal health spending in metropolitan economies. Washington, DC: The Brookings Institution. Retrieved from http://www.brookings.edu/research/reports/2004/09/labormarkets-gitterman

Grayson, M. S., Newton, D. A., & Thompson, L. F. (2012). Payback time: The associations of debt and income with medical student career choice. *Medical Education, 46,* 983–991.

Green, L. V., Savin, S., & Lu, Y. (2013). Primary care physician shortages could be eliminated through use of teams, nonphysicians, and electronic communication. *Health Affairs, 32*(1), 11–19.

Greiner, A. C., & Knebel, E. (Eds.). (2003). *Health professions education: A bridge to quality.* Washington, DC: National Academies Press.

Hallock, J. A., Christensen, J. A., Denker, M. W., Hochberg, C. J., Trudeau, W. L. & Williams, J. W. (1977). A comparison of the clinical performance of students in three- and four-year curricula. *Journal of Medical Education, 52,* 658–663.

Hauer, K. E., Durning, S. J., Kernan, W. N., Fagan, M. J., Mintz, M., O'Sullivan, P.S., … Schwartz, M. D. (2008). Factors associated with medical students' career choices regarding internal medicine. *Journal of the American Medical Association, 300*(10), 1154–1164.

Hayden, J. (2010). Use of simulation in nursing education: National survey results. *Journal of Nursing Regulation, 1*(3), 52–57.

Hayden, J. K., Smiley, R. A., Alexander, M., Kandong-Edgren, S., & Jeffries, P. R. (2014). The NCSBN National Simulation Study: A longitudinal, randomized, controlled study replacing clinical hours with simulation in prelicensure nursing education. *Journal of Nursing Regulation, 5*(2), S2–S64.

Horrocks, S., Anderson, E., & Salisbury, C. (2002). Systematic review of whether nurse practitioners working in primary care can provide equivalent care to doctors. *British Medical Journal, 324,* 819–823.

IHS, Inc. (2015). *The complexities of physician supply and demand: Projections from 2013 to 2025.* Washington, DC: American Association of Medical Colleges.

Institute of Medicine. (1972). *Educating for the health team.* Washington, DC: National Academy of Sciences.

Institute of Medicine. (2001). *Crossing the quality chasm: A new health system for the 21st century.* Washington, DC: National Academies Press.

Institute of Medicine. (2008). *Retooling for an aging America: Building the health care workforce.* Washington, DC: National Academies Press.

Institute of Medicine. (2011a). *The future of nursing: Leading change, advancing health.* Washington, DC: National Academies Press.

Institute of Medicine. (2011b). *Allied health workforce and services: Workshop summary.* Washington, DC: National Academies Press.

Institute of Medicine. (2011c). *Improving access to oral health care for vulnerable and under-served populations.* Washington, DC: National Academies Press.

Institute of Medicine. (2014). *Forum on medical and public health preparedness for catastrophic events.* Washington, DC: National Academies Press.

Interprofessional Education Collaborative. (2011). *Core competencies for interprofessional collaborative practice.* Washington, DC: Association of American Medical Colleges.

Ironside, P. M., & McNelis, A. M. (2009). Clinical education in prelicensure nursing programs: Findings from a national study. *Nursing Education Perspectives, 31*(4), 264–265.

Kane, R. L., Shamliyan, T. A., Mueller, C., Duval, S., & Wilt, T. J. (2007). The association of registered nurse staffing levels and patient outcomes. Systematic review and meta-analysis. *Medical Care, 45,* 1195–1204.

Kettel, L. J., Dinham, S. M., Drach, G. W., & Barbee, R. A. (1979). Arizona's three-year medical curriculum: A postmortem. *Academic Medicine, 54*(3), 210–216.

Kleiner, M. M., Marier, A., Park, K. W., & Wing, C. (2014). Relaxing occupational licensing requirements: Analyzing wages and prices for a medical service. National Bureau of Economic Research Working Paper 19906. Retrieved from http://www.nber.org/papers/w19906

Kleiner, M. M., & Park, K. W. (2010). Battles among licensed occupations: Analyzing government regulations on labor market outcomes for dentists and hygienists. National Bureau of Economic Research Working Paper 16560. Retrieved from http://www.nber.org/papers/w16560

Kochan, T., McKersie, R., Eaton, A., & Adler, P. (2009). *Healing together: The labor-management partnership at Kaiser Permanente.* Ithaca, NY: Cornell University Press.

Kohn, L. T., Corrigan, J. M., & Donaldson, M. S. (Eds.). (2000). *To err is human: Building a safer health system.* Washington, DC: National Academies Press.

Kottek, A., Bates, T., & Spetz, J. (2017). *The roles and value of geriatricians in healthcare teams: A landscape analysis.* San Francisco, CA: UCSF Health Workforce Research Center on Long-Term Care.

Kurtzman, E., & Buerhaus, P. (2008). New Medicare payment rules: Danger or opportunity for nursing? *American Journal of Nursing, 108,* 30–35.

Ladden, M. D., Bodenheimer, T., Fishman, N. W., Flinter, M., Hsu, C., Parchman, M., & Wagner, E. H. (2013). The emerging primary care workforce: Preliminary observations from the primary care team: Learning from effective ambulatory practices project. *Academic Medicine, 88*(12), 1830e–1834.

Lammers, E. J., McLaughlin, C. G., & Barna, M. (2016). Physician EHR adoption and potentially preventable hospital admissions among Medicare beneficiaries: Panel data evidence, 2010–2013. *Health Services Research, 51*(6), 2056–2075.

Lang, T. A., Hodge, M., Olson, V., Romano, P. S., & Kravitz, R. L. (2004).Nurse-patient ratios: A systematic review on the effects of nurse staffing on patient, nurse employee, and hospital outcomes. *Journal of Nursing Administration, 34,* 326–337.

Laschinger, S., Medves, J., Pulling, C., McGraw, R., Waytuck, B., Harrison, M., & Gambeta, K. (2008). Effectiveness of simulation on health profession students' knowledge, skills, confidence and satisfaction. *International Journal of Evidence-Based Healthcare, 6*(3), 278–302.

Lenz, E., Mundinger, M., & Kane, R. (2004). Primary care outcomes in patients treated by nurse practitioners or physicians: Two-year follow-up. *Medical Care, 61*(3), 332–351.

Lindsey, P. (2009). Starting an accelerated baccalaureate nursing program: Challenges and opportunities for creative educational innovations. *Journal of Nursing Education, 48,* 279–281.

Liu, Q., Peng, W., Zhang, F., Hu, R., Li, Y., & Yan, W. (2016). The effectiveness of blended learning in health professions: Systematic review and meta-analysis. *Journal of Medical Internet Research, 18*(1), e2.

Maine, L. L., Knapp, K. K., & Scheckelhoff, D. J. (2013). Pharmacists and technicians can enhance patient care even more once national policies, practices, and priorities are aligned. *Health Affairs, 32*(11), 1956–1962.

Marcyjanik, D., & Zorn, C. R. (2011). Accessibility in online nursing education for persons with disability. *Nurse Educator, 36*(6), 241–245.

Martsolf, G. R., Auerbach, D. I., Spetz, J., Pearson, M. L., & Muchow, A. N. (2015). Doctor of nursing practice by 2015: An examination of nursing schools' decisions to offer a doctor of nursing practice degree. *Nursing Outlook, 63*(2), 219–226.

Matherlee, K. (2003). The U.S. health workforce: Definitions, dollars, and dilemmas. Washington, DC: National Health Policy Forum. Retrieved from http://www.nhpf.org/library/background-papers/BP_Workforce_4–03.pdf

McCutcheon, K., Lohan, M., Traynor, M., & Martin, D. (2015). A systematic review evaluating the impact of online or blended learning vs. face-to-face learning of clinical skills in undergraduate nurse education. *Journal of Advanced Nursing, 71*(2), 255–270.

McGaha, A. L., Schmittling, G. T., DeVilbiss Bieck, A. D., Crosley, P. W., & Pugno, P. A. (2010). Entry of U.S. medical school graduates into family medicine residencies: 2009–2010 and 3-year summary. *Family Medicine, 42*(8), 540–551.

Mertz, E. A., Spetz, J., & Moore, J. (2017). Pediatric workforce issues. *Dental Clinics of North America, 61*(3), 577–588.

Nash, D. A. (2009). Adding dental therapists to the health care team to improve access to oral health care for children. *Academic Pediatrics, 9*(6), 446–451.

National Resident Matching Program. (2017). *2017 Main residency match data.* Washington, DC: National Resident Matching Program.

Needleman, J., Buerhaus, P., Mattke, S., Stewart, M., & Zelevinsky, K. (2002). Nurse-staffing levels and the quality of care in hospitals. *New England Journal of Medicine, 346,* 1715–1722.

Nehring, W. M., & Lashley, F. R. (2004). Current use and opinions regarding human patient simulators in nursing education: An international survey. *Nursing Education Perspectives, 25*(5), 244–248.

Newhouse, R. P., Stanik-Hutt, J., White, K. M., Johantgen, M., Bass, E. B., Zangaro, G., … Weiner, J. P. (2011). Advanced practice nurse outcomes 1990–2008: A systematic review. *Nursing Economics, 29*(5), 1–21.

Nicholson, S. (2009). *Will the United States have a shortage of physicians in 10 years?* Princeton, NJ: Robert Wood Johnson Foundation.

Nicholson, S., Vujicic, M., Wanchek, T., Ziebert, A., & Menezes, A. (2015). The effect of education debt on dentists' career decisions. *Journal of the American Dental Association, 146*(11), 800–807.

Ormond, B. A., & Bovbjerg, R. R. (2011). *Assuring access to care under health reform: The key role of workforce policy.* Washington, DC: The Urban Institute.

Pahel, B. T., Rozier, R. G., Stearns, S. C., & Quiñonez, R. B. (2011). Effectiveness of preventive dental treatments by physicians for young Medicaid enrollees. *Pediatrics, 127*(3), e682–e689.

Palaganas, J. C., Epps, C., & Raemer, D. B. (2014). A history of simulation-enhanced interprofessional education. *Journal of Interprofessional Care, 28*(2), 110–115.

Pew Charitable Trusts Dental Campaign. (2016). States expand the use of dental therapy: Research and analysis. Retrieved from http://www.pewtrusts.org/en/research-and-analysis/analysis/2016/09/28/states-expand-the-use-of-dental-therapy

Phoenix, B., Hurd, M., & Chapman, S. A. (2016). Experience of psychiatric mental health nurse practitioners in public mental health. *Nursing Administration Quarterly, 40*(3) 212–224.

Raymond, J. R., Kerschner, J. E., Hueston, W. J., & Maurana, C. A. (2015). The merits and challenges of three-year medical school curricula: Time for an evidence-based discussion. *Academic Medicine, 90*(10), 1318–1323.

Richards, D. A., Hill, J. J., Gask, L., Lovell, K., Chew-Graham, C., Bower, P., … Barkham, M. (2013). Clinical effectiveness of collaborative care for depression in UK primary care (CADET): Cluster randomised controlled trial. *British Medical Journal, 347*, f4913.

Richmond, H., Copsey, B., Hall, A. M., Davies, D., & Lamb, S. E. (2017). A systematic review and meta-analysis of online versus alternative methods for training licensed health care professionals to deliver clinical interventions. *BMC Medical Education, 17*(1), 227.

Rosenthal, T. C. (2014). The medical home: Growing evidence to support a new approach to primary care. *Journal of the American Board of Family Medicine, 21*(5), 427–440.

Sandberg, S. F., Erikson, C., & Yunker, E. D. (2017). Evolving health workforce roles in accountable care organizations. *American Journal of Accountable Care, 5*(2), 9–14.

Schommer, J. C., Cline, R. R., & Larson, T. A. (2005). Pharmacy looks to the future. In M. I. Smith, J. E. Fincham, & A. Wertheimer (Eds.), *Pharmacy and the U.S. health care system* (pp. 417–443). London, UK: Pharmaceutical Press.

Seago, J. A., Spetz, J., Chapman, S., Dyer, W., & Grumbach, K. (2004). *Supply, demand, and use of licensed practical nurses.* Rockville, MD: Bureau of Health Professions, Health Resources, and Services Administration.

Sekscenski, E., Sansom, S., Bazell, C., Salmon, M. E., & Mullan, F. (1994). State practice environments and the supply of physician assistants, nurse practitioners, and certified nurse-midwives. *New England Journal of Medicine, 331*(19), 1266–1271.

Siler, W. L., & Randolph, D. S. (2007). A clinical look at clinical doctorates. *Audiology Today, 19*(1), 22–23.

Skillman, S. M., Snyder, C. R., Frogner, B. K., & Patterson, D. G. (2016). *The behavioral health workforce needed for integration with primary care: Information for health workforce planning.* Seattle: University of Washington Center for Health Workforce Studies.

Spetz, J., Fraher, E., Li, Y., & Bates, T. (2015). How many nurse practitioners provide primary care? It depends on how you count them. *Medical Care Research and Review, 72*(3), 359–375

Spetz, J., & Parente, S. T. (2013). Nurse practitioner scope of practice and cost savings from retail clinics. *Health Affairs, 32*(11), 1977–1984.

Spetz, J., Phibbs, C. S., & Burgess, J. F. (2012). What determines successful implementation of inpatient information technology systems? *American Journal of Managed Care, 19*(3), 157–162.

Stange, K. (2013). How does provider supply and regulation influence health care markets? Evidence from nurse practitioners and physician assistants. *Journal of Health Economics, 33*, 1–27.

Sumaya, C. (2012). Enumeration and composition of the public health workforce: Challenges and strategies. *American Journal of Public Health, 102*(3), 406–474.

Trzebiatowski, G. L., & Peterson, S. (1979). A study of faculty attitudes toward Ohio State's three-year medical program. *Academic Medicine, 54*(3), 205–209.

U.S. Bureau of Economic Analysis. (2017). Domestic product and income: Income and employment by industry (interactive data application). Retrieved from https://bea.gov/itable

U.S. Bureau of Health Professions. (2010). *The registered nurse population: Findings from the 2008 National Sample Survey of Registered Nurses.* Rockville, MD: Health Resources and Services Administration.

U.S. Bureau of Labor Statistics. (2014). Union members—2013. Retrieved from http://www
.bls.gov/news.release/pdf/union2.pdf

U.S. Bureau of Labor Statistics. (2017). Employment projections and occupational outlook
handbook. Retrieved from https://www.bls.gov/emp/tables.htm

U.S. Census Bureau. (2014). National population projections: Summary tables. Retrieved
from https://census.gov/data/tables/2014/demo/popproj/2014-summary-tables.html

U.S. Department of Education. (2018). College affordability and transparency center.
Retrieved from https://collegecost.ed.gov/catc/Default.aspx#

U.S. Health Resources and Services Administration. (2016a). *National and regional projections of supply and demand for primary care practitioners: 2013–2025*. Rockville, MD:
Author.

U.S. National Center for Education Statistics. (2015). Integrated postsecondary education
data system. Retrieved from http://nces.ed.gov/ipeds

U.S. National Center for Education Statistics. (2016). Digest of education statistics, 2015
(NCES 2016–014). Retrieved from https://nces.ed.gov/fastfacts/display.asp?id=76

Weiner, J. P., Yeh, S., & Blumenthal, D. (2013). The impact of health information technology and e-health on the future demand for physician services. *Health Affairs*, *32*(11),
1998–2004.

Willard, R., & Bodenheimer, T. (2012). *The building blocks of high-performing primary care:
Lessons from the field*. Oakland: California HealthCare Foundation.

Wing, P., O'Grady, E., & Langelier, M. (2005). Changes in the legal practice environment of
nurse practitioners. *American Journal for Nurse Practitioners*, *9*(2), 25–39.

Wishner, J. B., & Burton, R. A. (2017). *How have providers responded to the increased demand
for health care under the Affordable Care Act?* Washington, DC: Urban Institute.

Wittich, C. M., Agrawal, A., Cook, D. A., Halvorsen, A. J., Mandrekar, J. N., Chaudhry, S., …
Beckman, T. J. (2017). E-learning in graduate medical education: Survey of residency
program directors. *BMC Medical Education*, *17*(1), 114.

Zacker, H. B. (2011). Creating career pathways for frontline health care workers. *Jobs to
careers: Transforming the front lines of health care*. Retrieved from http://beltline-
org.wpengine.netdna-cdn.com/wp-content/uploads/2013/07/J2C_CareerPath-
ways_011011.pdf

Ziv, A. Wolpe, P. R., Small, S. D., & Glick, S. (2006). Simulation-based medical education: An
ethical imperative. *Simulation in Healthcare*, *1*(4), 252–256.

10

Health Care Financing

James R. Knickman

LEARNING OBJECTIVES

▶ Understand trends in U.S. health care spending over time

▶ Explain the flow of funds into the health system (who pays) and the flow of funds through the system (how providers are paid)

▶ Understand the major categories of services purchased

▶ Differentiate between public and private spending and purchasing in addition to the categories of health plan types within the public and private systems

▶ Explain how 2010 federal health reform legislation is changing the health care financing system

▶ Describe the major reimbursement mechanisms for health care services

KEY TERMS

▶ accountable care organizations (ACOs)

▶ capitated payments

▶ consumer-driven health care

▶ diagnosis-related groups (DRGs)

▶ health maintenance organizations (HMOs)

▶ medical savings account

▶ payer mix

▶ preferred provider organizations (PPOs)

TOPICAL OUTLINE

▶ General overview of health care financing

▶ What the money buys and where it comes from

▶ How health insurance works

▶ How providers are paid for the health services they deliver

▶ Specialized payment approaches used by payers

INTRODUCTION

No matter what role an individual or an organization plays in the U.S. health care system, the complex way we pay for health services in this country influences what is done and how it is done. Most attempts to improve quality and efficiency or to shift resources from one type of health care to another (e.g., from hospital care to primary care or from acute care services to preventive services) also are shaped by how these services are funded.

> The Department of Health and Human Services estimates that within a few years as many as *1.4 million* people could be relying on short-term policies.*

This chapter explains the processes used to pay for health care in the United States. It sets the stage for the next chapter that focuses on the concepts of "costs" and "value" and addresses the difficult question: How much should we spend on health care?

Over the past 5 to 10 years, there has been substantial flux in our national approach to paying for care. The Obama administration's ambitious Patient Protection and Affordable Care Act (ACA) of 2010 has extended health insurance coverage to large numbers of Americans—perhaps as many as 24 million people—affecting both individuals and providers. But the Trump administration has made many changes that have undone key parts of Obamacare and set a path that likely will reduce the number of people covered by Obamacare. In addition, ongoing national concern about the affordability of medical care has led to much activity among payers—especially government payers—to find new payment approaches that moderate expenditure growth trends. Even the Trump changes are reactions in part to affordability; the newest changes likely will decrease the price of insurance for healthy Obamacare enrollees but increase insurance prices for unhealthy enrollees. Clearly, national opinion about affordability and financing challenges vary substantially in America.

This chapter considers the types of care that are paid for, how individuals go about paying for care, and how providers are paid. The chapter also explains the types of insurance and how each works, how the 2010 federal health reforms changed financing, and how reimbursement systems have evolved for paying providers and creating incentives for quality and efficiency. Finally, it describes emerging approaches for limiting the growth of health expenditures in the years to come.

---

*To hear the podcast, go to https://bcove.video/2DZzYso or access the ebook on Springer Publishing Connect™.

GENERAL OVERVIEW OF HEALTH CARE FINANCING

What do we mean by the "financing of health care"? This overarching question includes not only how we pay for care, but also who pays for care, how transactions between users and providers are handled, and how many total dollars are spent on care by an individual and by the entire American population. If we think of health care as a service that people need to purchase, we find that the approach used to purchase this service is far different from the typical approach for purchasing other kinds of services or commodities in our economy.

> If we think of health care as a service that people need to purchase, we find that the approach used to purchase this service is far different from the typical approach for purchasing other kinds of services or commodities in our economy.

For most goods and services other than medical care (such as an automobile or a massage), we use a simple payment system: If you want an item, you pay money for it directly to the person producing the item or the service. Suppliers of goods and services set prices they think make sense; if a purchaser/consumer is willing to pay the price (sometimes there may be a bit of haggling), the transaction happens and the purchaser buys the service. In the U.S. market-based economy, the consumer needs only to have enough money to make the purchase, and the transaction occurs with little intervention from the government or anybody else.

Health care is not a normal commodity or service, however, because of two features:

- The need for health care varies starkly from one individual to another: 20% of Americans use 80% of all health care dollars expended in any given year.
- The cost of health care is very high, and many people could not afford it if they had to pay cash each time they needed a service. For example, in 2011 a typical stay in a hospital routinely costs more than $10,000 and can cost much more than that. An MRI to diagnose the presence of a tumor could cost anywhere between $1,000 and $12,000, depending on where it is done and who is paying for it.

To overcome the obstacle of high costs, the United States has developed an insurance system that allows us to pay for services collectively. Put most simply, we pool our risks for needing health care. In essence, each individual pays what is called a premium to an insurance company, which is representing the average annual costs of health care across the group of people covered by the insurance company with an addition of a payment to cover the costs and profits necessary for the insurer. When these premiums are pooled across a population of people (often employees of a company), there is enough money to pay the expenses of the minority of people who need costly health care. In most years, the majority of people who have health insurance use a blend of services that cost much less than the dollars they put into the pool. In a year when someone has high health care needs, however, that person benefits from being able to tap many more resources from the insurance pool than he or she contributed that year.

This description greatly oversimplifies how the financing system really works across a range of dimensions. In fact:

- There are many types of health insurance; some are publicly paid for through taxes, some are paid for by employers, and others are paid for by individuals directly.
- Insurance does not pay for the entire costs of an individual's health care. Usually, insurance pays only a share of the costs and the individual pays the rest. How this copayment arrangement is structured varies greatly from insurance plan to insurance plan and can be quite complex.
- When insurance becomes involved in the transaction between a service provider and a user of the service, there are rules regarding which services the insurer will pay for and how much it will pay for them. These insurance reimbursement rules also can become incredibly complex and confusing and lead to conflict between insurers and the providers who get paid by the insurers.
- When people do not directly and fully pay for services, economists worry that they will use more services than they need or that a provider will deliver more care than needed. An insurance system must create incentives to avoid overuse and oversupply, or systemwide expenditures could skyrocket.

The U.S. health care financing system has evolved since World War II, when the first health insurance products began to be marketed. In the 1960s, wide-scale public insurance programs were enacted: Medicare, which is insurance for the elderly and the permanently disabled, and Medicaid, which is an insurance-type system for low-income Americans paid for in part by the federal government and in part by state governments.

The U.S. system of financing health care is quite distinct from those used in other developed nations (see Chapter 4). Most other developed countries have a system that involves a set of services to which every citizen is entitled, which is paid for substantially by the central government. In these situations, private insurance companies either help to manage the government-financed system or offer supplementary or alternative coverage.

The emergence of insurance in the United States in the 1940s occurred as new, more effective types of health care technology and practices were being developed. The combination of insurance and rapidly expanding clinical advances led to an expenditure explosion in the 1970s, which has continued ever since. In 1970, U.S. health expenditures totaled $74.9 billion and represented 7.2% of the nation's gross domestic product (GDP)—that is, 7.2% of all goods and services purchased in our economy were health related. By 2020, health expenditures are expected to reach nearly $4.4 trillion, or 19.2% of GDP (see Table 10.1 and Figure 10.1).

The health care financing system described above and that exists today largely acts as if health care is an economic commodity essentially like other commodities and services that people buy with their income. This perspective leads experts and policy makers to explore how an "economic" market for health care needs to be shaped, regulated, and nurtured.

TABLE 10.1 NATIONAL HEALTH EXPENDITURES (IN $ BILLIONS), SELECTED CATEGORIES AND YEARS: 1970–2020

TYPE OF EXPENDITURE	ACTUAL		PROJECTED
	1970	2013	2020
Total national health expenditures	$74.9	$2,914.7	$4,416.2
Total of all personal health care	63.1	2,452.3	3,717.8
Hospital care	27.2	929.0	1,397.4
Physician and clinical services	14.3	588.8	890.4
Prescription drugs	5.5	262.3	397.9
Program administration and net cost of private health insurance	2.6	217.1	339.1

Sources: 2005–2015 data from Centers for Medicare & Medicaid Services; 1970 and 2000 data (Levit, K., Smith, C., Cowan, C., Sensenig, A., Catlin, A., & The Health Accounts Team. (2004). Health spending rebound continues in 2002. *Health Affairs, 23,* 147–159); 2020 data from National Health Expenditures Projections, 2017–2026 (Cuckler, G. et al. Despite uncertainty, fundamentals primarily driving spending growth. (2018). *Health Affairs, 37*[2].)

Many Americans—but not a politically effective majority to date—take a very different perspective. They see health care services as an inherent right, and they see health care as such a complex service to provide that using economic market thinking will never result in an effective system capable of keeping people healthy and getting people better when they face health challenges.

At the current time, however, this idea is an aspiration that does not fundamentally currently shape the health financing system (Swendiman, 2010). However, many publicly financed health care programs described below do address the idea that we need to facilitate access to care for people who have low incomes and/or very serious illnesses.

FIGURE 10.1 U.S. NATIONAL HEALTH EXPENDITURE AS A SHARE OF GROSS DOMESTIC PRODUCT: 1970–2020

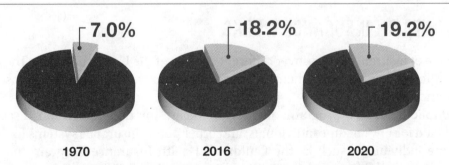

1970	2016	2020
7.0%	18.2%	19.2%

Sources: 2005–2016 data from Centers for Medicare & Medicaid Services; 1970 and 2000 data (Levit, K., Smith, C., Cowan, C., Sensenig, A., Catlin, A., & The Health Accounts Team. (2004). Health spending rebound continues in 2002. *Health Affairs, 23,* 147–159); 2020 data from National Health Expenditures Projections, 2017–2026 (Cuckler, G. et al. Despite uncertainty, fundamentals primarily driving spending growth. (2018). *Health Affairs, 37*[2].)

WHAT THE MONEY BUYS AND WHERE IT COMES FROM

If we consider all types of expenditures in the health system, the total national bill in 2016 was $3.3 trillion, which represented 18.2% of the national GDP that year (see Figure 10.1). The overwhelming share of this money ($2.8 trillion, or 85%) paid for personal health care services to individuals, whereas the balance paid for public health services, research, and administrative costs associated with running the delivery and financing system (see Table 10.1). Among personal health care services, 73% of expenditures focus on three types of care: (a) hospital care, the largest type by far; (b) physician and other clinical services; and (c) prescription drugs. Administrative costs associated with running the health insurance and other regulatory systems represent 9% of expenditures for personal health care services.

How Individuals Pay for Health Care

We begin with basics, considering how individuals pay for health care when they become ill or injured. In essence, there are two main ways an individual pays for a service: (a) through the person's insurance coverage or (b) with out-of-pocket cash from income or savings. For people who are uninsured and have no money, there is a third option: They can attempt to obtain the service free, as a charity case, often through a safety-net provider. States have various laws about when providers must give charity care, and the insurance system—especially public insurance—gives providers some money to help reimburse them for the charity care they deliver.

People who have either a public or a private insurance policy usually can receive services after showing their insurance card. The provider then bills the insurance company directly, although some providers demand that the individual pay the bill when the service is provided, in which case the individual must seek reimbursement from the insurer. If a person's insurance will pay for only part of the bill, the individual is usually responsible for paying the balance at the time services are delivered.

HOW HEALTH INSURANCE WORKS

A range of insurance types cover different subsets of the U.S. population. The first key differentiation among them is public programs versus privately sponsored insurance products.

Public insurance programs include Medicare for the elderly and disabled; Medicaid for low-income individuals; and other public insurance systems for low-income individuals, such as the Children's Health Insurance Program (CHIP), which covers children who are ineligible for Medicaid. Other public insurance programs cover veterans, public employees, members of the armed services and their families, and Native Americans.

Private insurance coverage varies depending on who pays for it. Small employers can purchase coverage for their workers through commercial companies (such as insurance companies like UnitedHealthcare, Aetna, or Kaiser Permanente).

Individuals who work for employers that offer no coverage or who are self-employed or unemployed may buy insurance through commercial companies. Individuals also can buy insurance through the insurance exchanges established by the ACA. These exchanges link individuals to a range of commercial insurance offerings, and the federal government subsidizes the premiums charged within the exchange for families with earnings between 138% and 400% of the federal poverty level (FPL). Large employers can buy coverage from commercial companies, or they can self-insure. Large employers often can save substantial costs by self-insuring, which they can do because they have so many employees that the risks balance out. When an employer does self-insure, it usually engages a commercial insurance company to manage the plan, make payments to providers, and enforce its rules.

Publicly Financed Programs

Medicaid

Medicaid originally was designed to assist recipients of public assistance—primarily single-parent families and low-income people who are aged, blind, or disabled (see Chapter 3). Over the years, Medicaid has expanded to include additional groups and now covers poor children, their parents, pregnant women, the disabled, and very poor adults (including those 65 and older). Much public attention is given to Medicaid's role in covering children's care; in reality, however, 64% of its expenditures support care for the 35% of enrollees who are elderly or disabled (see Figure 10.2).

Medicaid is administered by the states, and state and federal governments both finance the program. Except for requiring coverage for certain types of services, the federal government gives states flexibility in implementing and administering Medicaid to best meet the needs of their residents. As a result, there are many seemingly arbitrary differences in eligibility, coverage, and provider payment rates across states.

The ACA has provisions to expand the range of services covered by each state through the Medicaid program. The ACA also uses federal funds to expand the income eligibility for Medicaid to all individuals living in families with incomes below 138% of the FPL. However, court challenges to this provision have led to allowing states to opt out of accepting federal funds to expand coverage. In 2018, 14 states had chosen not to expand Medicaid eligibility (Kaiser Family Foundation, 2018).

A major change in Medicaid occurred when many states adopted a managed care approach in the early 1990s. In this payment strategy, the state usually pays a fixed, or "capitated," payment to an insurer, who then is responsible for keeping average costs for Medicaid patients below this fixed payment level. It has been difficult, however, for many states to accrue savings using a managed care approach. In most states, Medicaid already paid providers rates that were below (sometimes significantly below) commercial levels, and it was difficult for managed care insurers to reduce them further. Additional reductions would have squeezed safety-net providers, which largely depend on Medicaid revenues, jeopardizing their financial viability.

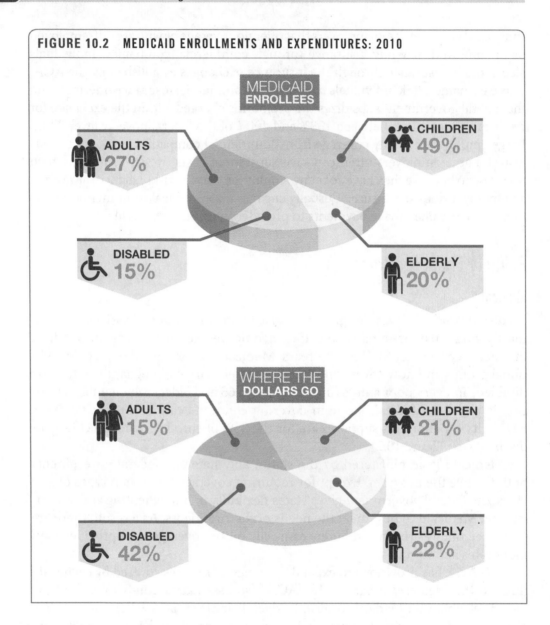

FIGURE 10.2   MEDICAID ENROLLMENTS AND EXPENDITURES: 2010

Medicare

Administered by the federal government, Medicare originally targeted people aged 65 and over, but it was quickly expanded to cover people with disabilities and severe kidney disease. To qualify, an individual must be a U.S. resident for a specified number of years and pay the Federal Insurance Contributions Act (FICA) payroll tax for at least 10 years. The entitlement was expanded in 1972 to allow people who did not meet the latter requirement to pay a premium for coverage. Even though enrollment in Medicare has doubled since its passage, annual expenditures have increased about 40-fold, making the federal government the nation's single largest payer of health care expenses.

Medicare has three key parts: Part A, which is hospital insurance; Part B, which is supplemental medical insurance covering physician services and outpatient care; and Part D, which pays for a substantial share of pharmaceutical costs. The Balanced Budget Act of 1997 established the Medicare+Choice program, designed to build on existing Medicare managed care programs and expand options under Part B to include plans that offer expansions in what services are covered in return for restricted panels of providers that enrollees can use.

In the 1980s and 1990s, Medicare experienced a series of changes to its payment mechanisms, which appear to have had at least temporary impacts on rising health care expenditures. In the 1980s, Medicare started paying hospitals under a payment system that set fixed prices (varying by region and the intensity of service required) for each stay in a hospital by a Medicare-covered patient instead of the traditional approach of paying for each day spent in a hospital. By the 1990s, Medicare also had started paying physicians differently, using fixed payment schedules for different types of physician services.

The George W. Bush administration added pharmaceutical coverage to Medicare through the Medicare Modernization Act, passed in December 2003. This coverage was expanded for Medicare enrollees as a part of the ACA of 2010.

Other Public Programs

In addition to Medicaid and Medicare, the United States has a patchwork of government health care programs for special populations: active duty and retired military personnel and their families, Native Americans, and injured and disabled workers.

PROGRAMS FOR ACTIVE DUTY AND RETIRED MILITARY PERSONNEL Historically, most health care needs of active duty military personnel have been handled in military facilities, where retirees and families also could receive free treatment on a space-available basis. U.S. Department of Defense spending on medical care more than tripled from 1988 to 2005, rising from $14.6 billion to $49 billion.

The Veterans Health Administration, the health care system of the Department of Veterans Affairs (VA), operates the largest integrated health care system in the United States, providing primary care, specialized care, and related medical and social support services to U.S. veterans and their dependents. In recent years, the VA has faced stiff criticism for its waiting lists for services due to a large number of returning veterans from the Iraq and Afghanistan conflicts as well as the aging of many veterans who served during the Vietnam War. There have been expanded initiatives to allow veterans to use community-based services when they find it difficult to gain access to services provided directly by VA-run health care facilities.

THE INDIAN HEALTH SERVICE In 1921, the Snyder Act established a program of health services for Native Americans, known today as the Indian Health Service (IHS) and administered by the U.S. Department of Health and Human Services (DHHS). Eligible participants are members of federally recognized Indian tribes and their descendants. The program's budget is approximately $4 billion to $5 billion annually, and it serves approximately 2.2 million of the nation's estimated 3.7 million American Indians and Alaska Natives (DHHS, IHS, 2016).

WORKERS' COMPENSATION Workers' compensation is an insurance system intended to protect workers against the costs of medical care and loss of income resulting from work-related injuries and, in some cases, illnesses. Underlying workers' compensation is the premise that all job-related injuries, regardless of fault, are a result of the risks of employment, and the employer and employee should share the burden of loss. Workers' compensation programs are operated by the states, each with its own authorizing legislation and requirements. The first such law was enacted in New York in 1910; by 1948, all states had a workers' compensation program.

Privately Financed Health Care

The private share of health care expenditures is made up of direct payments by individuals (representing 11% of total expenditures) and payments made by private insurance companies (representing 34% of expenditures). Public payments represent the balance at 55%.

Employer-Based Insurance

During the Great Depression, hospitals found that most Americans could not afford to pay their bills. The hospital industry, through the American Hospital Association, supported the growth of the first major health insurers: the Blue Cross plans in each state that pay for hospital care and the Blue Shield plans that pay for physician and other outpatient services. Over time, these nonprofit insurers had to compete with for-profit insurance companies, which emerged during World War II when unions began fighting for medical insurance to be part of employee benefits packages.

Growth in the health insurance market was a by-product of wartime wage and price controls; because wages couldn't be increased, enhanced benefits packages were one way unions and employees could obtain increased compensation. Growth accelerated after a decision by the Internal Revenue Service that employers could take a tax deduction for the cost of employee health insurance. The growing costs of health care, of course, would have led to increased private or public insurance coverage eventually.

During the next several decades, the employer-based health insurance system became increasingly entrenched. By the end of 2002, more than 64% of Americans received health insurance through their employer (Glied & Borzi, 2004). Since then, the percentage of Americans obtaining employer-based health insurance has slowly but steadily decreased, reaching 61% in 2008 and 49% in 2016.

The Individual Insurance Market

Although employer-based insurance dominates the private health insurance sector, a significant number of people must arrange and pay for health insurance on their own. The Employee Benefit Research Institute found that, in 2014, even though more than 160 million nonelderly Americans were covered by employment-based health benefits, about 34 million purchased coverage for themselves and family members in the individual market (Fronstin, 2015). As implementation of insurance exchanges supported by the ACA began in 2014, however, individual coverage grew quickly—totaling 8 million people the first year of the exchanges, with an expectation that this number could grow to 24 million by 2024. This growth is due in part to the substantial premium subsidies supported by the ACA and to a mandate that, until redesigned by the Trump administration, imposed tax penalties on people who did not have insurance coverage. The ACA offers substantial subsidies for many Americans to purchase insurance as individuals. Almost 14 million people purchased subsidized private insurance after the law was implemented in 2014 and the number is expected to grow to at least 16 million.

Consolidated Omnibus Budget Reconciliation Act

The Consolidated Omnibus Budget Reconciliation Act (COBRA) of 1985 attempts to reduce gaps in insurance coverage for individuals who are between jobs. The act requires employers to extend health insurance benefits to former employees for up to 18 months. Depending on qualifying circumstances, coverage may be extended for a spouse or dependent children for up to 36 months. Employees generally pay the entire premium for the coverage.

COBRA coverage can be expensive because many employers offer insurance that is generous in scope. It is likely that policies offered by the insurance exchanges will be less expensive than COBRA for many people, so COBRA might represent a diminishing share of insurance coverage over time.

HOW PROVIDERS ARE PAID FOR THE HEALTH SERVICES THEY DELIVER

Insurance Payments

Most services delivered by medical care providers are paid for through the complex insurance system described in the previous section. In the case of public payers (mostly Medicare and Medicaid), payment rates for providers are fixed by a complex set of rules and formulas set in place by public policy. The rates are in essence a "take it or leave it" offer from the federal government. In recent years, as public insurance rates have either decreased or not increased as fast as health care inflation, a number of providers have stopped serving Medicare or Medicaid patients.

> In recent years, as public insurance rates have either decreased or not increased as fast as health care inflation, a number of providers have stopped serving Medicare or Medicaid patients.

Private insurers go through a negotiation process with hospitals, physicians, and other providers to establish what will be paid by the insurer for each type of service. These negotiations can be quite complex and quite heated as both the payer and the provider seek favorable rates. Physicians often have less clout in these negotiations than hospitals unless they are organized into large groups or are in communities with physician shortages. In most areas, there are enough physicians to give insurers the upper hand in bargaining. The difficulty of negotiating good rates is one factor driving physicians to either join **preferred provider organizations** (PPOs) or to take salaried positions within hospital systems or in large corporate medical practices.

The various approaches to paying physicians used by Medicare, Medicaid, and private insurers have resulted in decreased payments to many physicians and falling or static incomes for many types of physicians over the past 5 to 10 years. In addition to tighter payment approaches, the recession of 2008–2010 decreased the demand for physician services. More people were uninsured and very price sensitive during the difficult economic times, and volumes have not recovered since that period.

Hospitals, by contrast, often have good negotiation positions because there are fewer hospitals in each community, and many people insist on having access to hospitals they perceive as high in quality. Smaller hospitals or community hospitals that are not academic medical centers sometimes have substantially less negotiating power. Just like physicians, however, hospitals have felt intense pressure on revenues since the recession of 2008–2010.

Any provider that does not negotiate rates with an insurer through a contract is considered an out-of-network provider by that insurer. Often, insurers do not reimburse patients who use out-of-network providers, or they provide only a specified amount and make the patient responsible for the difference between this amount and a hospital's charges.

In general, actual payment rates vary markedly across types of payers. Private insurers often pay the best rates because of the negotiation process; Medicare pays the second-highest rates generally, and Medicaid payment rates tend to be lowest. One exception to this pattern is federally qualified health centers, which often care for low-income people and have high reimbursement rates paid by public payers. These high rates reflect a priority to ensure access to care for low-income people and to compensate for what is often higher-than-average health care complexity for populations served by community health centers.

The financial viability of any given hospital, physician, or other provider often is crucially associated with the **payer mix** among the provider's patients. Providers that do not have a healthy share of patients covered by private insurance sometime have a difficult task covering costs.

Payments Made Directly by Patients

The other key source of reimbursement in health care comes directly from payments made by individuals. Individuals without insurance must pay cash for services, and individuals who use out-of-network providers also must pay cash and then seek reimbursement from their insurers. In recent years, an increased number of physicians have decided to be out-of-network providers, putting more payment responsibility on individual patients. This is particularly the case for specialty physicians in urban markets who serve wealthy patients and even more so for physicians who have reputations for high quality.

> In recent years, more and more physicians have decided to be out-of-network providers, putting more payment responsibility on individual patients.

On the payer side, insurers also are contributing to the growth in out-of-network providers as insurers move to so-called narrow networks of providers with whom they contract. Insurers are finding that they can offer lower rates if they concentrate their business among a small set of providers. Increasing numbers of consumers and employers seem willing to trade the right to select from a large network of providers for the opportunity to pay less for insurance. Most notably, the insurance products offered in the insurance exchanges set up by the ACA most often offer only access to narrow networks.

The prices charged by providers, especially hospitals, have become increasingly controversial. Many hospitals set very high rates for the relatively few patients who pay out of pocket for hospital care. In addition, these rates are rarely transparent; most patients are not told what care will cost until after they have received the care. Such practices have spurred a movement pushing for more transparency of prices charged by hospitals and more logic to the basis for setting prices.

SPECIALIZED PAYMENT APPROACHES USED BY PAYERS

Over the past 30 years, many new payment approaches have been developed in the attempt to achieve two goals: (a) reduce the high rate of year-to-year cost inflation in health care and (b) create incentives for providers to deliver higher-quality care and to use more efficient practices to manage patient care. The elusive sweet spot in the design of payment approaches is to pay providers adequately to deliver high-quality, needed services but to create incentives for both providers and patients to avoid overusing care and to devote attention and resources to keeping people healthy.

This chapter describes some of the historical and current approaches to reimbursement of providers. Chapter 11 describes many of the current new approaches to reimbursement that are being tested and tried around the country.

The approaches to reimbursement that have evolved historically over the years fall into three broad categories: (a) managed care; (b) consumer-driven care and high deductibles; and (c) fixed payment approaches—diagnostic groups, prospective payments, and bundled payments.

Managed Care

The biggest change in the privately financed portion of the U.S. health care system over the last three decades is the shift toward various forms of managed care: prepaid health plans, PPOs, and **accountable care organizations** (ACOs). Large businesses and government payers steered this shift in an attempt to reduce their health insurance costs.

Prepaid Health Plans

Managed care plans structure and reimburse care differently than conventional insurance. Very strict managed care plans, such as **health maintenance organizations** (HMOs), receive **capitated payments** and control which providers participate in their network. Capitated payments are fixed monthly or annual payments for each person for whom an insurer and/or a provider is responsible to deliver care, regardless of the amount and kinds of services eventually needed.

> The theory was that capitation would encourage providers to think more carefully about the necessity of costly tests and procedures and discourage unnecessary referrals to expensive specialists.

HMOs also often require primary care physicians to be gatekeepers to other types of services by requiring referrals for diagnostic tests and specialty care.

The theory was that capitation would encourage providers to think more carefully about the necessity of costly tests and procedures and discourage unnecessary referrals to expensive specialists. After all, in a world of capitated payments, providers actually lose money every time they deliver a service rather than making additional money. Despite capitation's limits on reimbursement, providers were expected to participate because they would have a captive audience of patients—in other words, they could make up any reimbursement shortfall by having increased numbers of patients. Patients, in return for giving up the freedom to use whichever physician or hospital they chose, would receive more organized care, with specialist and primary care more effectively coordinated. And, they often face fewer deductibles and copayments when they use providers in a prepaid health plan.

HMOs often act as both the insurer and the provider of services. However, HMOs use a range of approaches to providing services. Some employ physicians and own hospitals, whereas others contract with networks of physicians and with local hospitals. The best known HMO, Kaiser Permanente, uses a defined network of salaried physicians and owns its hospitals.

In the late 1990s, after a period of high-cost inflation, less-organized approaches to managed care began to spread widely. Consumers began to dislike these approaches, however, because they perceived many features as overly restrictive. They wanted to choose their own physicians, resented specialty care gatekeeping and other managed care hassle factors, and demanded more plan options. Consumers complained loudly to employers, who eventually moved toward offering less tightly controlled plans, which were not capitated for providers. This trend was in stark contrast to Medicaid managed care, which enrolls about two-thirds of Medicaid recipients nationwide into capitated programs in order to control spending. Similarly, some states are moving toward using managed care plans exclusively for Medicaid recipients.

Today, most consumers choose not to enroll in HMO plans. Only in California and, to a lesser extent in the other West Coast states, do HMOs represent a significant share of the insurance and service delivery market. In many areas of the country—including most of the eastern half—HMO penetration is minimal. Many seniors, however, enroll in Medicare Advantage insurance options that often operate like HMOs or tightly organized managed care plans.

Preferred Provider Organizations

At the unstructured end of the managed care spectrum are PPOs, rapidly growing organizations that encourage plan members to use a list of physicians with whom they have negotiated discounts and who sometimes work collaboratively as affiliated physician practices. Narrow networks are an offspring of the PPO concept and generally involve little if any coordination across providers in what, in essence, is a list of providers that have accepted an insurer's payment rate offer. Insured members who use a PPO or a narrow network are rewarded with lower out-of-pocket costs (deductibles, copays, and coinsurance). Patients who use an out-of-network provider often pay the difference between the insurer's reimbursement rate and whatever the physician charges. In strict forms of narrow network plans, an insurer pays nothing if an out-of-network provider is used by a covered patient.

Consumer-Driven Health Care and High Deductibles

Approaches to insurance that focus on making consumers sense price signals when they purchase health care is often called **consumer-driven health care**. This reimbursement idea generally involves setting a high deductible that individuals must pay before they receive insurance benefits. In some cases, costs of care during a deductible period can be paid by a **medical savings account** that employers or employees set up for health-related costs.

In many ways, consumer-driven health care—which puts individuals at risk to pay the bulk of everyday health care and pharmaceutical needs—offers a stark alternative to the managed care option. In consumer-driven health care, patients have free choice about who they receive care from but face sizable personal financial risk for deductibles and high prices of health care. This financial risk is particularly difficult for people with chronic health conditions.

Another form of copayment that represents consumer-driven health care is called reference pricing. This system involves a payer exploring the range of prices charged by different providers for a specific service in a given community.

The payer then identifies a subset of providers that charge a average or lower than average prices and have good health outcomes. The payer can set this price as the reference price and establish a rule that people covered by the insurance plan receive no more than the reference price as a reimbursement, even if they choose a provider that charges more than the reference price. The aim of this system is to force high-price providers to rethink how they manage the procedure in question and how they can reduce the costs of providing the service and to provide a strong incentive for consumers to choose an efficient provider. Providers that do not lower prices will lose business to the lower-cost providers—as happens in most markets for goods and services in our economy.

One final feature of consumer-driven health care is a set of efforts to make health care costs more transparent to the user of the services and to improve access to medical care. For example, in some cases this type of plan insists that payers set fixed prices, which enrollees can be made aware of, before a service is provided. Other features include greater use of email and phone calls to facilitate patient–provider interaction and walk-in hours that allow patients to see a provider on the same day they become ill. Many efforts to improve price transparency are not led by insurers or providers but by government and consumer-oriented organizations reacting to complaints from patients that they do not realize the price they will have to pay until after a medical care service is provided.

Fixed Payment Approaches

Diagnosis-Related Groups

One of the first examples of a reimbursement approach aimed at creating incentives for providers to be efficient was the 1981 Medicare hospital reimbursement system that dramatically altered the way hospitals were paid for the services they delivered. The **diagnosis-related group** (DRG) system set rates prospectively—that is, a payer said up-front that it would pay a fixed amount for the hospital stay of a patient with a specific diagnosis and no more (with some outlier exceptions), no matter how much the patient's care eventually cost or how long the hospitalization turned out to be. Fixed payments give hospitals a powerful incentive to increase efficiency, minimize unnecessary tests and services, and shorten patients' hospital stays.

Bundled Payment Rates

In concept, the early idea of DRGs is being expanded by the emerging concept of bundled payments, which pay both the physician and the hospital a fixed amount to provide an episode of care or, in the case of patients with chronic conditions, a specified time period of care. The details about how bundled payments are structured and about early evidence of how they reduce costs is covered in Chapter 11.

Prospective Payment Rates for Physicians and Other Providers

A companion idea to DRGs was the Medicare program's approach to using standardized principles to set rates for different specialists and for patients with different medical needs. The system is called the resource-based relative value scale (RBRVS) (Hsiao et al., 1988). Rates are determined through detailed research measuring the expected time and other resource inputs that physicians need to deliver a specific service.

Each state's Medicaid program also developed physician reimbursement rates, generally adopting the federal approach of using formulas to set rates rather than negotiate with physicians. Medicaid rates are often much lower than Medicare rates for the same services. The ACA mandates that state Medicaid programs raise physician reimbursement rates to at least 60% of the rates paid by Medicare. This provision is designed to increase the number of physicians willing to care for Medicaid patients.

CONCLUSION

The American approach to paying for health care has become incredibly complicated. It is complicated for consumers, for providers, and even for payers. The complexity is due to the difficult task of making sure payment approaches do not result in over- or underuse and supply of medical care by people with insurance. For almost 50 years, we have been constantly experimenting with new ideas for reimbursement approaches that work better for all of the parties involved.

But payment strategy is not the only challenge related to financing. Of equal concern is that 5% of people living in America have no insurance coverage, and this percentage could grow over the next few years if the ACA unravels. Our health system will continue to require a safety net for the vulnerable and the uninsured no matter what evolves. A world of tight reimbursements will make it increasingly difficult for hospitals and other providers to pay for safety-net care by shifting dollars from other payers and revenue sources.

What will happen if federal health reform does not achieve the anticipated expansions of access and control over the growth in health care costs? One of two radical options will most likely emerge: (a) collapse of the private approach to health care financing, which would lead to a single-payer public system like those in most other parts of the developed world (see Chapter 4), or (b) the emergence of a three-tiered system of care that maintains great access to care for wealthy Americans with comfortable incomes but restricts access moderately for middle-income Americans and rations care brutally for low-income Americans. Either option goes against fundamental principles engrained in U.S. history and politics: free enterprise on one hand and equality and equity on the other. The task of implementing a 21st-century financing system that will endure must engage new thinkers, new leaders, and new researchers who can reinterpret these principles in light of current realities.

▶ CASE EXERCISE—BECOMING AN ACCOUNTABLE CARE ORGANIZATION VERSUS NOT BECOMING AN ACCOUNTABLE CARE ORGANIZATION

You are the chief executive officer of a large, technology-intensive hospital in a community of 200,000 people. The community includes two other, smaller community hospitals and a wide range of physicians and other providers working in private practice. Currently, you are paid a fixed amount by Medicare—the federal insurance program for the elderly—for every eligible admission to your hospital, based on the severity of the patient's needs. Physicians and other providers in your community are paid fee-for-service.

The federal government has offered to form an accountable care organization (ACO) in your community that could accept a capitated annual payment for each person eligible for Medicare. Answer the following questions:

1. How would you go about deciding whether to accept the government's offer?
2. Would you want to lead the ACO or just be a part of it?
3. Would you argue for or against accepting the federal offer? Why?
4. If you wanted to proceed and lead the effort to form an ACO, how would you coordinate with the other local hospitals and providers?
5. How might you change the way care currently is organized in your community, given the new financial incentives embedded in a capitated rate?

DISCUSSION QUESTIONS

1. What complications does our current financing system cause for providers of care?
2. What complications does our insurance system cause for individual consumers?
3. What are some of the promising new approaches to changing our health system so that it has incentives to provide more efficient care?
4. Some people view increases in health care spending as a response to consumer demand, whereas others see these increases as potentially wasteful spending. When other industry sectors consume a rising share of GDP, it is viewed as a positive development. Should we be concerned about the rising cost of health care and its share of our GDP? What types of health care spending might be classified as valuable? As wasteful?

REFERENCES

Cuckler, G. et al. (2018). National Health Expenditures Projections, 2017–2026. Despite uncertainty, fundamentals primarily driving spending growth. *Health Affairs, 37*(2). https://doi.org/10.1377/hlthaff.2017.1655)

Fronstin, P. (2015, October). *Sources of health insurance coverage: A look at changes between 2013 and 2014 from the March 2014 and 2015 current population survey* (EBRI Issue Brief No. 419). Washington, DC: Employee Benefit Research Institute.

Glied, S. A., & Borzi, P. C. (2004). The current state of employer based health care. *Journal of Law, Medicine and Ethics, 32*, 404–409. doi:10.1111/j.1748-720X.2004.tb00150.x

Hsiao, W. C., Braun, P., Becker, E. R., Causino, N., Couch, N. P., DiNicola, M., & Douwe, B. Y. (1988). *A national study of resource-based relative value scales for physician services: Final report to the Health Care Financing Administration* (Publication 17-C-98795/1–03). Boston, MA: Harvard School of Public Health.

Kaiser Family Foundation. (2018). Status of state action on the Medicaid expansion decision. Retrieved from http://kff.org/health-reform/state-indicator/state-activity-around-expanding-medicaid-under-the-affordable-care-act

Levit, K., Smith, C., Cowan, C., Sensenig, A., Catlin, A., & The Health Accounts Team. (2004). Health spending rebound continues in 2002. *Health Affairs, 23*, 147–159. doi:10.1377/hlthaff.23.1.147

Swendiman, K. S. (2010) *Health care: Constitutional rights and legislative powers* (R40826). Damascus. MD: Penny Hill Press, Damascus, MD: Congressional Research Service.

U.S. Department of Health and Human Services, Indian Health Service. (2016). *IHS fact sheets, IHS Profile*. Washington, DC: Author.

11

Health Care Costs and Value

David C. Radley and John Marchica

LEARNING OBJECTIVES

- Understand contributing factors to the growth in health care costs in the United States over the past 60 years
- Explain value in terms of health care
- Recognize conflicts embedded within the health care delivery system that drive up costs and reduce value
- Identify why attempts at cost control have not succeeded

KEY TERMS

- accountable care organizations (ACOs)
- bundled payments
- electronic health records (EHRs)
- fee-for-service payment models
- overscreening
- waste

TOPICAL OUTLINE

- Spending levels and cost growth
- Defining and measuring value in health care
- Cost drivers and barriers to achieving value
- Initiatives to address expenditure/value tradeoffs
- Value-based payment models
- Delivery system reform
- State-driven value-based initiatives

INTRODUCTION

This chapter focuses on value—the intersection between spending, quality, and outcomes—in health care. Delivering high-quality health care at a cost that is sustainable over time is a pressing issue in the United States. In 2016, Americans spent $3.3 trillion, nearly one-fifth of all economic activity in the United States and equal to about $10,400 per person on health care (Hartman, Martin, Espinosa, Catlin, & National Health Expenditure Accounts Team, 2018). We spend more on health care in this country than other industrialized nations, yet the quality of the care delivered and subsequent patient outcomes are not notably better (Reinhardt, Hussey, & Anderson, 2004). As the U.S. population ages and new tests and treatments are developed, increased pressure to spend more will inevitably be passed along to federal, state, and local governments as well as to our nation's businesses and families. This chapter explores the idea of value in health care by describing health care spending levels and trends and discussing the implications of spending growth; discussing the reasons spending levels are high, sometimes to the detriment of care quality; and presenting ideas and current tactics to lower costs in ways that enhance the payoffs from our health spending.

> Life expectancy in the United States is up, as is the medical profession's ability to diagnose and treat disease, which are undeniable benefits. But other countries have experienced similar gains without incurring the same rising costs.*

SPENDING LEVELS AND COST GROWTH

In 1960, several years before the implementation of our major public insurance programs, national spending on health care totaled about $221 billion in current (2016) dollars. (Actual spending in 1960 was $27.2 billion, but there has been natural inflation in the economy over time. At today's inflation-affected prices, this $27.2 billion is equivalent to $221 billion. We present the inflation-adjusted figures when referring to 1960 expenditures in order to focus on "real" changes in spending.) On a per capita basis, this 1960 spending equaled $1,184 per person in inflation-adjusted dollars. Per capita spending grew 775% in real terms between 1960 and 2016, reaching nearly $10,348 per person in 2016. Importantly, the average annual growth in health care spending between 1960 and 2016 was about 9%, whereas nominal gross domestic product (GDP) growth during this period was 6.5%—meaning that health care spending grew substantially faster than other economic activity over the past five decades.[1]

---

[1]Analysis of historical National Health Expenditure (NHE) data, prepared by Centers for Medicare & Medicaid Services (CMS), Office of the Actuary, National Health Statistics Group, and available at https://www.cms.gov/Research-Statistics-Data-and-Systems/Statistics-Trends-and-Reports/NationalHealthExpendData/index.html. Inflation adjustments made using 1960 and 2016 CPI-U (Consumer Price Index for Urban Consumers) estimates, available at https://www.bls.gov/cpi/tables/supplemental-files/historical-cpi-u-201804.pdf

*To hear the podcast, go to https://bcove.video/2PnH2kM or access the ebook on Springer Publishing Connect™.

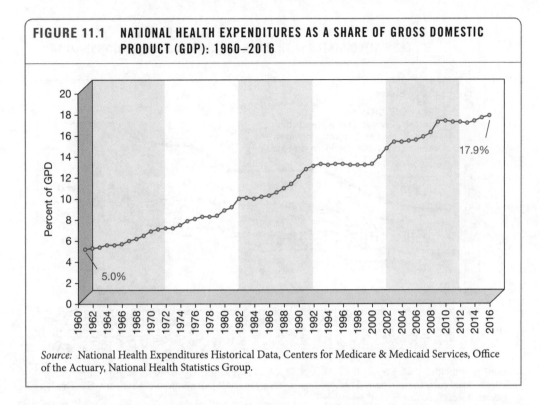

FIGURE 11.1   NATIONAL HEALTH EXPENDITURES AS A SHARE OF GROSS DOMESTIC PRODUCT (GDP): 1960–2016

Source: National Health Expenditures Historical Data, Centers for Medicare & Medicaid Services, Office of the Actuary, National Health Statistics Group.

A common way to think about health care spending is to put it in terms of GDP. Health care spending currently accounts for almost one-fifth of all economic activity in the United States, or 17.9% of GDP. Since 1960, health spending as a share of GPD has more than tripled, with an overall steady rise marked by periods of flat and accelerating growth (Figure 11.1).

A key issue is whether we should be concerned about how health care spending has grown over the past half century. Life expectancy has also increased during that time, and we've seen staggering advancements in our ability to detect and treat disease—higher spending simply reflects the investment made to support progress. While the evolution in medical science is undeniable, it is not a uniquely American phenomenon.

Certainly other nations have experienced increased health care spending, but the United States is unique in the degree of its increase—far outpacing even the nation with the second largest growth. In 1980, the United States devoted more of its GDP to health care spending (9%) than other developed nations, but the difference was not extraordinary. The United States, however, was on a different trajectory, and by 2014, U.S. spending as a share of GDP far exceeded that for other comparable nations (Figure 11.2).

If the United States spent significantly more on health care and received significantly better health outcomes, then health care cost growth might not be considered problematic. However, according to the Organisation for Economic Cooperation and Development (OECD), the United States ranks 26th out of 35 member countries for life expectancy and just below the OECD average for life expectancy. Nolte and McKee (2012), in tracking deaths before age 75 from conditions largely treatable

FIGURE 11.2   HEALTH CARE SPENDING AS A SHARE OF GROSS DOMESTIC PRODUCT (GDP)
IN THE UNITED STATES WITH INTERNATIONAL COMPARISON: 1980–2014

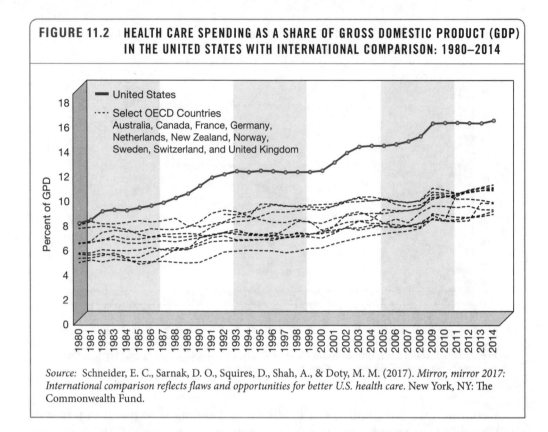

Source: Schneider, E. C., Sarnak, D. O., Squires, D., Shah, A., & Doty, M. M. (2017). *Mirror, mirror 2017: International comparison reflects flaws and opportunities for better U.S. health care.* New York, NY: The Commonwealth Fund.

with timely and effective health care—a measure called mortality amenable to health care—found that while deaths from health care treatable conditions have fallen in the United States, the rate of progress is slower than in three comparison nations: France, Germany, and the United Kingdom. And in a recent comparison of health system performance in 11 high-income countries,[2] Schneider and colleagues (Schneider, Sarnak, Squires, Shah, & Doty, 2017) found that the United States lagged significantly behind peer nations. The report looked at 72 performance metrics grouped into five dimensions and found that the United States ranked last or near last in *health care access, administrative efficiency, equity,* and *patient and population health outcomes,* and in its top-performing domain, *care processes,* the United States still only ranked in the in the middle of the pack (Schneider, Sarnak, Squires, Shah, & Doty, et al., 2017). On measures of outcomes and overall health system performance, therefore, it does not appear the U.S. system is getting results for its increased spending.

There are other reasons to be concerned about spending levels that hit closer to home. The federal government, state and local governments, and our nation's employers bear a great deal of the burden associated with high and growing health care costs. Increasingly, these costs are also being shifted to patients/consumers

---

[2]Australia, Canada, France, Germany, Netherlands, New Zealand, Norway, Sweden, Switzerland, United Kingdom, and United States.

in the form of higher insurance premiums and higher coinsurance, making even necessary care less affordable for many.

The federal government, each state government, and many local governments spend a great deal of their tax revenues on health care. The federal government finances (a) the Medicare program, which provides insurance for elderly and many permanently disabled Americans; (b) more than half of the Medicaid program, which pays for health care received by low-income Americans; (c) Veterans Affairs and Department of Defense health care expenses; and (d) the costs of extensive research, public health, and training activities. State governments pay for as much as half of the Medicaid program directly as well as for extensive activities in public health and regulation. Local governments generally support public health expenditures and some safety-net medical care. Governments at all levels are also purchasers, providing subsidized health insurance to millions of public employees across the country.[3]

In 1963, federal, state, and local governments financed only about $6 billion (equivalent to about $46 billion today) of total health care spending. This spending represented about 3% of total public spending. By 2012, governments were spending nearly $1.2 trillion (of the $2.8 trillion total) on health care, comprising more than 19% of total public spending. There are two key concerns with this growth in government costs. First, these costs are putting a great strain on taxes paid by workers and employers, and this strain is seen by many as decreasing the vibrancy of our economy. Second, the large share of tax dollars allocated to health care is crowding out expenditures on other important needs in our economy, such as education and infrastructure. This is especially true at the state and local levels, where government spending on health has increased by 154% over the past 40 years but expenditures on education have been "crowded out" and increased by just 74% over the same period.

> The large share of tax dollars allocated to health care is crowding out expenditures on other important needs in our economy, such as education and infrastructure.

Health care costs are not purely a public finance issue, however. Private businesses—which purchase health insurance for employees and their families—frequently cite increasing costs as problematic. For example, the cost of health insurance was cited as the top concern of small business owners in 2008 and 2012 (Wade, 2012). As a result, as health insurance costs have increased, employers provide fewer salary increases because resources are instead devoted to increased health insurance costs (again, health expenditures are "crowding out" expenditures on salaries). Additionally, fewer employers continue to offer group health insurance to employees—or they limit dependents of employees who can access coverage. For example, in August 2013, United Parcel Service began excluding

---

[3]Expenditures made to purchase insurance for public employees is counted in NHE estimates as private insurance costs, which are distinct from direct payments by federal and state governments for health care services received by Medicare and Medicaid beneficiaries.

health insurance coverage for spouses with access to health insurance at their own places of employment. Buchmueller, Carey, and Levy (2013) found that even though employers offered health insurance to more than 112 million employees in 2000, this number had declined to 108 million employees in 2011, or 4% fewer workers covered in one decade. Studies find that increasing health insurance costs decreases full-time employment and decreases hours worked for employees who work part time (Baicker & Chandra, 2005; Sood, Ghosh, & Escarce, 2009). Health care costs are implicitly part of national discussions about unemployment and job creation.

Health spending also is a burden on American families, which—despite the large expenditures by government and employers—also pay a sizable amount for health care in their family budgets. Table 11.1 shows how a typical family allocates its income across different types of expenditures. In 2016, total health care spending (including insurance premiums and direct medical costs) actually paid by the typical family was $4,612, which ranks it the fourth largest item consumed, only behind housing, transportation, and personal insurance/pensions (e.g., life insurance and retirement savings).

But the typical family is not every family. Families without insurance coverage, or even those with coverage but who remain underinsured—meaning they have health insurance that fails to provide adequate financial protection—and families that include someone with a chronic disease tend to spend a much larger share of after-tax income on health care. In 2015, the average single-person

TABLE 11.1   AVERAGE ANNUAL AFTER-TAX EXPENDITURES BY CONSUMER UNITS/HOUSEHOLDS: 2016

	AVERAGE ANNUAL EXPENDITURES IN DOLLARS: 2016	SHARE OF ANNUAL EXPENDITURES	CHANGE FROM PREVIOUS YEAR
Housing	18,886	33.0%	2.6%
Transportation	9,049	15.8%	−4.8%
Personal insurance and pensions	6,831	11.9%	7.6%
Health care	**4,612**	**8.0%**	**6.2%**
Food at home	4,049	7.1%	0.8%
Food away from home	3,154	5.5%	4.9%
Entertainment	2,913	5.1%	2.5%
All other	2,605	4.5%	0.0%
Cash contributions	2,081	3.6%	14.4%
Apparel and services	1,803	3.1%	−2.3%
Education	1,329	2.3%	1.1%
Total	57,312		

Source: 2016 Consumer Expenditure Survey, U.S. Department of Labor, Bureau of Labor Statistics.

deductible associated with employer-sponsored health insurance plans topped $1,500; average deductibles were more than $1,000 in every state but Hawaii and more than $2,000 in Maine and Montana (Collins, Radley, Gunja, & Beutel, 2016). On top of high deductibles, employees contributed an average of 21% of the total annual premium cost for a single policy and 27% of the cost of family plans. While the share of employees contributions has been fairly consistent in recent years, employees' costs have gone up in absolute terms. An employee's share of a single-person plan in 2006 was $788, compared to $1,255 in 2015. Coupled with slow wage growth, employees' total potential out-of-pocket costs—that is, their premium contributions plus their deductible—rose from 6.5% of median income in 2006 to 10.1% of median income in 2010 (Figure 11.3).

To sum up, health care spending levels in the United States are higher than in other developed countries, and they account for an increasingly disproportionate share of our nation's total economic activity. The burdens associated with growing costs are shared by federal, state, and local governments and by the public. Increasingly, American families are pinched by rising insurance and out-of-pocket medical costs. Despite high levels of spending and growth that's disproportionate with that of other sectors of the U.S. economy, health outcomes in the

FIGURE 11.3   EMPLOYEE PREMIUM CONTRIBUTION AND DEDUCTIBLE AS PERCENT OF MEDIAN HOUSEHOLD INCOME: 2006–2015

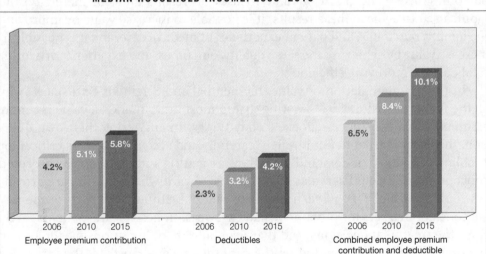

Note: Single and family premium contributions and deductibles are combined and weighted for the distribution of single-person and family households. Estimates of median household income used in the denominator for this ratio come from the Current Population Survey (CPS), which revised its income questions in 2013. The denominator in our ratio estimates prior to 2014 is derived from the traditional CPS income questions, while ratio estimates from 2014 are derived from the revised income questions. Household incomes are averaged over 2 years and have been adjusted for the likelihood that people in residence purchase health insurance together.

Sources: Medical Expenditure Panel Survey–Insurance Component (employee premium share and deductible, 2006, 2010, and 2015); Current Population Survey (median income, 2006-07, 2010-11, 2015-16), as reported in Collins, S. R., Radley, D. R., Gunja, M. Z., & Beutel, S. (2016). *The slowdown in employer insurance cost growth: Why many workers still feel the pinch.* New York, NY: The Commonwealth Fund.

United States are not keeping pace with progress made in the other countries, and on many measures of care quality, the United States is at best on par with patients' experience in other parts of the world.

DEFINING AND MEASURING VALUE IN HEALTH CARE

A widely accepted definition of value in health care remains elusive. In the broadest sense, we know that value is the pot of gold at the intersection of health care spending, patients' experiences and outcomes, and the quality of the care that providers deliver.

> We know that value is the pot of gold at the intersection of health care spending, patients' experiences and outcomes, and the quality of the care that providers deliver.

In one of the most commonly cited definitions of value, Porter and Teisberg (2006) offer "health outcomes achieved per dollar spent." Patients are at the center in this vision of value. The numerator in this equation is the quantitative assessment of patients' desire for survival, fast and uncomplicated recovery, and the long-term maintenance of well-being; the denominator is the sum of the dollars spent—across all health care providers—in pursuit of optimal patient outcomes. This conception of value focuses on results and not merely on the inputs used to achieve these results. It is possible to increase value by improving the quality, outcomes, and patient experience of medical care, and it is possible to increase value by achieving the same quality, outcomes, and experience at a lower total cost by improving efficiency.

In their contemplation of value, Blumenthal and Stremikis (2013) ask "why all the fuss with defining it?"—noting that in most other markets, value is simply assumed when consumers choose to buy things. In answering their own question, they suggest that defining value "carefully and systematically" is critical for enabling patients to understand what they are getting and that a widely accepted concept of value could serve as a "north star toward which health care providers could navigate." Of course, health care cannot be thought of in the same way we consider markets for other goods and services. In health care, patients rarely drive the treatment decisions, and they generally are only responsible for a small fraction of the costs generated by the care they receive. Instead, they trust the expertise of their clinical providers to make decisions on their behalf and benefit from the financial protection afforded by health insurance.

A shared understanding of what is meant by value in health care can also help address potentially competing interests in its pursuit. Porter (2010) acknowledges that the myriad stakeholders in health care often have conflicting goals. Patients want access to the services that will ensure the best possible outcome; they are interested in receiving care that is safe, as convenient as possible, and delivered in a way in which they feel respected and dignified. Providers, while likely acting in their patients' clinical interests, are also necessarily concerned with profitability, and payers are interested in lowering costs. These interests are often at odds with one another under the payment schemes that dominate U.S. health care today. For example, it is commonly misunderstood that cutting cost is the central way of producing value. Third-party payers often argue that the "value" they add is reducing payments to health care providers, thereby reducing the cost of health care to the employer, taxpayer, or individual who is the actual payer. Lowering payment alone won't necessarily enhance value if it results in providers cutting back in ways that limit patients' access to effective health care services. In contrast, many health care professionals who think about and work on quality issues focus on ensuring that consumers get the best treatment available at the correct time and may not even be aware of the associated costs because, as we describe in the next section, of opaque pricing structures (Robert Wood Johnson Foundation, 2013).

A key challenge in the value movement is the ability to meaningfully measure patient-centered outcomes and the costs associated with achieving those outcomes. There is no shortage of quality measurement frameworks (e.g., HEDIS [Healthcare Effectiveness Data and Information Set]; CMS [Centers for Medicare & Medicaid Services] star ratings; Agency for Healthcare Research and Quality [AHRQ]'s prevention, inpatient, safety, and pediatrics quality indicators), but current measurement tools fail to capture the information needed to adequately complete the value equation. Existing quality measures tend to focus on care processes and track the extent to which physicians adhere to accepted standards of care—for example, diabetic patients receiving appropriate blood sugar testing, adults receiving age- and gender-appropriate cancer screenings, or heart attack patients receiving appropriate upon arrival at a hospital. These are understandably important but, by focusing too keenly on care processes, our delivery systems risk shifting attention away from the things that matter most to patients.

Just as existing quality measurement strategies face limitations in a modern value-based care framework, so too do existing notions of "patient outcomes." By some measures, health outcomes are improving markedly in the United States (see Chapter 12). Deaths associated with stroke and heart disease are down substantially, and most would agree this is due to improvements in medical know-how, pharmaceuticals, and emerging technology. Cancer mortality also is improving due to better treatment approaches. Longevity after age 75 is higher in the United States than in many other countries, again perhaps due to the health services associated with medical care. Disparities in health outcomes between people of color and White Americans decrease after age 65, and most experts associate this with the near-universal accessibility of medical care that happens when people become eligible for Medicare.

While the importance of such gains cannot be overstated, these "outcomes" do not fully align with our understanding of patient outcomes in an evolving notion of value. Rather than thinking of outcome measurement in narrow terms, limited primarily to things that happen to patients (e.g., mortality or rehospitalization rate), achieving value in health care requires an acknowledgement that patient outcomes are subtle and multidimensional. Patient-centered outcomes must capture the nuances of patients' functional and psychological status, as well as perceptions and valuations of their care and their goals for recovery. Perhaps a more nuanced way to think of value in health care is that value is achieved when the health care that gets delivered helps patients achieve what matters most to them.

Take, for example, two patients with knee pain. Both are age 73, relatively healthy, and free from major chronic illness, but both have a diagnosis of osteoarthritis in their knee—a painful degenerative condition that is often an indication for total knee replacement (TKR) surgery. In this example, Patient A cares most about being pain free and maintaining as active of a lifestyle as possible. In discussing treatments options with her physician, she decides that she is willing to accept the risks associated with TKR surgery (e.g., infection, joint failure) if this is the treatment that will help her achieve her goal of being active with her grandchildren. Patient B is also interested in reducing his level of pain. However, Patient B recently lost a sibling who died from a surgical site infection following a routine operation and is very concerned about infection risk (even though he can acknowledge that chances of getting a surgical site infection are small). He is willing to tolerate some level of pain and loss of function if it means he can avoid the risks associated with surgery. Would our health care system be delivering high-value care if both patients received the same treatment? What if Patient A has a successful surgery (total cost $65,000) and Patient B is treated pharmacologically for pain and participates in physical therapy (total cost of $9,000), but both patients feel that they got what mattered most to them—would it be fair to say that Patient B received higher-value care because the overall cost was lower?

There does not appear to be a near-term solution for reconciling both sides of the value equation. For starters, patient-centered outcomes research (PCOR) and development of patient-reported outcome measures (PROMs) are still new scientific endeavors. While progress is being made to develop methods and establish scientific standards (Shah & Spinks, 2017), our nation's health care infrastructure is still a long way away from being able to meaningfully operationalize patient-centered outcome measures and use the data to inform treatment decisions. Doing so will require developing new processes to routinely solicit information directly from patients on their perceptions and values. Information systems will need to be adapted (or developed) such that they can combine clinical assessment data (including functional and psychological status) and qualitative information collected from patients with administrative records of the care they received and the costs they incurred. And most important, mechanisms need to be developed to get this information, in a usable form, in front of clinical care providers at the point of service.

COST DRIVERS AND BARRIERS TO VALUE

So far we have learned that health care is costly in the United States. This section discusses some of the key factors behind high spending levels and how those factors are actually working against efforts to achieve better value.

Recall from your introductory economic classes that *spending = quantity × price.* The same is true in health care. There are factors that influence how much health care gets delivered, some portion of which is considered duplicative, wasteful, or otherwise unnecessary, and the prices are often high and idiosyncratic, in that the same service could have difference prices, depending on who is paying. Compounding the pressures from high utilization and price, the predominant payment models in the United States create incentives that are misaligned for delivering high-value care.

> There are factors that influence how much health care gets delivered, some portion of which is considered duplicative, wasteful, or otherwise unnecessary, and the prices are often high and idiosyncratic, in that the same service could have difference prices, depending on who is paying.

Fee-for-Service Payment

Most experts agree that the **fee-for-service payment models** that finance the majority of care delivered in this country are themselves a major driver of high spending. In a fee-for-service (FFS) system, providers are compensated for each service performed, which can lead to unnecessary care being provided (and therefore unnecessary costs). As late as 2016, 86% of physicians reported being reimbursed predominantly under an FFS model (Morris, Abrams, Elsner, & Gerhardt, 2016) despite a widespread and longstanding acknowledgement that the model adds to overall cost.

The FFS reimbursement model dates back to a time when health care providers mainly saw patients to treat acute problems. FFS made a lot of sense in these scenarios. It was straightforward for a provider to charge a single fee to offer treatment from a relatively narrow set of therapeutic options at a time before prices put treatment out of reach for average Americans. But modern health care is different. The majority of health care spending now is devoted to treating chronic illnesses (including acute exacerbation of chronic problems) over long periods of time. Care is now rarely provided by a single physician; rather, team-based medicine is the modern norm. And where there used to be a relatively narrow set of treatment options available, new technologies and therapeutic innovations have vastly expanded the number of tools that clinicians have to choose from when diagnosing and fighting disease. While the delivery of medicine has changed in the last half century, the predominate financing mechanism hasn't kept pace. Instead, FFS payment has enabled, even supported, many of the factors we point to as current cost drivers.

Berwick and Hackbarth (2012) offer one of the more insightful examinations of health care spending in the United States, estimating 20% to 46% of health care expenditures are potentially wasteful and categorizing six discrete types of **waste**. By "keep[ing] processes, products, and services that actually help customers and systematically remov[ing] the elements of work that do not," they estimate that the U.S. health care system stands to save an average of $910 billion (in 2011 dollars). The remainder of this section discusses cost implications of each of Berwick and Hackbarth's categories.

Failure of Care Delivery

Failures in care delivery can generate excess cost in several ways. Most directly, patients receive services that do little in the way of advancing their treatment but that nonetheless generate charges. In a more concerning scenario, a patient may receive services that cause harm, which in turn initiates a set of services and charges associated with treating the damage. They can also generate charges over a longer term if foregoing effective and low-cost care leads to the use of more costly services later on.

Health care delivery systems should always be focused on providing the right care, to the right patient, at the right time—it seems almost too obvious to state. Yet, across the health care landscape, it's easy to find instances of suboptimal and, in some cases, outright poor quality and dangerous care being delivered. Classen and colleagues (2011), using a sophisticated and highly standardized process for retrospective patient chart review, found that adverse events capable of causing patients harm occurred in about a third of hospital admissions, with the majority related to medication use or linked to specific procedures. The Centers for Disease Control and Prevention (CDC) reports annually on hospital-acquired infection (HAI) rates and routinely finds wide variation in infection rates across hospitals on a number of infection types, with some hospitals reporting two-and-a-half times the national incidence of infections for central line–associated bloodstream infections (CLABSIs), catheter-associated urinary tract infections (CAUTIs), ventilator-associated events (VAEs), surgical site infections (SSIs), methicillin-resistant *Staphylococcus aureus* (MRSA) bloodstream infections, and *Clostridium difficile* (*C. difficile*) events (CDC, 2017). Not all care delivery failure occurs in hospitals. In 2014, for example, 13% of Medicare beneficiaries nationally, but up to one in four in some states, received a high-risk prescription medicine that should never have been prescribed according to clinical guidelines. In 2016, a third of adults reported not having had all recommended age- and gender-appropriate cancer screenings—tests that have been proved to help detect treatable cancers early to help save lives and avoid more costly treatment later on (Radley, McCarthy, & Hayes, 2018).

To be sure, providing the right care, to the right patient, at the right time is not easy, and most experts acknowledge that progress is made with each passing year. Nonetheless, each instance of a care delivery failure represents an opportunity to lower spending.

Failure of Care Coordination

A large part of what leads to high health care costs in the United States is caused by the uncoordinated approach we use to take care of people with medical problems. Poorly coordinated care can result in duplication of services—this is common with medical testing and imaging, when providers are unaware or unable to obtain recent results; avoidable complications and rehospitalizations; and declines in patients' functional status, which may lead to additional downstream treatment costs. A commonly cited failure of coordination is 30-day hospital readmission. After a patient is discharged from a hospital stay, timely follow-up care along with a coordinated post-acute response should prevent most patients from having to return to the hospital. Hospital readmission rates among Medicare beneficiaries have been hovering around 16% to17% in recent years, since legislation was passed that penalized hospitals with high rates. Even though readmissions are down over the long term, the fact that one of every six hospital discharges results in a readmission still represents a huge economic burden (Barrett, Wier, Jiang, & Steiner, 2015).

There is no one for whom poorly coordinated care is more costly than for the most complexly ill patients. You've probably heard the statistic—just 5% of the total U.S. population accounts for 50% of all health care spending, and 10% accounts for 66% of spending, while the bottom 50% of the population accounts for just under 3% of spending (Figure 11.4) (Mitchell, 2016). Individuals in the top spending group tend to have multiple chronic illnesses and functional limitations. Coordination of services is critical for these complexly ill individuals. Unfortunately, today's care delivery systems too often fall short in ensuring a high degree of integration as these patients move among various specialists, hospitals, and post-acute and long-term care settings. Compared to other adults, they use the emergency department and are admitted to the hospital at much higher rates, they see many more providers during the year, and they are far more likely to incur high costs year over year (Hayes et al., 2016).

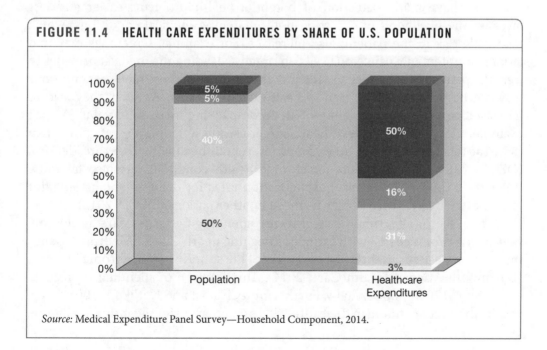

FIGURE 11.4   HEALTH CARE EXPENDITURES BY SHARE OF U.S. POPULATION

Source: Medical Expenditure Panel Survey—Household Component, 2014.

Overtreatment

Approximately 40 years ago, Wennberg published his first study of geographic variations in the use of medical care (Wennberg & Gittelsohn, 1973). Since then, hundreds of academic and journalistic articles have explored the causes and consequences of regional differences in how health care resources are used. The key finding to emerge from this work is: Where you live matters. There are big differences across the country in people's ability to access care, the quality of care they receive, and the outcomes they may expect to experience. More important, this research has also shown that more care isn't necessarily better. Fisher and colleagues demonstrated that despite significantly higher spending per Medicare beneficiary in some parts of the country, the quality of care received and patients' satisfaction and outcomes were not appreciably better, and in some cases they were worse, in regions where spending was high compared to lower cost areas (Fisher et al. 2003a, Fisher et al. 2003b).

One of the key implications of Fisher's et al. findings is that certain types of health care services, particularly those of little marginal benefit to patients, were used at lower rates in some places than in others without detriment to patients' health. Another way to say it is that some health care services were overused and generated cost and waste in the process. These findings were reinforced when the Institute of Medicine (IOM) estimated that waste accounted for about one-third of all health care spending, citing unneeded procedures as one of the primary sources (IOM, 2012).

Emerick and Lewis (2013) cite **overscreening** and treatment as a fundamental aspect of waste in health care. As advances in technology and medical condition diagnoses have made detection of potential health problems easier and less invasive, the likelihood of detecting nonthreatening medical conditions, which pose little risk to the patient, also increases. For example, screenings may find lesions or potentially cancerous cells on organs—leading the medical provider to treat the patient (with surgery, medicine, and so on). Yet these medical conditions may not be problematic or lead to health complications. As such, they lead to increased costs with no certainty of an accompanying increase in value. As one example, U.S. patients receive heart surgeries and angioplasties at more than twice the rate for patients in other countries, yet our health outcomes are identical (OECD, 2013). Hospital visits for chronic health conditions are also far more frequent in the United States; hospitalization rates for diabetes and asthma, for example, are nearly twice as high as those in other nations (OECD, 2013).

A final factor affecting our health care spending patterns bears discussion. End-of-life care is costly, with estimates pegging nearly 32% of Medicare spending to those patients in their last two years of life suffering from chronic illnesses (Dartmouth Atlas of Health Care, 2014). This fraction of spending represents more than $170 billion annually. Furthermore, Hagist and Kotlikoff (2006) show that health care spending in the United States increases significantly after age 65.

Just as variation exists across the country in Medicare spending, end-of-life care spending by Medicare is not evenly distributed across the country. Patients receiving more aggressive end-of-life care (and, by extension, spending more resources) do not have improved survival or better quality of life than others. For example, many terminal cancer patients choose to undergo chemotherapy during the last 10 to 30 days of life, which is expensive and only marginally extends the patients' lives (see, e.g., Harrington and Smith [2008], who note that 43% of terminal lung cancer patients in the United States receive chemotherapy in the last month of life, compared with just 23% in Italy). However, patients, families, and doctors likely feel more satisfied that they tried everything.

Overuse is another challenge to achieving value for which there are no easy answers. As Woloshin and Schwartz point out, overuse is "about more than money—at its core it is about physicians wanting to do their best for individual patients and the quality and safety of health care" (Woloshin & Schwartz, 2018). With a number of factors driving the practice of medicine toward providing more care—things like patients' and physicians' anxiety over uncertainty, difficulty accounting for patients' preferences and values in treatment decisions, and patients' widespread belief that more health care must be better—it's unlikely that the debate over overuse will end anytime soon.

Administrative Complexity and Fraud

By now, you should appreciate the complexity in the U.S. health care system. At its best, our system is a hodgepodge of public and private insurers, operating under different federal and state laws and regulations and paying for services under different payment models. This complexity has a price. The IOM estimates that administrative complexity alone costs in excess of $360 billion annually (Yong, Saunders, & Olsen, 2010), which is more than total spending on heart disease and cancer combined (Cutler, Wikler, & Basch, 2012). Cutler and colleagues argue that substantial savings could be realized by standardizing key administrative processes. They estimate, for example, that approximately $11 billion could be saved annually if all payers, public and private, were to adopt a standardized system for electronic billing; almost $3 billion could be saved by standardizing and stabilizing enrollment rules and procedures for public insurance programs; and as much as $6 billion might be saved by adopting systems that standardize procedures for automating certain routine tasks (e.g., computerized physician order-entry systems).

As complex as it is, it's no wonder that dishonest actors have found ways to take advantage of gaps in our system, generating fake bills for services they did not provide. In the same IOM report, it is estimated that approximately $75 billion worth of fake claims were paid to fraudsters, while Berwick and Hackbarth (2012) estimate that the total cost of fraud, including efforts to detect and stop it, are between $82 billion and $227 billion.

Pricing Failures

So far, we've discussed the quantity side of our spending equation. What about prices? A popular health policy article has the provocative title "It's the Prices, Stupid: Why the United States Is So Different from Other Countries" (Anderson, Reinhardt, Hussey, & Petrosyan, 2003). In addition to the complexity of costs and value calculations in U.S. health care is this simple fact: Almost every actor in the health sector has managed to command very high prices for the role he/she/it plays. U.S. physicians earn higher salaries than those in almost every other country (Laugesen & Glied, 2011), pharmaceutical prices are much higher in the United States than in other countries, hospital prices are much higher, and hospital administrators earn more in the United States than elsewhere. Furthermore, until recently, what we've known about health service pricing has been spotty at best. In this section, we'll learn more about the ways prices are different in the United States than in other places, as well as more about the recent movement toward price transparency.

The International Federation of Health Insurance Plans (IFHIP) collects pricing information for common health care services in the United States and several international comparison nations (IFHIP, 2013). Table 11.2 highlights some of the comparisons from the IFHIP 2012 report, the most recent year of publicly available data. The United States is an outlier, with average prices at least 33% higher than the next highest price nation for most services.

One of the barriers to fully understanding just how important a role price plays in the driving overall costs has been a lack of information and transparency.

TABLE 11.2 AVERAGE PRICES FOR SELECT HEALTH CARE SERVICES IN THE UNITED STATES WITH INTERNATIONAL COMPARISON: 2012

SERVICE	U.S. AVERAGE PRICE	NEXT HIGHEST PRICE COMPARISON COUNTRY	LOWEST PRICE COMPARISON COUNTRY
CT scan: head	$566	$328	$82
MRI	$1,121	$1,072	$118
Hospital cost per day	$4,287	$1,472	$429
Maternity: vaginal delivery (hospital and physician charges)	$9,775	$6,846	$1,188
Total hip arthroplasty (hospital and physician charges)	$40,364	$27,810	$3,365
Diagnostic colonoscopy	$1,185	$893	$413
Routine office visit	$95	$38	$10

Source: International Federation of Health Insurance Plans.

For a long time, most of what we know about spending and utilization has come from analysis of Medicare claims data. Since prices are generally fixed through Medicare's prospective payment system, we've been able to learn very little about price differences between hospitals for non-Medicare populations. This is starting to change as new data become available that can shed light on the interplay between price—which is the result of negations between health insurers and health care providers—and utilization for the segment of the U.S. population who get health insurance from their employers.

In their recent analysis of data from the Health Care Cost Institute (HCCI), which compiles administrative insurance claims data from three large national insurers that provide coverage for working-age adults and their dependents, Cooper and colleagues (Cooper, Craig, Gaynor, & Van Reenen, 2018) find that roughly half of the spending variation seen across U.S. cities is attributable to how services are used, and about half can be attributed to the prices charged. Unlike in Medicare, where service prices are fixed (so spending variation is due mostly to differences in utilization), among the privately insured, prices for the same services differed as much as 10-fold across cities and as much as sixfold among hospitals within a single city.

One of Cooper's most interesting, though not entirely surprising, findings was that prices tended be about 12% higher in markets dominated by a single hospital system compared to markets with four or more competing hospitals—a potential cause for concern if provider consolidation trends continue (Cooper et al., 2018). As Atul Gawande (2015) puts it, "It's the cost conundrum squared. The bigger the hospital, the more it can adopt systems that deliver better-organized, higher-quality, less-wasteful care. But the bigger the hospital, the more power it has to raise prices."

So why have actors in the health system been able to charge such high prices for their services? And how is that our health care system has been willing to tolerate high prices and blatant price discrimination (meaning a provider can charge different payers different prices for the same service) for so long? One reason is patients cannot be thought of in same way as typical "consumers" are in other markets. The public are generally not consumers of health care until they become patients, at which point stakes are high (i.e., potentially life or death), and insurance protects patients from the high costs. Another reason is that insurers have long been able to pass high prices along to enrollees in the form of higher premiums. So long as firms continue to buy health insurance products for their employees and shift costs by raising premium contributions and deductibles, insurance firms have minimal incentive to negotiate substantially lower prices with local providers. Finally, as alluded to in the quote from Gawande above, certain health care providers can command a "must-have" status when insurers are defining networks for insurance products to sell to local employers. Even if an insurer is willing to exclude certain high-price providers from a network to help lower the premiums it charges employers, it's often true that firms would be unwilling to buy insurance products that limit their employees' access to the biggest, most recognized providers in the area.

INITIATIVES TO ADDRESS EXPENDITURE/VALUE TRADEOFFS

For decades, we've recognized the need to get better value out of health care. As health care costs swelled in the 1980s, employers reacted by starting to shift more of the cost-sharing burden onto their employees—a trend that has continued to today.

Back then, insurance companies saw an opportunity to address the problem by creating managed care organizations (MCOs), primarily through health maintenance organizations (HMOs) and preferred provider organizations (PPOs). To be sure, MCOs like Kaiser Permanente, Group Health Cooperative, and Henry Ford Health System had been around for decades. But employers were looking for something to address their immediate needs, and by the 1990s, traditional indemnity health insurance had become a thing of the past.

The promise of MCOs was short-lived. Why? It is true that for a period of time MCOs held the line on costs. Yet there was a lack of focus on quality and patient satisfaction. Health plans that solely focused on costs—particularly capitated arrangements—often led to penny-wise and pound-foolish decisions by gatekeepers making short-term decisions about the insurer's bottom line.

In an address in 1999 at the Mayo Clinic, economist Alain Enthoven captured the sentiment of the moment. "The 'managed care revolution of the 1990s' achieved an important, if temporary, success," he said. "But it now appears to be failing. We see a great outpouring of anger, resentment, hostility, and frustration expressed in state and the federal legislatures as doctors, other providers, and many patients express strong dissatisfaction with managed care" (Stanford GSB Staff, 1999).

Managed health care continues to be the primary health insurance model today. But after the turn of the century, insurers began to experiment with new payment models to supplement their offerings. These models began to address the need for value—providing incentives to improve outcomes at lower costs. Blue Cross Blue Shield launched its Alternative Quality Contract for providers in 2009, at about the same time that Cigna was piloting its Collaborative Accountable Care model. Medicare began demonstration programs focused on quality and value, which eventually made their way into the Affordable Care Act; the establishment of **accountable care organizations** (ACOs); and the nation's first Medicare ACO program: the Pioneer Model ACO.

We will learn more about value-based payment models and attempts at health care delivery reform in the following sections, including bundled payments, ACOs, and more.

Value-Based Payment Models

Value-based payment models evolved from the present system because our primary funding models, FFS and capitation, each have perverse incentives that the accountable care model seeks to remedy (see previous section). In an

FFS system, providers are compensated for each service performed, which can lead to unnecessary services being provided (and therefore unnecessary costs). In a capitated model, providers are reimbursed at a fixed rate, usually on a per-member, per-month basis. In this reimbursement model, providers may have a disincentive to provide necessary treatments, which can lead to poor outcomes and, eventually, greater costs.

All value-based care models have the same three goals in mind: improve the patient experience (including quality and satisfaction), improve the health of populations, and reduce costs. In other words, the goal is to achieve the Triple Aim—the framework established by the Institute for Healthcare Improvement (IHI) to optimizing health system performance (Berwick, Nolan, & Whittington, 2008).

> All value-based care models have the same three goals in mind: improve the patient experience (including quality and satisfaction), improve the health of populations, and reduce costs.

Bundled Payments

In a **bundled payments** model, providers receive a lump sum payment for each episode of care they provide to patients. Bundled payments can align incentives for various providers, thereby encouraging collaboration across specialties and care settings.

Bundled payments are riskier for providers than some of the other arrangements because providers must service whatever health care needs the patient has during a given episode of care. They can benefit when patients require little care, but in complex cases or when complications arise, the cost of the care given can exceed the amount of the lump sum payment. For this reason, bundled payment programs are most effective where outcomes are more predictable, such as for total joint replacement procedures.

The bundled payments model has been implemented through a major initiative by the CMS and through commercial payers.

BUNDLED PAYMENTS FOR CARE IMPROVEMENT INITIATIVE Bundled Payments for Care Improvement (BPCI) providers voluntarily enter into payment arrangements that include financial and performance accountability for episodes of care. The initiative comprises four models of care: three retrospective bundled payment arrangements and a prospective bundled payment arrangement. "Convening organizations" are responsible for selecting bundled payment participants and managing the program. BPCI was initiated in 2013 (CMS, 2018).

In April 2016, CMS launched its first mandatory bundled payment model, the Comprehensive Care for Joint Replacement (CJR) program, in 67 geographic areas. Under the program, hospitals are accountable for the quality and cost of care provided to Medicare beneficiaries who undergo hip and knee replacements—not only during the patient's hospital stay, but also for the 90 days following discharge. Hospitals are eligible to receive an additional payment if they perform well on cost and quality measures. CMS later expanded this model to include surgeries for hip and femur fractures.

However, under the Trump administration, CMS was unwilling to continue with mandatory bundles, including another program expected to launch. In November 2017, CMS announced that it had finalized the cancellation of the hip fracture and cardiac bundled payment and incentive payment models, officially known as the Episode Payment Models and Cardiac Rehabilitation Incentive Payment Model, which were to be implemented on January 1, 2018 (CMS, 2017). The final rule also reduced the number of mandatory geographic areas participating in the CJR model from 67 to 34 and made participation voluntary for all low-volume and rural hospitals in all 67 geographic areas.

Had the CJR model continued to be mandatory in all 67 geographic regions, it was expected to save Medicare an estimated $295 million over the next three years, but with the reduced number of mandatory geographic areas, it will save about half that amount, or an estimated $189 million. The canceled cardiac payment models would have saved Medicare an estimated $170 million over five years.

In January 2018, CMS introduced a new voluntary bundled payment model: Bundled Payments for Care Improvement Advanced (BPCI Advanced). The new program includes 32 clinical care episodes, three of which are outpatient. Among the care episodes are major joint replacement of the lower extremity, spinal fusion, and percutaneous coronary intervention. Seven quality measures have been chosen for the new model, including the all-cause hospital readmission measure.

Bundled payments have been shown to reduce costs without affecting quality for joint replacement procedures. A study published online September 19, 2016, by the *Journal of the American Medical Association* compared the Medicare bundled payments and outcomes for lower extremity joint replacement episodes initiated during a 1-year period before the original BPCI model was launched versus similar episodes initiated during the first 21 months of the BPCI for participating and nonparticipating hospitals. The analysis showed that the average Medicare payment for the BPCI-participating hospitals decreased by $3,286 during the program's first 21 months, whereas the average Medicare payment for nonparticipating hospitals decreased by $2,119. The difference was attributed mostly to reduced use of institutional post-acute care. There was no significant change in quality outcomes (Dummiit, Kahvecioglu, & Marrufo, 2016).

COMMERCIAL BUNDLES Large commercial payers like Aetna, Humana, and United-Healthcare (UHC) have deployed the bundled payment model across specialties and procedures, in some cases achieving substantial cost savings without sacrificing quality.

For example, in May 2018, UHC reported that its bundled payment program for knee, hip, and spine procedures generated $18 million in savings for participating employers as a result of reduced readmissions and complications following surgery. UHC said its Spine and Joint Solution program helped reduce hospital readmissions by 22% and led to 17% fewer complications for joint replacement surgeries as compared with nonparticipating facilities. For spine surgeries, hospital readmissions were reduced by 10%, and there were 3.4% fewer complications as compared with nonparticipating facilities. UHC said the program includes 46 participating health care facilities, with more than 115 employers enrolled representing 3 million employees (UHC, 2018).

Bundled payment programs aren't limited to procedures. In April 2018, Humana announced the rollout of a national bundled payment model for maternity care. Humana said the program is for Humana commercial group members with low- to moderate-risk pregnancies. Humana's Maternity Episode-Based Model affects the entire perinatal episode of care, including prenatal care, labor and delivery, and post-delivery care. OB-GYNs are financially incentivized to achieve better outcomes. Five practices in Indiana, Kansas, Ohio, and Texas are the first to voluntarily participate in the model (Humana, 2018).

Medicare Access and CHIP Reauthorization Act

In 2016, CMS released the final rule for the Quality Payment Program under the Medicare Access and CHIP (Children's Health Insurance Program) Reauthorization Act (MACRA). The program replaces the sustainable growth rate formula, which was repealed in 2015. Providers who bill Medicare more than $90,000 per year or provide care for at least 200 Medicare beneficiaries qualify for the new payment program.[4]

The new payment program has two reimbursement tracks: the Merit-based Incentive Payment System (MIPS) for providers participating in traditional Medicare Part B and Advanced Alternative Payment Models (APMs) for those participating in a value-based care model.

Providers in the MIPS track will earn payment adjustments based on their performance in four categories: quality of care; cost of care, which will carry zero weight in the first performance year; clinical practice improvement; and "advancing care information," which is similar to meaningful use of **electronic health records** (EHRs). Those who do not submit a minimal amount of performance data for the first performance year will receive a 4% negative adjustment. Those who do submit data will receive a neutral to 4% positive adjustment, depending on the amount of data submitted. The adjustment gradually increases to a maximum of 9% in 2022.

---

[4]In November 2017, the $90,000 threshold was raised from the $30,000 threshold in the initial rule to give small practices a chance to ease into the Quality Payment Program. To that end, MACRA will provide $20 million annually for five years to help small practices (with up to 15 clinicians) and those in underserved areas prepare for participation.

Providers in an advanced APM can earn an annual 5% lump sum incentive payment from 2019 through 2024 and will not be subject to MIPS reporting or payment adjustments. Programs qualifying as Advanced APMs must use certified EHR technology, base payments on quality measures comparable to MIPS, and require providers to bear more than nominal risk.

Value-Based Pricing of Pharmaceuticals

Pharmaceutical pricing is complex. In fact, a major problem lies with the complexity of how drugs are priced and paid for in the United States—and a lack of transparency throughout the process.

When we pick up our prescription at the pharmacy, most of us pay a copay. The amount we pay has been negotiated in advance by a pharmacy benefit manager, or PBM, which earns rebates on each prescription dispensed. PBMs have a list of all prescription drugs, called a formulary, that they categorize into tiers. Drug plans vary, but typically lower-tier drugs are "preferred" and have a lower copay than higher-tier drugs. Drug manufacturers negotiate with PBMs to earn rebates and be the preferred drug in their category on the formulary.

This system of rebates and opaque PBM-manufacturer negotiations has drawn the ire of lawmakers and was recently highlighted by President Trump in his Blueprint to Lower Drug Prices. However, payers and drug makers have begun to experiment with value-based contracts for pharmaceuticals based on outcomes, often tied to real-world performance compared with what the drug demonstrated in clinical trials. In February 2016, for example, Cigna and Aetna reached outcomes-based agreements with Novartis for Entresto, a treatment for heart failure. Novartis agreed to a base price and a modest rebate, which would vary based on hospital admissions for heart failure and savings to the plan. The benchmark is set by Entresto's labeling, which states that in clinical trials the drug reduced the risk of death by 24% and hospitalization by 21% as compared with enalapril.

DELIVERY SYSTEM REFORM

Some efforts to meet the Triple Aim are related to how services are priced and how care is delivered. In this section, we will review two primary models of delivery innovation: patient-centered medical homes and ACOs. We'll also cover a hybrid program that borrows elements of these models, designed for patients with cancer.

Patient-Centered Medical Homes

In 2007, the major primary care physician associations developed and endorsed the Joint Principles of the Patient-Centered Medical Home (PCMH). PCMH is a primary care model that is patient centered, comprehensive, team based, coordinated, accessible, and focused on quality and safety. Adapted from the AHRQ's definition, the Patient-Centered Primary Care Collaborative describes the medical home as an approach to the delivery of primary care that is:

- *Patient-centered:* A partnership among practitioners, patients, and their families ensures that decisions respect patients' wants, needs, and preferences and that patients have the education and support they need to make decisions and participate in their own care.
- *Comprehensive:* A team of care providers is wholly accountable for a patient's physical and mental health care needs, including prevention and wellness, acute care, and chronic care.
- *Coordinated:* Care is organized across all elements of the broader health care system, including specialty care, hospitals, home health care, community services, and supports.
- *Accessible:* Patients are able to access services with shorter waiting times, "after hours" care, 24/7 electronic or telephone access, and strong communication through health information technology (IT) innovations.
- *Committed to quality and safety:* Clinicians and staff enhance quality improvement to ensure that patients and families make informed decisions about their health.

While being a governing philosophy of care, PCMHs are typically deployed for use in patients with chronic illnesses or comorbid conditions for which care coordination is essential. According to the National Committee for Quality Assurance (NCQA), its Patient-Centered Medical Home Recognition Program is the most widely adopted patient-centered medical home evaluation program in the country. More than 12,000 practices, including more than 60,000 clinicians, are recognized by NCQA, and more than 100 payers support NCQA recognition through financial incentives or coaching (NCQA, 2018).

Accountable Care Organizations

ACOs are groups of health care providers, such as physicians and hospitals, that collaborate to ensure the highest quality treatment possible for a segment of the population. Both providers and payers are incentivized to work together to improve the quality of care while reducing overall costs through efficient practices.

While the concept of an ACO may be elusive to some health care providers, it is actually quite straightforward. The entity responsible for the payment to the ACO for services, most commonly Medicare, establishes a prospective annual budget of expected expenditures based on the number of assigned beneficiaries and other factors. At the same time, Medicare (or other payer) sets forth quality measures to be monitored by the ACO, such as 30-day readmissions.

At the end of the year, Medicare compares the ACO's projected spending versus actual spending. If spending is less than what was budgeted, the ACO shares in some of the savings with Medicare—subject to maintaining quality standards for care and patient satisfaction. ACOs that have shared savings but poor quality receive reduced shared savings or no savings at all, which incentivizes the ACO to focus on both high-quality care and financial performance.

Most Medicare ACOs have what is referred to as one-sided or upside risk, meaning if they exceed their budget, they are not penalized for doing so. There is little risk in such an agreement. More experienced providers enter into two-sided or downside risk agreements, which means that if they spend more than what was prospectively budgeted, they must pay Medicare back a portion of the excess. Two-sided agreements confer not only more risk to the ACO, but also greater reward through increased shared savings.

Stemming from the Affordable Care Act, ACOs are the core test beds designed for the process of innovation toward systemic solvency, aligned incentives, and cost containment. Since their inception in 2011, ACOs have spread beyond the purview of CMS to commercial payers, employers, cities, and state Medicaid programs.

MEDICARE ACOs   There are five primary ACO programs and models offered by Medicare: the Medicare Shared Savings Program (MSSP), Pioneer ACO, Next Generation ACO, Investment Model ACO (AIM), and the Advance Payment ACO Model. To be eligible for shared savings, Medicare ACOs must provide CMS with performance data on 34 measures in four domains.[5] The first ACO experiment, the Pioneer ACO program, ended in 2016, with most participating providers having joined other ACO programs.

In December 2016, CMS announced a new Medicare-Medicaid ACO (MMACO) model that builds on the MSSP. Under this new model, MSSP ACOs that are currently accountable for assigned beneficiaries' Medicare expenditures can also take on accountability for the Medicaid costs of dually eligible enrollees.

Results for the Medicare ACO models have been mixed. For instance, in 2016, 31% of the ACOs participating in the MSSP, or 134 of 432, generated shared savings in 2016, the program's fifth performance year and fourth year of reporting results. For the year, participating ACOs collectively reduced Medicare spending by $652 million. Those that generated shared savings earned performance payments exceeding $700 million, CMS data show.

MEDICAID ACOs   Medicaid ACOs have arisen from a need for the delivery of integrated care, as well as to address social determinants of health. The common goals of these state-based initiatives is to improve the quality of care and curb costly and avoidable hospitalizations of Medicaid beneficiaries—especially those with multiple chronic conditions and behavioral health needs. States are leveraging existing investments in managed care and primary care to guide the development of their Medicaid ACO programs. As of March 2018, eight state Medicaid programs were operating ACOs, and at least nine more states were in the process of developing Medicaid ACOs.

---

[5]In 2011, CMS originally had 33 quality measures. In 2015, the agency added several more but also dropped some measures for a net total of 34.

COMMERCIAL ACOs The commercial ACO model consists of commercial insurance companies that encourage providers to enter into contracts in which payment is based on the value of their care. Today, employers are familiar with the concept of value-based health care and are amenable to offering an ACO option to their employees. Cigna, Aetna, Humana, UHC, and Blue Cross Blue Shield affiliates all have some form of accountable care initiative due to demand in the marketplace.

For example, as of February 2018, Cigna has more than 200 collaborative care agreements with primary care providers, covering 2.4 million commercial plan members in 31 states (Cigna, 2018a). Cigna also has specialty collaborative care programs in cardiology, gastroenterology, obstetrics-gynecology, oncology, and orthopedics (Cigna, 2018b).

EMPLOYER-DRIVEN ACOs Several large, self-insured companies have embraced the ACO concept. One well-known example is the Boeing-Providence Health Services (now Providence St. Joseph Health) ACO. Beginning in 2014, the multiyear agreement has set goals for company medical costs annually—if costs exceed projections, Providence pays the excess; if it beats the budget, it keeps the savings.

The contract stipulates patient satisfaction improvements and quality measures, such as having short appointment wait times and tracking population measures in diabetes and cardiovascular disease. Employees are incentivized to select the "preferred partnership" option by offering lower paycheck deductions, larger company contributions to health care savings accounts, no copayments for primary-care doctor visits (in most cases), and 100% coverage for generic drug prescriptions.

Oncology Care Model

The Center for Medicare and Medicaid Innovation (CMMI, or Innovation Center), launched its first specialty-specific, multipayer alternative payment model, the Oncology Care Model (OCM), on July 1, 2016. The first performance period of the 5-year initiative started on January 1, 2017. More than 200 physician-led oncology practices are participating in the model—almost double what CMS anticipated—along with 16 private insurers across the country. The Medicare arm of the OCM includes more than 3,200 oncologists and will cover approximately 155,000 beneficiaries.

Similar to ACOs for primary care physicians, the OCM is intended to improve the quality of care and health outcomes while holding down costs. And as with ACOs, the oncology model is designed to reward the value of care rather than the volume of care. The model covers almost all types of cancer.

Providers participating in the OCM range from solo practices to large physician groups with hundreds of oncologists. While participation is voluntary, practices have agreed to provide beneficiaries who are undergoing chemotherapy with 24-hour access to practitioners, and they must create a patient-focused care management plan that follows nationally recognized treatment guidelines. They are also required to use EHRs.

Private insurers participating in the OCM have agreed to align their models with the OCM by providing monthly payments for enhanced services, such as care coordination and navigation, and payments for performance. They have also agreed to share data with participating practices to help improve performance, and align with a set of core quality measures.

All participating practices receive monthly care management payments of $160 per Medicare beneficiary per month during a 6-month episode of care that starts on the date of an initial Part B or Part D chemotherapy claim. The model also includes all Part A and Part B services a beneficiary receives during those 6 months, as well as certain Part D expenditures. If a beneficiary requires chemotherapy beyond the end of an episode, a new 6-month episode begins. Practices will also receive monthly payments from payers they have contracted with for providing enhanced services to plan members.

Other Novel Programs for Delivery Reform

END-STAGE RENAL DISEASE CARE MODEL The Comprehensive ESRD Care (CEC) Model is designed to identify, test, and evaluate new ways to improve care for Medicare beneficiaries with end-stage renal disease (ESRD). There are 37 ESRD seamless care organizations (ESCOs) participating in the CEC Model. For its first performance year—which was from October 2015 through December 2016—13 providers reported $75.1 million in shared savings, of which $51.2 million was earned by participating providers.

INDEPENDENCE AT HOME DEMONSTRATION This project is designed to test the effectiveness of home-based primary care in improving health outcomes, reducing hospitalizations, and lowering Medicare costs. During a 3-year period, physicians and nurse practitioners from participating primary care practices make in-home visits to Medicare beneficiaries who have multiple chronic conditions and functional limitations. Patients' care experience will be tracked through quality measures; practices that meet the quality measures and generate Medicare savings beyond a minimum requirement may receive incentive payments. Currently, 14 independent practices and three consortia are participating in the demonstration.

In the first year of the demonstration, practices saved CMS more than $25 million, at an average of more than $3,000 per beneficiary. CMS awarded $11.7 million in practice incentives. In the second demonstration year, Independence at Home practices saved, in aggregate, a net of $7,821,374, or an average of $89 per beneficiary. Seven participating practices earned incentive payments in the amount of $5,322,343 (CMS, 2016).

HOME HEALTH VALUE-BASED REIMBURSEMENT PILOT CMS has a value-based reimbursement pilot program for Medicare home health care agencies under way, as of January 2016. The model is part of the 2016 Home Health Prospective Payment

System proposed rule. CMS will increase or decrease the amount reimbursed for services depending on quality performance. Payment adjustments will start at 5% and will increase to 8% in later years. According to the rule, the goals of the incentive program are to improve the patient experience and quality of care and to weed out poorly performing agencies.

Nine states were randomly selected to be part of the pilot program; the proposed states are Arizona, Florida, Iowa, Maryland, Massachusetts, Nebraska, North Carolina, Tennessee, and Washington. Performance data are not yet available.

STATE-DRIVEN VALUE-BASED INITIATIVES

Innovation is taking place at the state and local levels across the country, with efforts to improve value in specific patient populations, such as behavioral health programs for people with mental illness. Often these programs are funded through grants awarded by the CMS Innovation Center or are state Medicaid pilot programs.

There are two examples in which health care delivery and payment reform: the Maryland All-Payer Model and the Vermont All-Payer ACO.

Maryland All-Payer Model

Since the 1970s, Maryland has been the only state in the United States to have an all-hospital rate-setting system. On January 1, 2014, Maryland instituted an all-payer model for hospitals, in which an annual global budget is established for all inpatient and outpatient hospital expenses. Through an agreement with CMS, Maryland hospitals are exempt from the Inpatient Prospective Payment System (IPPS) and Outpatient Prospective Payment System (OPPS).

In May 2018, CMS renewed Maryland's request to renew and expand the state's all-payer model. Starting in January 2019, physician practices and nursing homes can voluntarily participate in the program. Maryland hopes to better coordinate care in the community for nonhospital services, such as for behavioral health and long-term care services. For patients with chronic illnesses, Maryland will pay physician practices a management fee for care coordination and other services.

According to a review of the Maryland All-Payer Model in 2018, Medicare saved $679 million in the first 3 years of the program—more than double the $330 million it had expected to save prior to the model's implementation (Haber, Beil, Amico, & Morrison, 2018).

Vermont All-Payer ACO

In December 2017, Vermont state lawmakers approved a budget of $620.8 million for OneCare Vermont, the state's multipayer ACO that includes several hospitals within Vermont and two in New Hampshire, hundreds of physicians, rural health clinics, and other facilities. The Green Mountain Care Board, which approves hospital budgets and insurance prices in Vermont, oversees the ACO.

The ACO is a 5-year experiment designed to revamp the way in which health care is delivered. Primary care providers at participating hospitals and clinics receive a monthly fee of $3.25 per patient for all covered patients. Providers involved in the care of the sickest patients receive an extra $15 to $25 per month.

Hospitals are responsible for a total of $21.5 million in financial risk, and if the ACO performs well on a specific set of quality measures, all participating providers will share a $4.3 million bonus. An estimated one in every five Vermont residents will receive care under the OneCare ACO.

The goal is to hold annual growth in health care costs to no more than 3.5% for 5 years, starting in 2018. Payments to the ACO, in turn, will increase by a weighted average of 3.5% annually. The state expected to have approximately 30% of primary care physicians participating in the model by the beginning of 2018 and 80% participating by the fifth year (D'Ambrosio, 2017).

Prior to the program launch, Governor Peter Shumlin estimated that the all-payer system could save the state approximately $10 billion over a decade (Aloe, 2017).

CONCLUSION

Over the past several decades, health care spending in the United States has increased faster than general economic growth. This growth can be attributed to a financing model that has historically rewarded volume over value and that is fraught with waste; opaque pricing systems with few checks and balances; and a citizenry conditioned to demand limitless and immediate health care.

Attempts at slowing cost growth have largely focused on reducing payments to providers or on restraining services covered by insurance companies. These attempts ultimately end up being undone, in part because they often result in limiting access for patients.

The current movement toward value in health care seems to have two centers of gravity. The first can be seen in efforts to reimagine patient-centered outcome measurement, with the goal of providing health care that helps patients achieve the outcomes that matter most to them. The other is in redesigning care delivery systems to consider patients' needs more holistically over the course of a care episode.

While there are several innovative state-based programs currently under way, for example, in Maryland and Vermont, with bold ambitions to reimagine health and health care in very broad terms, efforts like this remain the exception rather than the norm. Much of the current, and likely near-term, payment and delivery system reform is rooted in federal innovation programs or in the private sector (sometimes with federal backing). Regardless of its source, the buzz and amount of activity in delivery system reform seems to be an acknowledgment that spending levels may be reaching a tipping point. Public and private innovators alike see high spending growth as an opportunity as much as they see it as a crisis.

To be sure, there will be no easy fixes to solve the value equation. Importantly, we need to gather data on ongoing programs designed to address the issue. Whether it is changing payment to reimburse for bundles of services, accountable care models, or the use of technology to reduce unnecessary treatments and procedures, better data will be needed to provide insights into what saves money without sacrificing value and what does not. Organizations such as Kaiser Permanente, in which the provider is the employer and the insurer, have led to cost reductions and improved outcomes for patients; such models of care should be analyzed for sustainability and scalability.

This chapter discussed on costs and value in the delivery of health care services. But what must be kept in clear focus is that spending on medical care does not address the key determinants of the overall health of a population. The best way to keep people healthy is through public health initiatives, prevention initiatives, and social policies that make healthy choices possible and likely. These strategies are not what the medical care enterprise is about; medical care restores health more than it ensures that a population is healthy over its life span. A key question for public policy is to think through how much should be spent to create population health and how much should be spent on recovery-oriented medical care (see Chapter 5).

▶ CASE EXERCISE—MONITORING OF VALUE

You are a senior manager at a major health care provider in a competitive environment. The CEO of the medical center informs you that the board of directors has asked that monthly reporting not be limited to financial projections and budget-to-actual reports. Rather, the board is becoming concerned with evaluating the medical center's performance on value. The board still has a fiduciary responsibility to ensure the financial health of the organization, but members are increasingly concerned with value provided and not just cost. The CEO asks you to advise her on what she should propose to the board for such monitoring of value.

As you draft your recommendations, consider the following questions:

1. Why might the board of directors want to monitor value?

2. What indicators would you recommend to the CEO?

3. How would you gather data and evidence that might suggest increasing value for cost?

4. How would you measure success in these value-for-cost efforts?

DISCUSSION QUESTIONS

1. Is the growth in health care costs a real concern for the United States? Why or why not?

2. Comment on the claim that "the U.S. health care delivery system is the finest in the world."

3. Recent legislation requires insurance companies that offer coverage for mental health or substance abuse to provide the same level of benefits as they do for medical treatments. What are the implications of this requirement for health care costs? What are the implications for value?

4. Pharmaceutical companies frequently advertise drugs that require a doctor's prescription. Consider how such advertising might affect drug costs and utilization of services by patients.

5. An August 4, 2013, a *New York Times* article described the role of nonmedical costs in driving up health care. European health care centers are described as "Spartan"—for example, a Belgian clinic was described as having metal folding chairs, bland wall colorings, and no gift shop. This was contrasted with a U.S. hospital that had a comfortable waiting room, a fancy lobby, and even newsstands to sell conveniences to patients and visitors. Discuss these differences in light of cost and value. What barriers might the United States face in making a transition to a more European-style system?

6. In India, doctors are usually consulted only for very difficult and complicated procedures. Routine procedures are typically handled by lower-skilled health care workers such as nurse practitioners, nurses, or paramedics. What barriers might the United States face in making a transition to a more Indian-style system?

7. Discuss three interventions at the provider level and at the state level (where much regulation occurs) that will increase value for costs in health care. Explain why the interventions will work. If they will work, why haven't we implemented them already?

REFERENCES

Aloe, J. (2017). Shumlin pushes new health care model. *Burlington Free Press*. Retrieved from https://www.burlingtonfreepress.com/story/news/politics/government/2016/10/06/shumlin-pushes-new-health-care-model/91531388

Anderson, G. F., Reinhardt, U. E., Hussey, P. S., & Petrosyan, V. (2003). It's the prices, stupid: Why the United States is so different from other countries. *Health Affairs*, *22*(3), 89–105.

Baicker, K., & Chandra, A. (2005). The labor market effects of rising health insurance premiums (Working paper no. 11160). Cambridge, MA: National Bureau of Economic Research. Retrieved from http://www.nber.org/papers/w11160

Barrett, M. L., Wier, L. M., Jiang, H. J., & Steiner, C. A. (2015). All-cause readmissions by payer and age, 2009–2013. Agency for Healthcare Reporting and Quality, HCUP Statistical Brief #199. Retrieved from http://www.hcupus.ahrq.gov/reports/statbriefs/sb199-Readmissions-Payer-Age.pdf

Berwick, D. M., & Hackbarth, A. D. (2012). Eliminating waste in U.S. health care. *Journal of the American Medical Association*, *307*(14), 1513–1516.

Berwick, D. M., Nolan, T. W., & Whittington, J. (2008). The triple aim: Care, health, and cost. *Health Affairs*, *27*(3), 759–769.

Blumenthal, D., & Stremikis, K. (2013, September 17). Getting real about health care value. *Harvard Business Review*. Retrieved from https://hbr.org/2013/09/getting-real-about-health-care-value

Buchmueller, T., Carey, C., & Levy, H. G. (2013). Will employers drop health insurance coverage because of the Affordable Care Act? *Health Affairs*, *32*(9), 1522–1530.

Centers for Disease Control and Prevention. (2017). The 2015 national and state healthcare-associated infection data report. Retrieved from https://www.cdc.gov/hai/surveillance/data-reports/2015-HAI-data-report.html

Centers for Medicare and Medicaid Services. (2016). Independence-at-home demonstration. Retrieved from https://innovation.cms.gov/initiatives/independence-at-home

Centers for Medicare and Medicaid Services. (2017). Bundled payments for care improvement initiative: General information. Retrieved from https://www.cms.gov/Newsroom/MediaReleaseDatabase/Press-releases/2017-Press-releases-items/2017-11-30.html

Centers for Medicare and Medicaid Services. (2018). Bundled payments for care improvement initiative: General information. Retrieved from https://innovation.cms.gov/initiatives/bundled-payments

Cigna. (2018a). UPMC and Washington physician hospital organization collaborate to improve care and costs in Western Pennsylvania. Retrieved from https://www.cigna.com/newsroom/news-releases/2018/cigna-upmc-and-washington-physician-hospital-organization-collaborate-to-improve-care-and-costs-in-western-pennsylvania

Cigna. (2018b). What is Cigna collaborative care? Retrieved from https://www.cigna.com/newsroom/knowledge-center/aco/

Classen, D. C., Resar, R., Griffin, F., Federico, F., Frankel, T., Kimmel, N., … James, B. C. (2011). "Global trigger tool" shows that adverse events in hospitals may be ten times greater than previously measured. *Health Affairs, 30*(4), 581–589.

Collins, S. R., Radley, D. R., Gunja, M. Z., & Beutel, S. (2016). *The slowdown in employer insurance cost growth: Why many workers still feel the pinch.* New York, NY: The Commonwealth Fund.

Cooper, Z., Craig, S. V., Gaynor, M., & Van Reenen, J. (2015, rev. 2018). The price ain't right? Hospital prices and health spending on the privately insured (Working paper no. 21815). Cambridge, MA: National Bureau of Economic Research. Retrieved from http://www.nber.org/papers/w21815

Cutler, D., Wikler, E., & Basch, P. (2012). Reducing administrative costs and improving the health care system. *New England Journal of Medicine, 367*, 1875–1878.

D'Ambrosio, D. (2017). Care board five-year experiment will focus on keeping patients healthy. *Burlington Free Press.* Retrieved from https://www.burlingtonfreepress.com/story/news/2017/12/21/care-board-five-year-experiment-focus-keeping-patients-healthy/957467001/

Dartmouth atlas of health care. (2014). End-of-life care. Retrieved from http://www.dartmouthatlas.org/keyissues/issue.aspx?con=2944

Dummiit, L. A., Kahvecioglu, D., & Marrufo, G. (2016). Association between hospital participation in a Medicare bundled payment initiative and payments and quality outcomes for lower extremity joint replacement episodes. *Journal of the American Medical Association,, 316*(12), 1267–1278.

Emerick, T., & Lewis, A. (2013). *Cracking health costs: How to cut your company's costs and provide employees better care.* Hoboken, NJ: Wiley.

Fisher, E. S., Wennberg, D. E., Stukel, T. A., Gottlieb, D. J., Lucas, F. L., & Pinder, E. L. (2003a). The implications of regional variations in Medicare spending. Part 1: The content, quality, and accessibility of care. *Annals of Internal Medicine, 138*(4), 273–287.

Fisher, E.S., Wennberg, D.E., Stukel, T.A., Gottlieb, D.J., Lucas, F.L., & Pinder, E.L. (2003b). The implications of regional variations in Medicare spending. Part 2: Health outcomes and satisfaction with care. *Annals of Internal Medicine, 138*(4), 288–298.

Gawande, A. (2015). Health care's price conundrum. *The New Yorker.* Retrieved from https://www.newyorker.com/news/news-desk/health-cares-cost-conundrum-squared

Haber, S., Beil, H., Amico, P., & Morrison, M. (2018). Evaluation of the Maryland all-payer model third annual report. RTI International. Retrieved from http://www.hscrc.state.md.us/Documents/Modernization/md-all-payer-thirdannrpt.pdf

Hagist, C., & Kotlikoff, L. J. (2006). Health care spending: What the future will look like (Policy report no. 286). Washington, DC: National Center for Policy Analysis.

Harrington, S. E., & Smith, T. J. (2008). The role of chemotherapy at the end of life: "When is enough, enough?" *Journal of the American Medical Association, 299*(22), 2667–2678.

Hartman, M., Martin, A. B., Espinosa, N., Catlin, A., & National Health Expenditure Accounts Team. (2018). National health care spending in 2016: Spending and enrollment growth slow after initial coverage expansions. *Health Affairs, 37*(1), 150–160.

Hayes, S. L, Salzberg, C. A., McCarthy, D., Radley, D. C., Abrams, M. K., Shah, T., & Anderson, G. F. (2016). *High-need, high-cost patients: Who are they and how do they use health care? A population-based comparison of demographics, health care use, and expenditures.* New York, NY: The Commonwealth Fund.

Humana. (2018). Humana launches national value-based model for maternity care: Bundled payment model aims to improve patient experience and outcomes for Humana commercial group members. Retrieved from https://www.businesswire.com/news/home/20180418005705/en/Humana-Launches-National-Value-Based-Model-Maternity-Care

Institute of Medicine. (2012). *Best care at lower cost: The path to continuously learning health care in America.* Washington, DC: Author.

International Federation of Health Insurance Plans. (2013). 2012 Comparative price report. Retrieved from http://hushp.harvard.edu/sites/default/files/downloadable_files/IFHP%202012%20Comparative%20Price%20Report.pdf

Laugesen, M. J., & Glied, S. A. (2011). Higher fees paid to U.S. physicians drive higher spending for physician services compared to other countries. *Health Affairs, 30*(9), 1647–1656.

Mitchell, E. (2016). Concentration of health expenditures in the U.S. noninstitutionalized population, 2014. Agency for Healthcare Research and Quality, Statistical Brief #497. Retrieved from http://www.meps.ahrq.gov/mepsweb/data_files/publications/st497/stat497.pdf

Morris, M., Abrams, K., Elsner, N., & Gerhardt, W. (2016). Practicing value-based care: What do doctors need? *Deloitte University Press.* Retrieved from https://www2.deloitte.com/insights/us/en/industry/health-care/physician-survey-value-based-care-models.html

National Committee for Quality Assurance. (2018). Patient-centered medical home recognition. Retrieved from http://www.ncqa.org/programs/recognition/practices/patient-centered-medical-home-pcmh

Nolte, E., & McKee, M. (2012). In amenable mortality—deaths avoidable through health care—progress in the U.S. lags that of three European countries. *Health Affairs, 31*(9), 2114–2122.

Organisation for Economic Cooperation and Development. (2013). *Health at a glance 2013: OECD indicators.* Retrieved from http://www.oecd.org/els/health-systems/Health-at-a-Glance-2013.pdf

Porter, M. E. (2010). What is value in health care? *New England Journal of Medicine, 363*(26), 2477–2481.

Porter, M. E., & Teisberg, E. O. (2006). *Redefining healthcare: Creating value-based competition on results.* Boston, MA: Harvard Business Review Press.

Radley, D. C., McCarthy, D., & Hayes, S. L. (2018). *2018 scorecard on state health system performance.* New York, NY: The Commonwealth Fund.

Reinhardt, U. E., Hussey, P. S., & Anderson, G. F. (2004). U.S. health care spending in an international context: Why is U.S. spending so high, and can we afford it? *Health Affairs, 23*(3), 10–25.

Robert Wood Johnson Foundation. (2013). Finding value in health care: How providers are addressing rising costs. Retrieved from http://www.rwjf.org/content/dam/farm/reports/issue_briefs/2013/rwjf405299

Schneider, E. C., Sarnak, D. O., Squires, D., Shah, A., & Doty, M. M. (2017). *Mirror, mirror 2017: International comparison reflects flaws and opportunities for better U.S. health care.* New York, NY: The Commonwealth Fund.

Shah, K. P., & Spinks, T. E. (2017, February 5). How a cancer center rapidly developed patient-centered outcome measures. *NEJM Catalyst*. Retrieved from https://catalyst.nejm.org/cancer-center-rapidly-developed-patient-centered-outcome-measures

Sood, N., Ghosh, A., & Escarce, J. J. (2009). Employer-sponsored insurance, health care cost growth, and the economic performance of U.S. industries. *Health Services Research*, *44*(5), 1449–1464.

Stanford GSB Staff. (1999). Managed care: What went wrong? Can it be fixed? Retrieved from https://www.gsb.stanford.edu/insights/managed-care-what-went-wrong-can-it-be-fixed

UnitedHealthcare. (2018). UnitedHealthcare's value-based care program for knee, hip and spine procedures demonstrates improved health outcomes and reduced costs. Retrieved from https://www.businesswire.com/news/home/20180509005151/en/United HealthcaresValue-Based-Care-Program-Knee-Hip-Spine

Wade, H. (2012). *Small business problems & priorities, 2012*. Nashville, TN: The National Federation of Independent Business. Retrieved from http://www.nfib.com/Portals/0/PDF/AllUsers/research/studies/small-business-problems-priorities-2012-nfib.pdf

Wennberg, J., & Gittelsohn, A. (1973). Small area variations in health care delivery. *Science*, *182*(4117), 1102–1108.

Woloshin, S., & Schwartz, L. M. (2018). Overcoming overuse: The way forward is not standing still. *British Medical Journal, 361*, k2035.

Yong, P. L., Saunders, R. S., & Olsen, L. (Eds.). (2010). *The healthcare imperative: Lowering costs and improving outcomes—workshop series summary*. Washington, DC: National Academies Press. Retrieved from https://www.ncbi.nlm.nih.gov/books/NBK53920/pdf/Bookshelf_NBK53920.pdf

12

High-Quality Health Care

Carolyn M. Clancy and Irene Fraser

LEARNING OBJECTIVES

▸ Explain why quality measurement is important in health care
▸ Explain how health care quality in the United States compares to that in other countries
▸ Understand methods used to improve quality
▸ Understand the extent to which economic incentives have influenced quality improvement
▸ Describe recent trends in quality improvement
▸ Discuss the core competencies for health administrators that impact quality

KEY TERMS

▸ handoff
▸ outcomes
▸ pay-for-performance (PFP)
▸ performance measurement
▸ professionalism

TOPICAL OUTLINE

▸ Defining quality in health care
▸ The current state of quality in the United States
▸ Approaches to improving quality
▸ Creating incentives for providers to improve quality
▸ Recent developments affecting quality
▸ The role of managers in promoting quality

INTRODUCTION

TG is a 55-year-old man with diabetes, high blood pressure, and arthritis in both knees. As one knee becomes increasingly painful (and sometimes buckles), he is advised to have a total knee replacement. Surgery goes well, but TG develops a serious infection. For months, he's unable to put any weight on the operated leg, and for weeks he is forced to take antibiotics and miss work. TG then has a second surgery to remove the joint replacement and have a new one placed. This time, the operation and recovery both go smoothly. TG's spouse and family are delighted that their long odyssey is over, but they wonder: Could they have done something differently? Should they have searched for information on quality and safety about the physician and hospital, and would doing so have made a difference?

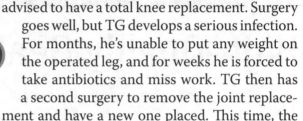

Recent research confirms that a sizable gap exists between the *best* medical care and the care that is routinely provided.*

Historically, an individual having surgery relied on a physician's recommendation—or that of a family member or friend—regarding a surgeon and/or hospital. Today, there are numerous sources of online information regarding performance for hospitals and other health care organizations. Websites also provide condition-specific information to help people understand what a diagnosis means, the options for treatment, and questions to ask when exploring those options. This plethora of information, however, is not easy to navigate, and many areas have yet to be addressed.

As a result of numerous studies, prestigious reports, and media accounts, Americans now know that high-quality, safe care is not automatic. Furthermore, the past 20 years have been marked by widespread efforts to assess and improve health care quality. Passage of the 2010 Patient Protection and Affordable Care Act (ACA) and the American Recovery and Reinvestment Act of 2009 (ARRA) created greater momentum toward ensuring quality care by (a) accelerating interest in linking payment for services to results and (b) creating multiple provisions that put providers on a path to high-quality, affordable health care. The momentum is likely to persist whatever the future is for the ACA.

This chapter describes the current state of health care quality (including avoidable harms from care); reviews selected efforts to conceptualize, measure, and improve quality; describes how measures are used to guide improvements in care; addresses promising initiatives to improve care; and predicts how the health care landscape will evolve in the coming years.

DEFINING QUALITY

Quality is defined by the Institute of Medicine (IOM) as "the degree to which health services for individuals and populations increase the likelihood of desired

The views expressed in this chapter are those of the authors and are not intended to represent official policy of the Department of Veterans Affairs or the U.S. government.

The authors gratefully acknowledge the expert assistance of Louise Arnheim and Brent Sandmeyer.

*To hear the podcast, go to https://bcove.video/2zJpdY8 or access the ebook on Springer Publishing Connect™.

health outcomes and are consistent with current professional knowledge" (Lohr & Schroeder, 1990). Implicitly, this definition covers both individuals and patient groups, including those who seek care and those who do not. Furthermore, the definition was intended to focus on outcomes or end results important to individuals and to recognize that medical knowledge evolves. The IOM identifies six dimensions of quality: Health care should be safe, effective, patient centered, timely, efficient, and equitable (IOM, 2001). A frequently used shorthand definition of quality is "the right care for the right patient at the right time."

HOW ARE WE DOING?

Throughout the 20th century, impressive successes in biomedical science and public health—including dramatic reductions in cardiovascular diseases, the transition of HIV infection from a death sentence to a highly manageable chronic condition, and significant reductions in the percentage of Americans who smoke— resulted in substantial increases in life expectancy by as much as 30 years.

However, multiple studies indicate that there is much room for improvement, especially in the care of people with chronic illnesses. Research during the past decade confirms a sizable gap between best possible care and that which is routinely provided. In addition, international studies comparing health and health care in the United States with other countries are sobering. A recent Commonwealth Fund study (Schneider, Sarnak, Squires, Shay, & Doty, 2017) of 11 countries (Australia, Canada, France, Germany, the Netherlands, New Zealand, Norway, Sweden, Switzerland, the United Kingdom, and the United States) found that the United States ranked dead last, as it did in the 2014, 2010, 2007, 2006, and 2004 editions of the study. At the same time, the study shows, the United States spent far more on health care than any of the other 10 countries.

> Numerous studies examining the processes and outcomes of care have shown substantial variations in clinical practice and have resulted in a movement to develop better methods for determining the relationship between care processes and outcomes.

Numerous studies examining the processes and outcomes of care have shown substantial variations in clinical practice (itself an indicator of questionable quality) and have resulted in a movement to develop better methods for determining the relationship between care processes and outcomes. A recent study, for example, proposed four criteria by which to assess outcome measures (Baker & Chassin, 2017). These efforts also have revealed underuse, overuse, and misuse of services as well as the substantial time lapse for new scientific findings to be translated into practice—a problem that persists to this day.

Most troubling, a growing body of research has shown that medical care too often fails to deliver the first requirement of quality: safety. The past two decades have seen increased attention paid to avoidable harms that occur as a result of receiving care such as health care–associated infections (HAIs), surgical complications, and errors in prescribing and dispensing medications. One analysis, using death rates reported in studies since 1999 and extrapolating to the number of hospital admissions in 2013, identified medical errors as the third leading cause of death in the United States (251,000 lives) after heart disease (611,000) and cancer (585,000) (Makary & Daniel, 2016). The data do not include deaths from medical errors in other settings—only hospitals.

On a more promising front, research also has shown that conscious, concerted, evidenced-based interventions to improve safety and quality can have a positive impact. There has also been increasing recognition of how factors external to direct care—including reimbursement, organizational structure, and leadership—influence safety and quality. The U.S. Agency for Healthcare Research and Quality (AHRQ), which is mandated by Congress to report annually on the state of health care quality and health care disparities, has found statistically significant increases in a selected set of quality measures across all settings and populations since 2003. However, the magnitude of improvement has most often been modest, and disparities in care associated with individuals' race, ethnicity, age, education, income, and other factors remain pervasive. The following sections explore strategies and approaches for making these—as well as other, larger—improvements.

HOW DO WE IMPROVE QUALITY?

As noted above, health care quality in the United States is by no means optimal. Moreover, it varies considerably across communities, providers, and even departments in the same facility. How do we improve it? There is no easy, simple answer, and no switch that can be flipped. Figure 12.1 provides a framework for identifying the intersection of several major factors in quality improvement. For starters, we know there are several critical steps that providers or administrators can take:

- Measure what you are doing—and with what result.
- Know what works clinically, and make sure you are doing it.
- Look at how care is organized and delivered and what process improvements might be made.
- Prioritize quality and safety. (This is especially important for those in leadership positions.)

Measure What You Are Doing

Human beings are fascinated with measuring things, and this fascination starts at an early age. First-grade students are given a ruler and asked to measure the length of the kitchen table, the heights of their parents, or the size of their television. Children tackle such assignments with great enthusiasm, usually surpassing the basic number of items on a teacher's list. As we grow older, many of us remain fascinated with measuring things, especially if they are important to us. Golfers, runners, bowlers, and cyclists, for example, frequently keep

FIGURE 12.1   IMPROVING CARE THROUGH SYSTEM REDESIGN

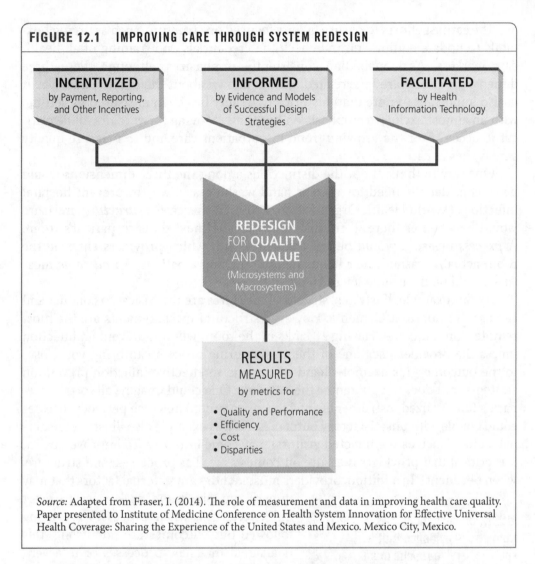

Source: Adapted from Fraser, I. (2014). The role of measurement and data in improving health care quality. Paper presented to Institute of Medicine Conference on Health System Innovation for Effective Universal Health Coverage: Sharing the Experience of the United States and Mexico. Mexico City, Mexico.

meticulous records on the events in which they have participated to track their own improvement.

Similarly, health care providers or leaders who seek to improve the quality and safety of their care start by measuring what they are doing and with what effect. Obviously, health care is more complicated than running or bowling and is growing increasingly more complex. As a result, determining *what* to measure is no easy task. (And, as discussed later in this chapter, the provider is not the only person who is measuring.)

A good starting point is with the definition of quality provided by Avedis Donabedian (1988). According to Donabedian, quality consists of three important dimensions: structure, process, and outcomes.

- Structure refers to facilities and health care professionals providing care.
- Process refers to the set of services provided.
- **Outcomes** refer to the end results that people experience and care about.

The earliest efforts to ensure quality focused on structure, such as urging hospitals to update equipment and check the credentials and training of all health care workers. As Donabedian consistently emphasizes, although these three dimensions clearly are interrelated, little is known about their causal linkages. It is also important to note that, historically, quality has been measured by setting, with an almost exclusive emphasis on hospitals. Moving forward, it will be critical to account for the growing trend in outpatient care and to measure quality across sites of care.

One way to think about the distinctions among the three dimensions would be to consider the need for regular hand washing as a way to prevent hospital infections (World Health Organization, 2009). In this case, a *structural* measure would be whether there were sinks in, or located next to, each patient's room. A *process* measure would be the frequency with which providers entering the room actually washed their hands before touching a patient. An *outcome* measure would be the frequency of HAIs.

As this example illustrates, structural measures are the easiest to conduct and can assess important elements. However, structural measurements are the most remote from outcome. Having 10 sinks in the room will not prevent an infection unless the provider uses one of them. Measuring process can bring you closer to the outcome—for example, hand washing is an effective infection prevention strategy—but does not guarantee the outcome. One could imagine all sorts of scenarios (unsterilized instruments, infected visitors, etc.) in which perfect processes could couple with unsatisfactory outcomes. As this example also illustrates, external factors (such as the infected visitors) may come into play. To improve quality, it is critical that providers measure outcomes as well as processes (and structure, when pertinent). In addition, providers must identify any external factors that may imperil outcomes and seek ways to exert influence. And, when processes are being followed but outcomes are not strong, this is a signal that new processes or interventions need to be identified that will improve outcomes.

> Ideally, process measures derive from strong evidence that a specific service results in an improved outcome.

Ideally, process measures derive from strong evidence that a specific service results in an improved outcome. These measures typically are derived from clinical research that shows a particular act or intervention. For example, giving beta blockers to patients who have suffered a heart attack—*all things being equal*—will achieve better outcomes.

Process measures are commonly expressed as a percentage of eligible patients who received a particular service or action (the beta blocker or the washed hands). Monitoring process measures very closely can be critical to quality improvement. But it is equally important to monitor outcomes to make sure that there are no other, unmeasured factors intervening to produce poor outcomes, even with good process scores. As discussed later in this chapter, consumers and payers are particularly interested in outcomes. Further, policy makers also are moving in the direction of outcome measures. One particular area of current interest is development and expansion of patient-reported outcomes (PROs). In effect, this growing interest recognizes that clinical outcomes measured now may not always represent all of the things that matter to patients (www.qualityforum.org/Projects/n-r/Patient-Reported_Outcomes/Patient-Reported_Outcomes.aspx).

While each health care provider measures structures, processes, and outcomes individually (and in his or her own way), there is a growing national effort to be more strategic and aligned in the selection and specification of measures. This effort will enable patients, payers, and policy makers to more meaningfully compare performance across providers and over time. In 1999, the National Quality Forum (NQF) was established as a public–private partnership charged with setting standards for health care quality. NQF began by establishing a Strategic Framework Board to develop a measurement strategy and set of priorities. Since that time, it has served as the consensus-based standard-setting organization (Burstin, Leatherman, & Goldmann, 2016; NQF, 2018). The NQF uses a multi-stakeholder consensus process to review and endorse proposed measures. It now has about 300 endorsed measures used by the federal government, states, and private entities in public reporting and payment initiatives (www.qualityforum.org/about_nqf/work_in_quality_measurement). Over the years, the NQF has worked to better align similar but competing measures and expand the proportion of outcome measures, now at more than 30% (Burstin et al., 2016).

In addition to this greater interest in outcomes, there is growing interest in measuring the quality of an entire episode of care rather than each individual service. After all, what a patient cares about is the quality of the entire treatment plan, not just how well each individual piece was performed. Payers moving from fee-for-service to some type of bundled payment or capitation system also will want to measure the whole—rather than just the sum—of the

> What a patient cares about is the quality of the entire treatment plan, not just how well each individual piece was done.

parts. While achieving evidence-based, credible, and reliable measures that cut across services and even sites of care is a major challenge, it is one that must be met in order to move the quality agenda forward.

Even though good measures are important, they are meaningless without good data. The definition of what constitutes good data varies depending on the purpose the data will serve. For quality improvement, data ideally are (a) readily available as a by-product of the care process itself, (b) recent enough to permit analysis and improvement in close to real time, and (c) detailed enough to enable the posing and testing of hypotheses about which factors were responsible for current levels of quality or recent changes in quality. External benchmarks and, especially, examples of high performers can also be useful to prod continuous improvement and guard against complacency.

Just as measures are meaningless without good data, the utility of both is limited by poor communication. It is often said that health care is data rich but information poor. In other words, every encounter involves information collection, but the information is not easily shared by the multiple providers involved in a patient's care. Indeed, most physicians effectively "fly blind," with little (if any) information about how their practices compare to their peers' and with limited capacity to quickly identify all patients in their practice with a specific condition or treatment. Important clinical details are most often recorded on paper, whereas billing is almost universally electronic.

Major data sources for quality assessment include billing data, medical charts (which are more detailed but expensive and laborious to review), and patient surveys. Provisions in the ARRA requiring broad adoption of electronic health records (EHRs) that can be shared among providers should make the task of data collection easier. These provisions should also facilitate more timely feedback to providers to accelerate improvements in care where needed (see Chapter 14).

Fundamentally, at the front lines of care delivery, the process of measurement itself remains very much a work in progress. For example, a study focusing on primary care practice use of EHR data to assess quality improvement found that current functionality "may be insufficient to support federal initiatives tying payment to quality measures" (Cohen et al., 2018). The heterogeneity of the U.S. health care system means that most hospitals experience separate demands for information on quality from states, public payers, private-sector payers, accreditors, and others. Advances in measurement science have enhanced our capacity to assess dimensions of care and identify opportunities for improvement. For example, various tools, such as AHRQ's State Snapshots, allow care providers to compare their quality scores with other providers in their region or state and allow states to compare themselves on numerous quality measures with other states (www.ahrq.gov/research/data/state-snapshots/index.html). Given this enhanced focus, coordination of priorities for quality measurement among multiple payers will be required.

Measurement of care is the first practical step toward improving care. Determining *what* to measure and *how* to measure are critical to gathering the right information that will help to improve organizational processes of care and transform health care delivery for the better.

Know What Works Clinically

At its core, health care quality is the sum of multiple individual interactions between clinicians and patients; hence, most widely used process measures derive from scientific evidence about which treatments work best and for whom. In practical terms, valid measures reflect both strong evidence and professional endorsement; a specific treatment or approach represents what should be done for most individuals with a specific condition. The usual approach occurs when clinical professional organizations develop and disseminate practice guidelines from which measures are derived; these measures, in turn, are recognized by independent private-sector organizations. This supply chain is highly dependent on three factors: scientific funding, the capacity of professional organizations to conduct technical work and update both guidelines and measures to reflect scientific advances, and the degree to which data can be obtained to apply the measure. Policy efforts to promote adoption of EHRs and other applications of health information technology should be a game changer, making it easier to collect requisite data and to include reminders and decision support that help to improve care in real time.

Since publication of the IOM report, *To Err Is Human*, which identified avoidable harms to patients as a result of medical care as a leading cause of death (IOM, 1999), there has been increased emphasis on identifying what works clinically to prevent avoidable harms. For example, hospitalized patients who are immobilized for long periods because of injury, surgery, or other factors are at increased risk for blood clots. Anticipating this risk and administering prophylactic blood thinners reduces the risk dramatically. Similar strategies have been developed and implemented for common preventable harms. The IOM report also directed health care organizations to establish and nurture environments that encourage all staff members to speak up with concerns about actual or potential patient harms.

Improve Organization and Delivery

Although it is critical to perform those services with proven effectiveness, doing so will not ensure quality or good outcomes. Human bodies are complex, and health care organizations are also complex. In the past, health care primarily consisted of a visit between one patient and one doctor or other provider. Today, most health care is delivered by increasingly large, complex organizations. High-quality health care requires that all providers—physicians, nurses, receptionists, technicians—do excellent work as both individuals and as part of collaborative teams at all organizational levels.

One way to think about this organizational component is to consider a set of concentric circles with the patient and physician (or other provider) at the center. At the bedside or in the exam room, it is obviously essential that there be a correct diagnosis and appropriate treatment. Much recent research and quality improvement effort has been directed toward improving safety and quality at this micro level. As noted earlier, however, clinicians seldom act in a vacuum.

Outside the clinician–patient circle is a "team" circle. This team might include, for example, a surgeon and others in the intensive care unit, or one or more primary care clinicians and their other staff, such as nurses, nutritionists, and a receptionist. A patient's quality of care depends on the talents of individual team members and the quality of the members' interactions as a team. Based on early research related to teams, there are now sophisticated tools and training materials to help improve team performance. One example is TeamSTEPPS®, developed jointly by the Department of Defense and AHRQ, which includes modules on primary care, nursing homes, and care for patients with limited English proficiency (www.ahrq.gov/teamstepps.index.html).

When looking at ways to improve quality, it is also important to look at the care processes themselves, both at the team level and across teams (the so-called meso level of the organization) that might be involved in the care of a particular patient. This meso level is the next circle out in the set of concentric circles. Many industries have spent years working to improve their production processes by closely examining each of the steps involved, seeing how they fit together or do not fit together, and then asking whether those processes can be improved to reduce the number of defects or the range of variations. As noted in the final section of this chapter, however, health care has come late to this type of analysis and improvement.

Finally, to truly achieve quality of care for a patient, it is important to look at the macro level; that is, how different health care organizations relate to each other and to the external environment. Because multiple organizations may be involved in a single patient's care, patients may still encounter safety and quality problems even when treated by a talented and coordinated team of professionals.

For example, the patient **handoff** (e.g., hospital discharge) is a time of particular vulnerability at the macro level. Discharge is frequently a difficult and confusing time for all concerned. Patients and their families have a lot of conversations and receive a lot of paperwork. They either return home or go to a post-acute care facility, where they may have few or no follow-up conversations with hospital staff. For patients with little English proficiency or health literacy, or those without easy access to follow-up care, any gap can be especially troublesome. For example, the discharge planner may not ask the right questions, the patient may have no regular source of primary care or social support, or the patient may even be homeless. A patient with these issues may develop complications or require hospital readmission. Although some readmissions might be planned or result from an unrelated problem, many readmissions result from complications of care during a recent hospital stay, a problem with discharge planning, problems with post-acute care, or a lack of necessary follow-up care. Recognition of these issues has prompted the Centers for Medicare & Medicaid Services (CMS) to use readmission rates as a quality metric (Centers for Medicare & Medicaid Services, n.d.,b). It also has led to development of discharge planning toolkits, which have had much success in reducing such rates.[1] A nationwide public–private partnership—the Partnership for Patients—has used such toolkits as part of a nationwide campaign to reduce readmission rates (www.partnershipforpatients.cms.gov).

Recently, there has been considerable experimentation with efforts to improve care through other macro-level interventions. A prominent example is the emergence of primary care medical homes (PCMHs, also called patient-centered medical homes) as a way to achieve coordination of care for patients

---

[1] For an example of a discharge planning training program, see AHRQ's Project RED (www.ahrq.gov/professionals/systems/hospital/red/index.html).

across multiple organizations, with the primary care provider playing an essential role. The growth of accountable care organizations (ACOs), in which a single entity is held accountable for care across the spectrum, provides another example of a macro-level approach. Finally, some organizations recognize that, in the final analysis, nonmedical services may play an even greater role in health than medical care. Safety net providers, for example, include many nonmedical services into their mix. Such services may include nutrition counseling, transportation, or even housing.

Of all of these approaches, micro-level quality improvement is undoubtedly the easiest and the closest to most clinicians' comfort zone. Improvements in care are most immediately visible for services under the direct control of a clinician or a health care organization (such as ordering the right tests for patients with diabetes or heart disease). Control of cholesterol, diabetes, or asthma, on the other hand, may require changes not only in patients' lifestyle choices, but also in their communities, and achieving these improvements requires coordination with multiple external organizations.

Prioritize Quality and Safety

As the above discussion makes clear, achieving safety and quality is not easy and requires that everyone involved look outside the box of their own job description, continually seeking ways to achieve more systemic improvements. Here, the single most important determinant of that happening is whether organizational leadership deems quality a top priority. Each day, leaders of health care organizations—including their boards—convey priorities to staff by the questions they ask, the outcomes they reward, and so on. Effective leaders nurture a culture of safety and quality, which lays the groundwork for quality improvement (Jiang, Lockee, Bass, Fraser, & Norwood, 2009). Furthermore, organizations differ substantially in terms of scores on safety culture surveys, such as those compiled by AHRQ at www.ahrq.gov/professionals/quality-patient-safety/patientsafetyculture.

Culture is also one of the five C's essential to prioritizing quality and safety within a given health care organization (see Figure 12.2). Together, they serve as a framing mechanism for health care leaders to consider, as follows:

- *Culture:* Is the organization one in which employees feel supported in speaking up if they see something that might lead to potential patient harm? Additionally, does the health care organization promote continuous learning and improvement?
- *Capacity:* Does the organization have the right mix of clinicians, providers, and specialties?
- *Capability:* Do clinicians have the right tools (data) to do their jobs?
- *Consistency:* Does the organization promote the use of evidence-based research and best practices to ensure consistency in care?
- *Candor:* Do providers encourage patients to ask questions about their care and work to promote a truly interactive doctor–patient dialogue? Does the organization promote transparency and access to information?

FIGURE 12.2   THE FIVE C's

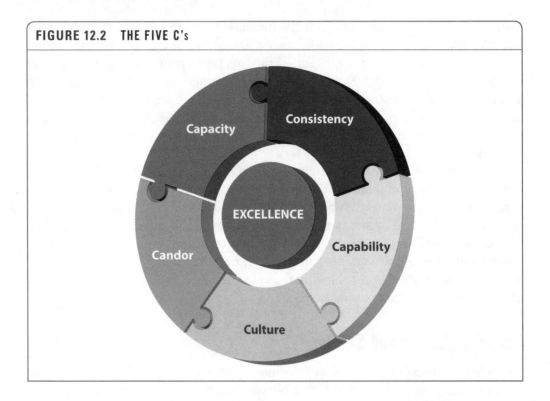

HOW DO WE INCENTIVIZE QUALITY CARE?

The health care environment is replete with financial, policy, and other drivers that influence provider behavior. Improving the quality of health care therefore means finding ways to harness these drivers to maximize and align positive incentives to the provision of quality and to eliminate perverse incentives. Because these incentives occur within the complex human and organizational environment in which care is provided, the effect of particular incentives varies from institution to institution, over time, and within institutions. To complicate matters further, we lack strong evidence of when, how, how much, and why most potential incentives will be effective in achieving their intended outcomes while avoiding unintended ones (e.g., manipulating metrics to achieve expected results).

As a starting point, six drivers are discussed: professionalism, public reporting, payment, national and regional quality improvement initiatives, consumerism, and regulation.

Professionalism

Professionalism refers to the conduct, aims, or qualities that characterize members of a given profession. People choose to enter health care over banking, engineering, law, or another profession for a reason. It is important to recognize that most clinicians strive to provide the right care to the right patient at the right time and take great pride in doing so. In addition, most people who develop measures recognize the importance of using metrics that are credible for their scientific content and recognized by the profession as important. Similarly, when health plans, employers, and community quality collaboratives use private performance reports as a way to encourage quality improvement, it is important that they use measures that resonate with physicians and other providers (Shaller & Kanouse, 2012). In short, efforts to improve quality that build on current science and clinicians' desire to do well by their patients are far more likely to succeed than those perceived as "counting the countable" but overlooking the important aspects of care.

> Efforts to improve quality that build on current science and clinicians' desire to do well by their patients are far more likely to succeed than those perceived as "counting the countable," but overlooking the important aspects of care.

Virtually all licensed professionals are required to document a commitment to continuing medical education—an enterprise that is increasingly linked to the challenges confronting clinicians in daily practice. Whereas in the past, continuing education focused almost exclusively on knowledge (what to do in specific circumstances), far more attention is currently paid to expanding the focus to include specific skills (how to provide specific services). In a similar manner, the medical boards that certify physicians based on their knowledge have shifted their process to include an explicit link to quality improvement processes, thereby establishing a direct link between knowledge and actual performance.

An early example of this approach focused on pediatric practices in North Carolina. Practices were randomized to receive focused coaching to improve the delivery of clinical preventive services; all clinicians received continuing education credits in exchange for participation (Margolis et al., 2004).

Major specialty boards are now partnering with large health care organizations to encourage and support physicians to continually refresh their skills and knowledge. A clear and tangible connection between pride in one's work and the tools for assessing quality can be a potent, nonfinancial driver of high-performing organizations.

Public Reporting

Another potential driver for quality is creation and dissemination of comparative public reports for consumers. Smith and colleagues (Smith, Saunders, Stuckhardt, & McGinnis, 2012) noted that "transparency of process, outcome, price, and cost information, both within health care and with patients and the public, has untapped potential to support continuous learning and improvement in patient experience, outcomes, and cost and the delivery of high-value care."

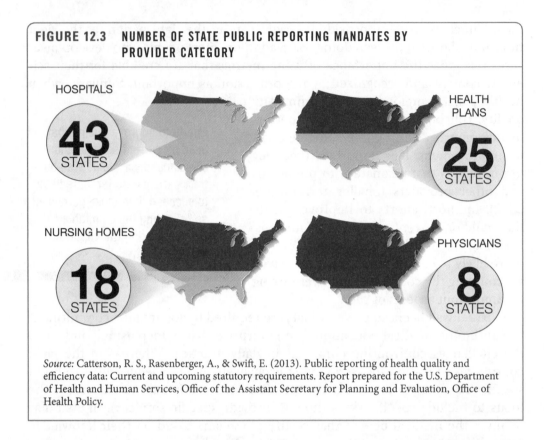

FIGURE 12.3   NUMBER OF STATE PUBLIC REPORTING MANDATES BY PROVIDER CATEGORY

HOSPITALS

43 STATES

HEALTH PLANS

25 STATES

NURSING HOMES

18 STATES

PHYSICIANS

8 STATES

Source: Catterson, R. S., Rasenberger, A., & Swift, E. (2013). Public reporting of health quality and efficiency data: Current and upcoming statutory requirements. Report prepared for the U.S. Department of Health and Human Services, Office of the Assistant Secretary for Planning and Evaluation, Office of Health Policy.

Reports comparing the quality—and sometimes the cost—of individual facilities or providers have proliferated in recent years. Part of the premise is philosophical, based on a consumer's right to know about his or her own care. However, the growing impetus behind publication of public reports is based on the premise that the availability and use of this information can be a force for improving quality.

Public reports have the potential to improve quality in three ways. First, public reports theoretically enable consumers to comparison shop for health care—just as they do for other products—selecting those with higher quality and/or lower costs (among other reasons, such as convenience). At the very least, an effective public report could help an individual consumer identify a hospital, physician practice, or nursing home with higher quality and/or better value. If enough informed consumers make these choices, the theory goes, the cumulative effect of individual informed decisions could potentially improve quality across the community, with high-quality providers gaining more business and low-quality providers losing business.

Second, employers, health plans, and others who contract with providers of care can favor high-scoring organizations when creating networks of care and can educate their employees or plan members about the quality differences.

Third, public reports enable health care providers to compare their performance with the performance of their peers. For reasons both professional and business related, providers do not want to be perceived poorly.

Public reports for consumers have increased significantly in the past several years, driven by state mandates and national legislation, as well as by national and regional quality improvement efforts and private transparency efforts, such as the Leapfrog Safety Grade, HealthGrades, Consumer Reports, and others. As Figure 12.3 shows, reports comparing hospital quality are the most common state mandate, but increasingly, states are requiring quality reports for health plans, nursing homes, and physicians as well. At the national level, CMS reports publicly on the quality of hospitals, nursing homes, physicians, and other providers. Additionally, the ACA ushered in a greater emphasis on public reporting. In particular, sections 3014 and 3015 of the ACA call for increased U.S. Department of Health and Human Services (DHHS) activity in quality measurement and public reporting.

What do we know about the effects of such reports? The evidence is fairly clear about the potential effect on provider behavior. While some providers undoubtedly ignore these reports, it is clear that others often take notice and take action (AHRQ, 2012a). A classic study in Wisconsin showed that hospitals with public reports were significantly more likely to initiate quality improvement activities than those with private reports (scores shared only with the individual hospital) or no reports. This finding was particularly true of low-scoring hospitals and the areas in which they had scored poorly (Hibbard, Stockard, & Tusler, 2003). Moreover, making data public brought actual improvements in the clinical areas reported (Hibbard, Stockard, & Tusler, 2005).

On the other hand, there is less evidence that public reports significantly change consumer behavior (AHRQ, 2012a). There are several reasons for this finding, and some of those reasons have nothing to do with the reports themselves:

- Consumers often are not in a position to choose between two providers. Their employer may offer only one health plan, or their plan may restrict their choice of hospital or medical group.
- Circumstances may not permit a choice: A patient suffering a heart attack is not in a position to research options for a hospital.
- Patients often rely on physicians for referrals and are not accustomed to seeking information from public reports.

In addition, several factors related to the reports themselves may account for this consumer behavior:

- *The measures:* Most of the information in public reports has not been developed in response to expressed consumer interest, but rather in response to what measure developers and report producers think should interest consumers and patients, and which they can easily measure.
- *Competing reports:* With policy interest in transparency growing and public reports on quality proliferating, confusion reigns regarding scores. Furthermore, the number of competing reports has resulted in tremendous discrepancy. There are two sources of apparent discrepancies: (a) minor differences in measure specifications and (b) summary rating systems ("star" systems, or systems focused on a specific dimension of

care, such as patient safety, among others). Multiple studies have documented that a hospital can get an "A" rating from one system while doing poorly on another (Rau, 2013).

■ *Information overload:* Consumers prefer to start with simple summary measures and icons and then drill down in accordance with their interests. Many report cards are designed as online versions of paper reports, with page after page of detailed tables.

■ *Clunky format:* Increasingly, consumers rely upon websites and social media for information. These venues support and link to sophisticated, fast search engines where consumers can prioritize their own preferences as part of the search process. For the most part, public reports on provider quality lag behind this technology trend.

In an effort to assess the state of public reporting, AHRQ partnered with The Commonwealth Fund to hold the Summit on Public Reporting. By bringing together major stakeholders and experts, including researchers, consumers, payers, providers, and policy makers, the Summit organizers sought to discuss the current state of the art in public reporting, identify major gaps, and to develop an agenda for the future. In preparation for the Summit, a contractor surveyed experts and stakeholders for their take on the current state of public reporting. The results were daunting: 81% said that even the best existing reports needed substantial improvement and redesign (AHRQ, 2011).

As a follow-up to the summit, AHRQ partnered in 2012 with CMS to launch a Science of Public Reporting initiative. The initiative's goal was to build the science and to accelerate adoption of proven improvements by CMS, states, and others developing public reports for consumers. To build the evidence base, AHRQ funded 17 grants in (a) effective design and presentation; (b) effective dissemination; and (c) strengthening the underlying data, measures, and methods (AHRQ, 2012b).

To help capture and disseminate the findings, AHRQ produced a special journal issue, *Medical Care Research and Review Supplement* (AHRQ, 2014). AHRQ worked directly with some of the report's developers, including CMS, to ensure that findings would be used as soon as the evidence became available. The AHRQ website links to publications from the grants and identifies findings on the use of public reporting for physicians and primary care, hospitals, nursing homes, and home health and hospice (https://www.ahrq.gov/professionals/quality-patient -safety/quality-resources/tools/sciencepubreport/index.htmlospice). To bolster take-up and dissemination of findings, AHRQ accelerated evolution of My Own Network Powered by AHRQ (MONAHRQ, available at MONAHRQ.ahrq.gov), a free, evidence-based website builder that enabled a state or other reporting entity to download free software from AHRQ (including Hospital Compare data), add locally available data (state hospital discharge data) to populate reporting fields, and create an almost instant public reporting website. While the agency is no longer investing in this work, many states and localities are still producing public reports based on this tool (www.ahrq.gov/professionals/systems/monahrq/ sites/index.html). In addition, evidence from this work has influenced CMS reporting efforts, such as Physician Compare, Hospital Compare, and Nursing Home Compare.

Public reporting faces several future challenges:

- *Linking cost information (ideally, consumer price information) to quality.* With the growing use of high-deductible health plans, consumer interest in price is likely to grow. Some health plans now produce reports for members that show out-of-pocket costs, and some states provide these data more widely as well.[2] One important caution from research to date is the need to display cost and quality information together; otherwise, a consumer is likely to draw the erroneous conclusion that the higher-cost service is better (Hibbard, Greene, Sofaer, Firminger, & Hirsh, 2012).
- *Incorporating social media.* With so many consumers—particularly younger ones— relying on social media to compare products, and so much of social media working to incorporate health care services, finding ways to incorporate the growing evidence base into these outlets will be an important challenge. On the other hand, understanding the importance of creating opportunities for consumers to self-identify what is important to them in terms of quality and amenities is important to the future of quality measurement and public reporting. Consumers often identify quality factors that experts overlook.
- *Increasing the timeliness and clinical robustness of public reports.* Consumers are becoming more and more accustomed to being able to access near real-time information, and providers are rightfully concerned about being judged on the basis of old information. Although there is hope that EHRs may eventually solve these problems, it is critical in the short term to take advantage of electronic capabilities to add clinical detail and speed to existing reports.

Payment

Payment incentives are another set of powerful drivers in the quality landscape. Any base payment structure brings inevitable incentives. The typical, traditional payment system for most providers in the United States has been fee-for-service, a system that typically has rewarded providers for more services rendered or longer hospital stays. In the 1980s, the Medicare program moved hospitals to a diagnosis-related group (DRG) system, in part as a way to reduce incentives for prolonging hospital length of stay. Under capitation, in which a health plan is responsible for the care of a defined population and is paid a fixed fee per member per month, the incentive is to reduce the number of high-cost services (such as hospitalization). (See Chapters 11 and 12 for more detail about payment approaches.)

In recent years, public and private payers have sought ways to create deliberate, targeted incentives—usually as an overlay on top of fee-for-service or other payment systems—to reward hospitals, physicians, and others for achieving particular quality or efficiency goals. This array of strategies, which variously are called **pay-for-performance (PFP)** or value-based purchasing, builds on the

---

[2] See, for example, the All-Payer Claims Database (www.apcdcouncil.org).

growing measurement enterprise, often using measures used in public reporting. One recent survey showed that 10.9% of current payments are value oriented (i.e., tied to performance or designed to cut waste), with traditional fee-for-service, bundled payment, capitation, and partial capitation making up the remaining 89.1% (Catalyst for Payment Reform, 2013). CMS is moving rapidly in the direction of value-based purchasing, with initiatives such as the Hospital Value-Based Purchasing program, performance bonuses for Medicare Advantage (MA) programs, and the Physician Value-Based Payment Modifier. In the private sector, insurers sometimes reward higher quality (and/or lower cost) by selectively contracting with only some providers in the marketplace or by tiering providers, thereby offering consumers lower copayments for some than for others.

Tracking the effect of such strategies is not easy, for several reasons:

- *Incentive size:* The incentive is often relatively small compared with the overall volume of business, and especially compared with the cost of making the improvements required to reap the reward. Consequently, if there is no effect, it is hard to tell whether a larger incentive might have worked.
- *Incentive confusion and fatigue:* CMS itself has many incentives applied to the same institutions. Hospitals, for example, have incentives related to readmission rates, adoption of "meaningful use" of certified EHR technology, and incidence of major patient safety events, in addition to more targeted incentives such as those in the Hospital Value-Based Purchasing program. In any particular market, these incentives may or may not be aligned with the incentives from private payers, or even Medicaid. In addition, sorting out the relative effects of public reporting and incentives is no easy matter.
- *No pure controls:* The ubiquity of differing incentives—coupled with public reporting efforts—makes it very difficult to find a control for purposes of evaluation.
- *Context and implementation:* The effect of payment incentives is likely to vary not only by provider (hospitals versus nursing homes versus physician groups), but also depending on how providers pass incentives along within the organization.

There has been some evaluation of the effect of financial incentives, but the wide-range of payment approaches and evaluation strategies complicates efforts to draw strong overall conclusions, particularly for evaluations focused on private-sector strategies. A recent analysis of the 355 evaluations collected in "Payment Reform Evidence Hub" (McClellan, Richards, & Japinga, 2017) found that the preponderance of evaluations focused on Medicare and Medicaid, with less attention paid to commercial payment initiatives. The analysis also found that many evaluations that focused on private programs were "internal" in that they did not release detailed results or specifics of how the reform was evaluated.

On the other hand, the Medicare program recently has been ramping up its move to value-based purchasing in ways that the market has not seen before, so it is possible that future evaluations may show stronger and broader impact. For example, CMS now has a voluntary Shared Savings Program, under which physicians, hospitals, and others involved in patient care can create an ACO, which is in turn is held accountable for the quality, cost, and experience of care for an assigned Medicare population. There are several different tracks, each with their particular financial risk arrangements. However, the general idea is that the ACO can share in the savings achieved from better care (Centers for Medicare & Medicaid Services, 2018).

With the proliferation of new—and in many cases, stronger—payment incentives, it will be critical that research address the complex question of what *form* of incentives, in what *magnitude* and under what *circumstances*, have the power to produce *which* intended consequences, while *avoiding unintended consequences*. One critical, potential unintended consequence is exacerbation of disparities. Safety net providers, often financially fragile, care for many patients with medical and nonmedical problems (such as homelessness) that cannot yet be adequately incorporated into risk-adjustment methodologies. Finding a way to hold all providers to high standards for all patients while accounting for the greater challenges some face is a continuing goal.

> Finding a way to hold all providers to high standards for all patients while accounting for the greater challenges some face is a continuing goal.

National and Regional Quality Improvement Initiatives

While the strategies described above can increase the individual and corporate desire for improvement, change is difficult at any level. Some of the most dramatic improvements in quality have resulted from deliberate, well-organized, regional or cross-regional collaborative efforts. These collaboratives start with evidence about what can work—along with evidence about what facilitates and impedes implementation—and build and implement a deliberate change strategy.

An excellent example of how various stakeholders came together to successfully strategize and improve quality began with research findings by Pronovost and colleagues. In 2007, Dr. Peter Pronovost and his team at Johns Hopkins reported the substantial successes of a deceptively simple approach to reducing infections associated with central line infections (Pronovost et al., 2006).[3] The problem is self-evident; central line infections have a mortality rate of 25%, and the approaches deployed are straightforward: rigorous attention to hand hygiene sterile technique and avoidance of the lines when feasible. Yet rates of these infections appeared for many years to be persistently high. The research team partnered with Blue Cross in Michigan, all Michigan hospitals (including their chief executive officers), and the Michigan Hospital Association. They combined a straightforward set of practices with empowerment strategies (e.g., any worker could "stop the line" if procedures were not followed), involvement of senior leadership, and modest data collection to facilitate rapid feedback. All hospitals

---

[3] Central lines are used to administer treatments that frequently destroy peripheral veins, such as chemotherapy or high-dose nutrition for patients unable to eat. They are also used to monitor heart and lung function in severely ill patients.

in Michigan achieved dramatic reductions, and the approach has subsequently spread to hospitals across the country in collaboration with the American Hospital Association. The combination of identifying an important problem (HAIs are easy to understand and fear), engaging senior leadership, leveraging a facility with data, and using practical strategies for applying data was enormously successful. The relevant organizational structures were quite different, depending on hospital size and complexity, but the intervention was highly adaptable.

Some of the most significant examples of this approach include:

- *Partnership for Patients:* This public–private partnership, led by CMS, includes multiple other federal agencies, hospitals and national provider organizations, patient and consumer organizations, state governments, employers, and others. The aim is to work with participating hospitals to decrease all-cause patient harm and reduce hospital readmissions (partnershipforpatients.cms.gov/about-the-partnership/aboutthe partnershipforpatients.html; https://downloads.cms.gov/files/cmmi/pfp-interimevalrpt .pdf).

- *Institute for Healthcare Improvement (IHI):* The IHI, a not-for-profit organization based in Cambridge, Massachusetts, seeks to *organize and mobilize quality improvement* and transformation by organizing learning networks and collaboratives in projects to drive and sustain improvement.

- *Quality improvement organizations (QIOs):* QIOs are groups of health quality experts, clinicians, and consumers who work under the direction of CMS to (a) improve care for Medicare beneficiaries and (b) review quality concerns (Centers for Medicare & Medicaid Services, n.d.,a). As a result of recent legislation, QIOs doing quality improvement will be separate from those doing review.

- *Community quality collaboratives:* These multi-stakeholder, regional collaboratives around the country take an active role in *public reporting, encouraging community engagement*, and *facilitating quality improvement* at the regional level.

Consumerism

In the past 20 years, there has been a gradual but marked change in the public's expectations regarding health care. Many people are more interested in health and health care, but also more skeptical about advice that doesn't feel right for them. Advances in communication technology, which have reduced asymmetries in health information between health professionals and patients, have surely accelerated this trend. Moreover, surveys of Americans in the baby boomer age group have consistently demonstrated less trust in authority in multiple areas—including medicine—when compared with older cohorts.

As noted in the discussion of public reporting, consumers or patients also can play an important role in quality. However, the consumer incentive functions differently in the health care market for several reasons:

- Because of the private and public insurance system, the purchaser of care is generally not the actual consumer of that care.
- Consumers and patients often lack the information they need to act in their own interests.

- Consumers often do not feel empowered to question their medical care team on recommended services or drugs in the way they would question, for example, a car mechanic or a roofer. Shortened medical visits do not make it any easier for patients to ask questions.
- Medical care services are only one factor that affects health. Lifestyle factors (such as obesity, low activity levels, poor diet, and smoking) have a larger effect on health than medical care.
- Even though consumers have an incentive to be healthy, good health is a more distal goal that often cannot compete with immediate gratification.

To improve quality and outcomes, it is important to activate and align the incentives of patients, consumers, and providers. In the past few years, several developments have created steps in that direction:

- Increased transparency in quality and price is starting to provide some of the information needed for consumers to make better choices, and the increased availability of clinical information on the Internet and social media is also making useful information more accessible to patients.
- Higher copays and deductibles are creating an environment in which consumers are motivated to choose a better-value provider and to question services they will purchase out of pocket. Unfortunately, past research (Chernew & Newhouse, 2008) has shown that increasing out-of-pocket payments leads patients to reduce their use of both necessary and less necessary services.
- Value-based insurance design—in which copays for services of questionable utility are high and copays for critical services are low or nonexistent—is a recent effort to be more strategic in the use of consumer financial incentives.
- Another path for incentivizing consumers is to alter the price of insurance based on health habits—for example, by charging smokers more or providing a reward to smokers who successfully quit. This is a very common approach for employers.

Regulation

Periodic inspections of health care facilities through accreditation combined with explicit processes for verifying the credentials and skills of clinicians (often referred to as *credentialing*) have been mainstays of the regulatory approach to health care quality. Historically, accreditation was conducted periodically and represented basic competence in operations important to care quality, such as sterile processing and environment of care. In addition, concerns about whether requisite improvements were sustained could not be fully allayed. Recently, CMS has been placing increased emphasis on The Joint Commission and other accreditation organizations to prioritize issues according to potential or likely impact on patient safety and to apply more rigorous approaches to assuring sustained improvement. In addition, CMS has instituted periodic comparisons of accreditation findings to those found by their state inspectors (CMS, 2017). The application of this approach, however, has confirmed that accreditation and credentialing are necessary but far from sufficient to guarantee provision of high quality care. No site visit or process can guarantee that care will be high quality, but accreditation organizations are now using tougher approaches to following up identified problems, including multiple unannounced inspections.

WHAT ARE MAJOR RECENT DEVELOPMENTS AFFECTING QUALITY?

Achieving high-quality health care is a high priority for many stakeholders. For patients, quality can be a life-or-death matter. Some of the initiatives described earlier, such as public reporting and payment incentives, have been deliberate efforts to affect quality. In recent years, passage of the ACA has been the single most important development affecting quality. However, other new forces are also at work.

The Patient Protection and Affordable Care Act

The ACA, signed into law in 2010, is primarily recognized for its effects on health care coverage. The ACA has expanded access to health insurance to millions of Americans. It also provided patient and consumer protections (e.g., eliminating use of preexisting condition limitations and lifetime caps on covered expenses).

Far less attention has been paid to the law's explicit recognition that sustaining the promise of expanded health care coverage demands efforts to promote and incentivize high-quality, affordable care. Numerous provisions in the law address many aspects of quality, such as improving measure selection, testing new models of care, and supporting research about which treatments work for patients. In addition, the ACA requires the development and annual update of a first-ever National Strategy for Quality Improvement (www.ahrq.gov/working forquality). Selected examples are described here:

- *Building on current efforts:* In the past decade, there have been incremental policy steps encouraging or requiring performance transparency in selected domains. Starting with voluntary efforts, progressing through what has been termed "pay for reporting" (a small percentage of annual update tied to reporting on quality), to linking achievement of selected quality goals to reimbursement (value-based purchasing), this journey also has included expansion in the number and types of metrics, including surveys to assess patients' experiences of care. The ACA requires that this approach be expanded to other settings—including rehabilitation and skilled nursing facilities—and that the incentives be increased over time.

    Combined with subsequent legislation, the ACA has resulted in a strong focus on value-based payment through a broad array of initiatives that link some portion of payment to quality of care. The most common examples include payment penalties for avoidable hospital admissions within 30 days of hospital discharge, hospital payments influenced by both quality and patient experience assessments, and bundled payments. The latter approach incentivizes coordination across care settings and providers through the use of a set price for all services for a clearly defined episode of care, such as elective joint replacement. These initiatives, combined with similar private-sector programs, represent a fundamental foundation for transitioning to payments that reward value rather than volume.

Evidence to date indicates a reduction in potentially avoidable hospital readmissions and significant reductions in several common HAIs. Experience to date also suggests nontrivial challenges in organizing financial and clinical data around episodes of care rather than care setting. However, continued increases in health care expenditures make it highly likely that improving quality and safety through payment incentives will continue to expand (Chee, Ryan, Wasfy, & Borden, 2016).

- *Testing new approaches:* The ACA created a new Center for Innovation at CMS, which supports the development and application of new approaches to financing linked with quality requirements. Examples include bundled payments, in which one payment is made for a broad array of services provided within one discrete episode of care, as well as support for ACOs, which integrate services and payments across multiple settings and establish virtual integrated organizations. A unique feature of the ACA allows successful demonstrations or models to be continued and possibly incorporated into future policy updates.
- *Primary care (or patient-centered) medical home:* The PCMH is part of a professional movement to revitalize and reinvent the delivery of primary care. The ACA includes multiple provisions to support and evaluate this new approach to primary care, which includes a strong focus on care organized around the patient's needs and preferences, a reliance on care teams rather than on individual clinicians, integration of mental health services, and reliable after-hours care.

Although these models are still evolving, they are important because the combination of increased needs associated with an aging population and expanded access to insurance is expected to place high demands on the primary-care sector.

Role of Nongovernmental Organizations

Many nongovernmental organizations also play a significant and evolving role in quality and quality improvement by developing and endorsing measures, accrediting health care organizations, conducting research on quality improvement at the micro- and macro-levels, using market power to encourage change, and facilitating use of emerging evidence to bring about transformation. Below are some examples:

- *National Quality Forum:* The NQF, a not-for-profit, membership-based organization, has a major role in quality measurement. As noted earlier, it endorses standards for **performance measurement**. In particular, NQF reviews and endorses measures for use in public reporting and payment.
- *The Joint Commission and other accreditation organizations:* As noted above, The Joint Commission, another not-for-profit organization, *accredits and certifies* health care organizations and programs. This accreditation is critical to hospitals and other organizations because CMS requires accreditation as a condition of participation in the Medicare program. Since 2008, other accreditation organizations have been approved by CMS to fulfill that responsibility (www.cms.gov/medicare/provider-enrollment-and-certification/surveycertificationgeninfo/downloads/

accreditation-organization-contact-info.pdf). Historically, accreditation has been seen as ensuring minimal competence to provide safe, high-quality care. In recent years, CMS has required these organizations to develop and implement more rigorous standards and to demonstrate sustained improvements when problems are identified. In addition, CMS annually compares observed findings from accreditation organizations with findings from their state surveyors in a proximal time period (CMS, 2017).

- *National Committee for Quality Assurance (NCQA):* The NCQA also *accredits and certifies* health care programs. While its particular initial focus was health plans, NCQA has expanded its scope to include disease management organizations, PCMHs, and ACOs. It also originated, maintains, and updates Healthcare Effectiveness Data and Information Set (HEDIS) *measures* of health plan performance.

- *University research programs:* Research programs at major universities around the country, funded by the National Institutes of Health, AHRQ, and private foundations, develop *measures* of quality and safety as well as *evidence* on how to improve quality and safety at both the micro and macro levels.

- *Employers and employer organizations:* Large employers and employer organizations, such as the National Business Group on Health and the National Business Coalition on Health, have a stake in both employee health and health care costs. Individually and as a group, they seek to *incentivize higher quality and value.*

- *Catalyst for Payment Reform:* The Catalyst for Payment Reform is an independent nonprofit, member-based organization of about 30 employers. Formed in 2009 with the goal of helping employers get better value for their health care dollar, the group aims to move health care payment from volume based to value based and to use purchaser power to improve the health care system (www.catalyze.org/about-us).

- *Leapfrog:* The Leapfrog Group is a national nonprofit organization founded in 2000 to drive a movement designed to achieve "giant leaps forward in the quality and safety of American health care." A major initiative is the Leapfrog Hospital Safety Grade, which uses nationally available data on hospital safety and data from the organization's annual survey of hospitals to assign patient safety letter grades to hospitals (www .leapfroggroup.org/about).

- *Patient groups:* Increasingly, patient groups are advocating for additional research on quality, particularly as it relates to a specific disease or condition. Some groups, such as the National Breast Cancer Coalition (NBCC) and the Arthritis Foundation, are leading national initiatives in this regard.
  - For nearly 20 years, NBCC has been a national leader in health care quality, beginning with its Quality Care Initiative (a "patient-centered, evidence-based vision of quality care" for those with breast cancer) and including its landmark publication, *Framework for a Health Care System Guaranteeing Access to Quality Health Care for All* (www.breastcancerdeadline2020.org/about-nbcc/quality-care/nbcc-health-care -framework.html).
  - The Arthritis Foundation has combined forces with several other groups (including the Childhood Arthritis and Rheumatology Research Alliance and the Dartmouth Institute for Health Policy and Clinical Practice) to pilot the Rheumatology Learning Health System (RLHS), a model that integrates self-reported patient information, data from a patient's clinical visit, and data from arthritis patient registries to create the foundation for a "personalized patient–doctor dialogue" (http://blog .arthritis.org/news/tag/rheumatology-learning-health-system/).

Lean

Lean, a tool developed by the automotive industry in Japan, is gaining increased interest as a way to improve health care quality and efficiency in the United States. Lean provides this five-step process for improving quality:

1. Specify value from the standpoint of the end customer by product family.
2. Identify all the steps in the value stream for each product family, eliminating wherever possible those steps that do not create value.
3. Make the value-creating steps occur in tight sequence so that the product will flow smoothly toward the customer.
4. As flow is introduced, customers pull value from the next upstream activity.
5. As value is specified, value streams are identified, wasted steps are removed, and flow and pull are introduced, begin the process again and continue it until a state of perfection is reached in which perfect value is created with no waste. (Lean Enterprise Institute, n.d.)

Lean has been used successfully to redesign health care. For example, Denver Health implemented a Lean system redesign in 2005, and between 2006 and 2008 achieved the following results: a 50% lower registration time in eight federally qualified health centers, lower patient cycle times and no-show rates, 25% higher provider productivity in clinics, $14 million in cumulative savings, and $3.5 million in increased clinic revenues (AHRQ, 2007).

Even though examples such as Denver Health show promise, there has been little systematic evaluation of whether, and under what circumstances, interventions such as these can achieve similar success across a wide variety of systems. While there have been some reviews of publications on Lean in health care, these reviews and most of the underlying studies concentrate on a narrow band of project outcomes, such as quality or efficiency. Although it is clear from this work that Lean *can* be successful, less is known about the factors necessary for such success: for example, the organizational processes supporting implementation, characteristics of implementing organizations, or interactions between Lean and other features of the organizational context. A recent study by AHRQ (Harrison et al., 2016) provides an understanding of how context shapes Lean implementation.

Patient and Family Engagement

As noted earlier, many local and regional efforts to promote transparency in quality performance have developed through the establishment of multi-stakeholder coalitions that include consumers, employers, health care providers, insurers, and other parties. In a similar vein, an increasing number of health care organizations have sought the experiences of patients and families to inform their efforts to deliver services focused on patients' needs and preferences. Studies have revealed that patients and families often observe aspects of care not immediately visible through other sources; capturing those observations and experiences can provide important insights about the care experience through the patient's eyes. Some observers have labeled patient engagement the "blockbuster drug" of the 21st century.

Even though many governing boards have long included at least one public representative, Massachusetts now requires all hospitals to have a formal patient and family advisory council. AHRQ also has supported an effort to develop and evaluate a survey tool that builds on patient and family experiences of care to improve patient safety.

Finally, it is critical to note the role of social media in consumer engagement. Whether via Facebook post, online review (including Yelp), or Tweet, consumer engagement via social media is far-reaching in terms of audience and immediate in impact. Often, however, there is no credible, third-party mediator. The "good news" is that social media generates greater information sharing and dialogue; the "bad news" is that social media generates information sharing and greater dialogue that may amplify misleading and erroneous information. Nevertheless, it is clear that the patient's voice represents a vital component of current and future efforts to continuously improve health care delivery.

CORE COMPETENCIES FOR HEALTH ADMINISTRATORS

Until recently, administrators have not necessarily made assessing and improving the quality of care a top priority. Yet, increasingly, the bottom line for all health care facilities—and therefore the priority for administrators—will be an explicit focus on care quality, that is, quality that is transparent and verifiable, rather than simply reputed. As a result, health care administrators need a solid grounding in quality measurement and in the design and evaluation of interventions and programs to improve quality (Lloyd, 2010a, 2010b).

Pragmatically, the function and structure of quality improvement have evolved considerably in the past 20 years in response to policy, regulatory, and other initiatives. It is also fair to acknowledge, however, that the constellation of disciplines, skills, and triggers for action is still quite dynamic. One fundamental consideration is the extent to which functions are centralized (e.g., a quality department) or distributed (quality is everyone's job), focused on improvement versus minimizing or avoiding risk, and internal to a health care organization versus external to it (e.g., payers writing requirements into contracts).

The steady expansion of policy initiatives—especially growing requirements for performance transparency and value-based purchasing—has prompted multiple formal activities, initiatives, and an emerging critical mass of organizations offering technical assistance and tools to advance internal improvements. At the same time, it is clear that external demands from payers, regulators, and consumer groups for enhanced transparency remain important to help drive improved performance. Moreover, continued increases in health care spending are also motivating increased demands for demonstrating value as well as quality.

The example described earlier regarding the prevention of central line infections is illustrative of several key competencies. First, it demonstrates the need to be aware of the evidence on quality shortfalls as well as improvement potential. Second, it underscores the importance of both a willingness and an ability to engage with other stakeholders. Third, it shows how the ability to utilize and apply data is vital to success.

It is eminently clear that a health administrator's facility with performance data—including the capacity to present the information in different ways to different audiences (e.g., standardized infection rates versus days since there's been no infection in a given unit)—is, and will continue to be, a core competence. Note that this implies a full grasp of the application of data to identify and solve problems rather than simply conducting the requisite analyses, though a grounding in statistics is also imperative (e.g., how often should hand-washing rates be assessed?). Nurses have arguably led the way in monitoring compliance with regulations and policies as a core component of quality assessment, but the full team required now includes clinicians from multiple disciplines. The ability to motivate, persuade, and communicate effectively is also a clear prerequisite.

Since publication of the results by Pronovost and colleagues (2006), an increasing number of payers now require reporting of different HAIs and/or incorporate HAI rates in their payment strategies. In light of this payer role in quality, many health administrator positions are now in insurance companies, large employers, or public payers. Improving quality from the payer side requires many of the skills described earlier, but because the specific actions are one step removed from actual delivery, improvement from this side also requires the ability to specify requirements, share results with employees/consumers/patients to inspire them to choose high-quality care, and recognize when reported results don't add up.

Addressing near-term challenges specified by the ACA—including the prevention of HAIs, avoidable hospital readmissions, and avoidable patient harms— also requires a new vision for understanding how individual health care facilities relate to others in the community or region.

For example, policies that promote decreased payments for higher-than-average readmission rates will motivate hospitals to work with community partners in very different ways to address the cause of the poor performance (e.g., limited primary care capacity, limited after-hours care, poor health literacy among patients in the community, or something else). Similarly, the ACA's provisions to promote health (e.g., addressing the upstream causes of disease and illness) will also blur traditional hospital boundaries. In other words, the hospital administrator's job will no longer be confined within hospital walls, but will require working with community partners—perhaps via health education and disease prevention programs.

While inpatient care has been the major focus of efforts to promote improved quality, steady declines in hospital discharges for the past 8 to 10 years (due, in part, to advances in technology that enable ambulatory delivery of services that once typically required hospitalization; i.e., a growing number of surgical procedures) mean that ensuring quality and value will require the same skills applied to assessing quality of care in ambulatory settings. Indeed, many current initiatives such as bundled payments require attention to developing data streams that permit easy linking of care across sites. A recent study of Veterans Health Administration (VHA) care for patients with congestive heart failure is illustrative. The authors found that mortality rate over time for all veterans with heart failure, independent of where care was provided, varied substantially across facilities in the veterans' health care system (Groeneveld et al., 2018). These results stand in sharp contrast to a study comparing hospital quality for veterans over age 65 seen in VHA facilities with that for patients seen in private-sector hospitals over a 10-year period. In this study, VHA patients over age 65 had better outcomes on all quality measures, including mortality, than did Medicare patients (Nuti et al., 2016). This apparent discrepancy underscores limitations in current measurements and the importance of linking care processes to outcomes (Heidenreich, 2018).

In short, a focus on improving quality and safety cannot be outsourced to the quality department or team. To succeed and thrive, every department within a health care organization must make improving quality and safety a strategic imperative. The success of current and future health administrators will likely depend on their willingness and skill to engage clinical colleagues, payers, and the broader community to achieve shared goals.

CONCLUSION

Success in the years ahead will depend on the ability of administrators to implement change and continuously enhance environments that meet the following goals: (a) promote excellence in response to individual patient needs and preferences, (b) promote effective teamwork, and (c) celebrate efforts to identify innovations that make the right thing to do the *easy* thing to do. In short, one hopes that today's status quo will be unrecognizable in a few short years, as health care delivery overall responds to public and policy incentives for superb care and links that response closely to broad efforts aimed at promoting health and reducing the need for high-intensity services. The public should expect no less.

▶ CASE EXERCISE—USING DATA TO SUPPORT SUSTAINABILITY

You are the CEO of a 200-bed community hospital that serves an increasing number of older patients. Your top priority is the quality and safety of care. Given the recent economic downturn and decreased Medicare reimbursement to your facility, you are increasingly concerned about the hospital's ability to stay open and continue serving all of the community.

You have heard that Medicare hospital payments will continue to be trimmed for patients who experience harms considered to be largely preventable: for example, blood clots, surgical infections, ventilator-associated pneumonias, health care–acquired infections (HAIs), and others. You want to ensure your hospital takes every precaution to prevent all possible avoidable harms to patients.

With the help of your assistant, you summarize the challenges before you as follows:

- Medicare-denied payments focus exclusively on the additional care required to treat injury or condition arising from a preventable harm (such as when a second procedure is required to retrieve a surgical instrument).

- To date, the denied payments have pertained only to hospital care. However, you also know that some analysts are recommending that the same policy be applied to physician payments.

- One measure your hospital already has taken is to require that all workers who interact with patients wash their hands in order to prevent HAIs. Although this would seem a simple and obvious initiative, its success has been limited.

- You also learn that your hospital's patient safety department isn't tracking the kinds of events for which the hospital may be financially penalized.

- Finally, you are aware that the ACA affects hospital payment in another way: by trimming reimbursements for potentially avoidable hospital readmissions. As noted earlier, your hospital serves a high proportion of older patients. Many of them currently have multiple admissions for acute exacerbations of chronic illnesses, such as congestive heart failure and diabetes. In the future, these multiple admissions could become very costly.

Consider how you would address these leadership challenges. Be sure to address the following questions:

1. Who on your senior team should lead this effort?
2. Who else should be involved?
3. What precisely are you charging the team to do?
4. Who will help to communicate this effort to all front-line staff?
5. What kinds of systems need to be created to track progress?
6. What external resources could be utilized?
7. What are three items you'd like to measure?
8. How do you set up a system in such a way as to increase the likelihood of sustainability?

DISCUSSION QUESTIONS

1. Why is it important to measure both processes and outcomes? What are the opportunities and challenges for each type of measure?
2. What is the range of factors beyond the patient–physician (or other clinician) dyad that can affect quality of care for the patient?
3. What are the most promising new developments likely to improve health care quality?

4. How do public reporting and payment incentives affect the quality of care by hospitals, physicians, and others?

5. How can a health care leader best mobilize the power of professionalism as a force for quality? How can such strategies align with other incentive systems such as public reporting and payment?

REFERENCES

Agency for Healthcare Research and Quality. (2007). *Managing and evaluating rapid-cycle process improvements as vehicles for hospital system redesign: Continued.* Rockville, MD: Author. Retrieved from http://archive.ahrq.gov/research/findings/final-reports/rapidcycle/rapidcycle1.html

Agency for Healthcare Research and Quality. (2011, March 23). *National summit on public reporting for consumers.* Washington, DC: Author.

Agency for Healthcare Research and Quality. (2012a). *Public reporting as a quality improvement strategy: A systematic review of the multiple pathways public reporting may influence quality of health care.* Rockville, MD: Author.

Agency for Healthcare Research and Quality. (2012b). *Building the science of public reporting: Research grants.* Rockville, MD: Author. Retrieved from http://www.ahrq.gov/professionals/quality-patient-safety/quality-resources/tools/sciencepubreport/index.html

Agency for Healthcare Research and Quality. (2014). *State snapshots.* Rockville, MD: Author. Retrieved from http://www.ahrq.gov/research/data/state-snapshots

Baker, D. W. & Chassin, M. R. (2017). Holding providers accountable for health care outcomes. *Annals of Internal Medicine, 167*(6), 418–423. doi: 10.7326/M17-0691

Burstin, H., Leatherman, S., & Goldmann, D. (2016). The evolution of healthcare quality measurement in the United States. *Journal of Internal Medicine, 279*(2), 154–159.

Catalyst for Payment Reform. (2013). National scorecard on payment reform. Retrieved from http://www.catalyzepaymentreform.org/images/documents/NationalScorecard.pdf

Catterson, R. S., Rasenberger, A., & Swift, E. (2013). Public reporting of health quality and efficiency data: Current and upcoming statutory requirements. Report prepared for the U.S. Department of Health and Human Services, Office of the Assistant Secretary for Planning and Evaluation, Office of Health Policy.

Centers for Medicare & Medicaid Services. (n.d.,a). Quality improvement organizations. Retrieved from http://www.cms.gov/Medicare/Quality-Initiatives-Patient-Assessment-Instruments/QualityImprovementOrgs

Centers for Medicare & Medicaid Services. (2017). FY 2016 report to Congress (RTC): Review of Medicare's program oversight of accrediting organizations (AOs) and the Clinical Laboratory Improvement Amendments of 1988 (CLIA) validation program.

Centers for Medicare & Medicaid Services. (n.d.,b). Hospital quality initiative. Outcome measures. Retrieved from https://www.cms.gov/Medicare/Quality-Initiatives-Patient-Assessment-Instruments/HospitalQualityInits/OutcomeMeasures.html.

Centers for Medicare & Medicaid Services. (2018). Medicare Shared Savings Program. Retrieved from https://www.cms.gov/Medicare/Medicare-Fee-for-ServicePayment/sharedsavingsprogram/about.html

Chee, T. T., Ryan, A. M., Wasfy, J. H, & Borden, W. B. (2016). Current state of value-based purchasing programs. *Circulation, 133*(22), 2197–2205. doi:10.1161/CIRCULATIONAHA.115.010268

Chernew, M. E., & Newhouse, J. P. (2008). What does the RAND health insurance experiment tell us about the impact of patient cost sharing on health outcomes? *American Journal of Managed Care, 14*(7), 412–414.

Cohen, D. J., Dorr, D. A., Knierim, K., DuBard, C. A., Hemler, J. R., Hall, J. D., ... Balasubramanian, B. A. (2018). Primary care practices' abilities and challenges in using electronic health record data for quality improvement. *Health Affairs, 37*(4), 635–643. doi:10.1377/hlthaff.2017.1254

Donabedian, A. (1988). The quality of care: How can it be assessed? *Journal of the American Medial Association, 260*(12), 1743–1748.

Fraser, I. (2014). The role of measurement and data in improving health care quality. Paper presented to Institute of Medicine Conference on Health System Innovation for Effective Universal Health Coverage: Sharing the Experience of the United States and Mexico. Mexico City, Mexico.

Groeneveld, P. W., Medvedeva, E. L., Walker, L., Segal, A. G., Richardson, D. M., & Epstein, A. J. (2018). Outcomes of care for ischemic heart disease and chronic heart failure in the Veterans Health Administration. *Journal of the American Medical Association Cardiology, 3*(7), 563–571. doi:10.1001/jamacardio.2018.1115

Harrison, M. I., Paez, K., Carman, K. L. Stephens, J., Smeeding, L., Devers, K., & Garfinkel, S. (2016). Effects of organizational context on Lean project implementation in five hospital systems. *Health Care Management Review, 41*(2), 127–144.

Heidenreich, P. A. (2018). In pursuit of better measures of quality care. *Journal of the American Medical Association Cardiology, 3*(7), 553–554. doi:10.1001/jamacardio.2018.1204

Hibbard, J., Greene, J., Sofaer, S., Firminger, K., & Hirsh, J. (2012). An experiment shows that a well-designed report on costs and quality can help consumers choose high-value health care. *Health Affairs, 31*(3), 560–568.

Hibbard, J., Stockard, J., & Tusler, M. (2003). Does publicizing hospital performance stimulate quality improvement efforts? *Health Affairs, 22*(2), 84–94.

Hibbard, J., Stockard, J., & Tusler, M. (2005). Hospital performance reports: Impact on quality, market share, and reputation. *Health Affairs, 24*(4), 1150–1160.

Institute of Medicine. (1999). *To err is human—Building a safer health system.* Washington, DC: National Academies Press.

Institute of Medicine. (2001). *Crossing the quality chasm: A new health system for the 21st century.* Washington, DC: National Academies Press.

Jiang, H. J., Lockee, C., Bass, K., Fraser, I., & Norwood, E. P. (2009). Board oversight of quality: Any differences in process of care and mortality? *Journal of Health Care Management, 54*(1), 15–30.

Lean Enterprise Institute. (n.d.). Principles of Lean. Retrieved from www.lean.org/whats-lean/principles.cfm

Lloyd, R. (2010a). Helping leaders blink correctly: Part 1. *Health Care Executive, 25*(3), 88–91. Retrieved from http://www.ache.org

Lloyd, R. (2010b). Helping leaders blink correctly: Part 2. *Health Care Executive, 25*(4), 72–75. Retrieved from http://www.ache.org

Lohr, K. N., & Schroeder, S. A. (1990). A strategy for quality assurance in Medicare. *New England Journal of Medicine, 322*(10), 707–712.

Makary, M. A., & Daniel, M. (2016). Medical error—the third leading cause of death in the U.S. *British Medical Journal, 353*, i2139.

Margolis, P. A., Lannon, C. M., Stuart, J. M., Fried, B. J., Keyes-Elstein, L., & Moore, D. E., Jr. (2004). Practice-based education to improve delivery systems for prevention in primary care: Randomised trial. *British Medical Journal, 328*(7436), 388. Retrieved from http://www.ncbi.nlm.nih.gov/pubmed/14766718

McClellan, M., Richards, R., & Japinga, M. (2017). Evidence on payment reform: Where are the gaps? *Health Affairs* blog. Retrieved from https://www.healthaffairs.org/do/10.1377/hblog20170425.059789/full

National Quality Forum. (2018). Patient-reported outcomes: The opportunity. Retrieved from https://www.qualityforum.org/Projects/n-r/Patient-Reported_Outcomes/Patient-Reported_Outcomes.aspx

Nuti, S. V., Qin, L., Rumsfeld, J. S., Ross, J. S., Masoudi, F. A., Norman, S. T., … Krumholz, H. M. (2016). Association of admission to Veterans Affairs hospitals vs. non–Veterans Affairs hospitals with mortality and readmission rates among older men hospitalized with acute myocardial infarction, heart failure, or pneumonia. *Journal of the American Medical Association, 315*(6), 582–592. doi:10.1001/jama.2016.0278

Pronovost, P., Needham, D., Berenholtz, S., Sinopoli, D., Chu, H., Cosgrove, S., … Goeschel, C. (2006). An intervention to decrease catheter-related bloodstream infections in the ICU. *New England Journal of Medicine, 355*(26), 2725–2732.

Rau, J. (2013). Hospital ratings are in the eye of the beholder. *Kaiser Health News.* Retrieved from https://khn.org/news/expanding-number-of-groups-offer-hospital-ratings

Schneider, E. C., Sarnak, D. O., Squires, D., Shah, A., & Doty, M. M. (2017). *Mirror, mirror 2017: International comparison reflects flaws and opportunities for better U.S. health care.* New York, NY: The Commonwealth Fund.

Shaller, D., & Kanouse, D. (2012). *Private "performance feedback" reporting for physicians: Guide for community quality collaboratives.* Rockville, MD: Agency for Healthcare Research and Quality.

Smith, M., Saunders, R., Stuckhardt, L., & McGinnis, J. M. (Eds.). (2012). *Best care at lower cost: The path to continuously learning health care in America.* Washington, DC: National Academies Press.

World Health Organization. (2009). *WHO guidelines on hand hygiene in health care.* Geneva, Switzerland: Author. Retrieved from http://whqlibdoc.who.int/publications/2009/9789241597906_eng.pdf

13

Health Care Management

Anthony R. Kovner and Christy Harris Lemak

LEARNING OBJECTIVES

▶ Discuss what board members do
▶ Describe challenges that boards face
▶ Understand what managers do and how they behave
▶ Discuss challenges managers face
▶ Understand how organizational performance is measured
▶ Understand the constraints and opportunities for managers of evidence-based practice

KEY TERMS

▶ accountability
▶ evidence-based management
▶ governance
▶ management
▶ self-perpetuating governance boards
▶ stakeholders

TOPICAL OUTLINE

▶ Governance, performance, and accountability
▶ The complex tasks of leadership and management
▶ Evidence-based management
▶ Challenges managers face

INTRODUCTION

Excellent managers sometimes fail in meeting new challenges. And sometimes they succeed in dramatically turning organizations around. Impact on organizational performance depends on circumstances and timing. In baseball, there is an old saying that "managers are hired to be fired." We have seen that managers make a difference in the performance of organizations. Health care organizations (HCOs) obtain inputs from society, such as workers and medical devices, and add value, such as treatments, to make unhealthy people healthy again or to keep people healthy. Managers are in charge of allocating resources to most effectively create valued services based on evidence about how to do this well. Managers are accountable to those who own or govern HCOs. The owners are responsive to stakeholders, who include persons and organizations affected by the performance of HCOs, and most important, to the patients they serve and the people living in the communities they serve.

> The role of health care managers is to obtain *inputs* from society—such as funding, technology, and the expertise of medical professionals—and to add *value*—such as research and treatments—to keep people healthy and help them when they are ill.*

For complex organizations like hospitals, large physician practices, and other health-related enterprises to perform effectively, it is essential to develop organizational attributes that ensure effective governance, accountability, stakeholder involvement, and leadership.

This chapter describes how HCOs are governed and managed and the process of evidence-based management.

We start by defining key terms. **Governance** is the process for making and reviewing strategic decisions made by HCOs, such as whether and how to finance a new hospital wing, how to evaluate the quality of patient care, and whether to hire nurse practitioners to provide primary care. **Management** shapes and implements governance decisions. **Accountability** means being responsible for making informed and wise decisions that affect health outcomes and processes of care at a given level of quality and a given level of cost. **Stakeholders** are individuals and groups who will be influenced by or have an interest in the decisions that HCOs make. HCO stakeholders include, among others, regulators and accrediting bodies, payers and financers, clinicians and support staff, local community leaders and donors, patients and their family members, taxpayers, beneficiaries, vendors, and many others.

GOVERNANCE, PERFORMANCE AND ACCOUNTABILITY

The Concept of the Governing Board

HCOs can function under nonprofit, public, or for-profit ownership. In a nonprofit organization, the organization is owned by a nonprofit board of directors.

---

*To hear the podcast, go to https://bcove.video/2QEW0ri or access the ebook on Springer Publishing Connect™.

Most nonprofits are regulated by the state in which the organization was founded. Nonprofit boards are often **self-perpetuating**; that is, the existing board members select new members when openings arise. Public HCOs, such as a state-owned medical school or a public hospital, are owned by and accountable to elected public officials or to boards appointed by elected public officials. For-profit health systems are corporations owned by and accountable to investors, who are typically stockholders, whose interests generally are represented by a governing board elected by the investors. HCO boards may be subject to ultimate control by remote owners, such as a church, whose officials appoint board members, or a large corporate entity that may own many separate companies.

HCO governing boards may include physicians and others knowledgeable about health care delivery, experts who understand finance and banking, individuals who can help raise resources to support the organization, and others who represent patients and community interests.

The goals of boards and those who appoint boards can differ widely. For example, a church-owned hospital may place a higher priority on complying with doctrines regarding abortion than on achieving a high rate of return on investment. Investor owners may reverse these priorities. Boards dominated by patients and community members may care most about quality and access to care among members of the community.

What Boards Do

According to Bowen (2008), boards have eight principal functions:

- Select, encourage, advise, evaluate, compensate and, if need be, replace the chief executive officer (CEO).
- Discuss, review, and approve strategic directions.
- Monitor performance of management in achieving agreed-upon goals.
- Ensure that the organization operates responsibly and effectively.
- Act on specific policy recommendations and mobilize support for decisions taken.
- Provide a buffer for the president or CEO and "take some of the heat."
- Ensure that the necessary resources will be available to pursue strategies and achieve objectives.
- Nominate suitable candidates for election to the board and establish and carry out an effective system of board governance.

Most board members are not employees of the organization, and many have limited previous experience in making HCO decisions. As a board, directors must exercise the duties of care (acting as prudent persons), obedience (staying focused on the mission of the organization), and loyalty (making sure to avoid conflicts of interest). The board is considered the conscience of the organization and is accountable to stakeholders for protecting and achieving the mission.

Board members are not liable for a bad business decision as long as it can be shown that a (hypothetical) "prudent board member" could have made the same decision in the same situation. Fundamentally, board members' decisions must serve their HCO's mission. For example, a board of a nonprofit nursing home would rarely find it logical to advance its mission by investing in a race track. Board members must also be attuned to potential conflicts of interest. For example, when a board is considering a banking relationship, a board member who works for a bank must acknowledge that interest and be absent from the discussion.

Little is known about the relationship between what nonprofit boards do and HCO performance, though studies have begun to find positive relationships between board attention to quality of care and hospital performance (Tsai et al., 2015). Most HCOs have no formal accountability mechanisms for their board.

What is the value added of the board relative to its cost to the organization? There are costs of governance such as the time the manager must spend with board members—planning meetings, listening to board members' views inside and outside of meetings, and negotiating priorities and accountabilities. On the benefit side, boards add energy and considerable resources, have a more balanced view of organizational situations than the CEOs, and can take a longer view of establishing and accomplishing the organizational mission. The board ensures that "the main thing is the main thing," which means keeping the HCO focused on accomplishing the mission, which can include earning revenue, ensuring jobs or access to care for low-income populations.

In practice, the governing board selects the CEO, who in turn selects the other managers. The board delegates much of the organizational decision making to the CEO. The board establishes the organization's strategic direction through a periodic strategic planning process and review of stakeholder perspectives and market information. The board establishes the organization's mission, vision, and values and is accountable for keeping these statements aligned with the HCO's current and future situation. (For an example of a hospital's mission, vision, and value statement approved by an HCO board, see Exhibit 13.1.)

Challenges That Boards Face

HCO boards must respond to many organizational challenges, which vary by institution and over time. Some relatively constant challenges, however, include making sure the organization has revenues that cover operating costs, ensuring services are delivered with high quality, and ensuring health outcomes for patient

---

EXHIBIT 13.1   MISSION, VISION, AND VALUES: 2013 STATEMENT FOR UCHealth

UCHealth was created through the partnership of the University of Colorado Hospital and Poudre Health System.

Mission: We improve lives. We do this in big ways through learning, healing, and discovery. We do this in small ways through human connection. But in all ways, we improve lives.

Vision: From health care to health

Values: Patients first, integrity, and excellence.

EXHIBIT 13.2 WHICH HOSPITAL IS BEST?

Assume a grandmother has asked you to help her select a hospital for her hip surgery. For a community you know well, consider how you would help her evaluate the local hospitals and make recommendations.

What measures are most important? Is there a single "best" hospital? Why is this so difficult? What sources, such as the following, would you use to determine which hospital is best?

care are as positive as possible. In order to do its job addressing these challenges, a board sets and reviews metrics that measure HCO performance.

Measuring the performance of health care providers has become complex and more sophisticated in recent years as there are a variety of measures of "success"—including financial performance, patient satisfaction and "experience" ratings, and clinical quality ratings, to name a few. Increasingly, comparative data are being made available by payers and regulators that allow the board and others to assess HCO performance (Figueroa, Feyman, Blumenthal, & Jha, 2017; www .Hospital Compare.gov). For an example of how stakeholders can determine "which hospital is best," see Exhibit 13.2.

Of course, there are other organizational goals that an HCO and its board can set. For example, the board might push the organization to improve the health of the community's population, rather than just focusing on patients who use their services. For an example of linking performance to values, see Exhibit 13.3. Or the board might set a goal of growing or shrinking the size of the organization in response to changing community needs.

A key responsibility of the board of a community-based health care delivery organization is to understand the needs of the community and be proactive in meeting these needs. Increasingly, boards may feel pressure to think in terms of broader outcomes—such as maintaining the health of the community—rather than the narrower outcomes of technical quality and outcome improvement. These changes are driven by changing approaches to reimbursing delivery

> A key responsibility of a board of a community-based delivery organization is to understand the needs of the community and be proactive in meeting these needs.

EXHIBIT 13.3 LINKING PERFORMANCE TO VALUES

Concentra, a subsidiary of Humana Inc., is a national health company with 320 medical centers in 38 states (www.concentra.com).

Managers at Concentra link performance in each of its clinics to values of being Welcoming, Skillful, and Respectful. Measures of performance are tracked and monitored relative to goals and benchmarks, such as metrics for Welcoming (e.g., clinic appearance), Respectful (e.g., follow-up calls made), and Skillful (e.g., wait times, communication, and patient satisfaction). Clinic and other staff personnel who consistently achieve benchmark performance receive bonuses and other awards.

organizations and increased integration of organizations within a community (e.g., see Chapter 11 on financing and Chapter 12 on quality improvement).

Boards can have a significant influence on HCO performance by setting and overseeing strategy for an institution. They can decide to close or merge hospitals or mental health clinics. They hold managers accountable for improving quality and transparency. They may drive organizations to cooperate with other community organizations to improve population health. They should ensure that managerial incentives are aligned with strategy.

The challenges are daunting for a board to be effective in making sure an HCO is performing well. To be effective, board members must spend enough time to learn how the HCO operates and what drives effectiveness.

Some current issues facing HCO boards have to do with board composition. For example, some boards require members to make financial contributions or to convince others to make contributions. This may be done to increase board member engagement with the HCO or to raise money for special projects, even if the amounts are small relative to the total HCO budget. A main argument against this requirement is financial hardship that could discourage potential board members of modest means from joining a board. Another board composition topic is limiting the terms of board member service, often to two terms of 3 years each, sometimes with an age requirement (typically limiting election to members below 70 years of age).

Another important board composition requirement refers to HCO board diversity and the desire for board members who are representative of the community served in terms of race, ethnicity, and gender. This is particularly relevant as HCOs move toward population health improvement strategies (Lemak, Paris, & McDonagh, 2017). There is room to improve in this area. The American Hospital Association's Institute for Diversity and Health Equity recently reported that only 14% of hospital board members in the U.S. were racial minorities and this percentage had not changed over the time period 2011–2015 (Livingston, 2018).

Healthy relationships between board members and senior staff of the HCO, clear goals and objectives, and timely measures of outcomes related to goals and objectives are essential for good board governance. Finally, to be effective, boards should understand what they should *not* do. Key among things not to do is meddling in ways that do not allow leaders to manage effectively.

THE COMPLEX TASKS OF LEADERSHIP AND MANAGEMENT

The first person who comes to mind in thinking about health care delivery is a clinician—a doctor, a nurse, a physical therapist, or an aide. But managers, who are often behind the scenes (and who sometimes have experience as clinicians), make it possible for much of appropriate clinical care to happen. Managers create and maintain the environment that supports clinicians in their work.

Managers create and maintain the environment that supports clinicians in their work.

To understand what managers do, we consider the wide range of roles they play, the factors that make managers effective, and some of the challenges managers face in leading HCOs to be effective and efficient and to achieve their mission and goals.

Managers play many roles in HCOs. Managerial work can vary from directing health information technology to sustaining diabetes prevention activities. Managers oversee accounts payable, fundraising and development, operational support for clinical departments, and human resources/labor relations. Managers function in interactive environments, working collaboratively with other managers and clinicians to achieve organizational goals.

Four useful ways of looking at what managers do are (a) the functions managers perform (e.g., planning or finance), (b) responsibilities they are accountable for, (c) what choices managers make in how they spend their time and effort, and (d) with whom they spend their time. According to Longest (1990), basic managerial functions include:

- *Planning*: determining goals and objectives
- *Organizing*: structuring people, dollars, services, and equipment to accomplish objectives
- *Directing*: motivating workers to meet objectives
- *Coordinating*: assembling and synchronizing diverse activities and participants
- *Controlling*: comparing actual results with objectives

In 2014, a young manager told one of the authors that in his large health system, key managerial functions included:

- Managing unit or area performance
- Coaching and mentoring associates
- Promoting employee and physician engagement—the internalization of mission as the person takes "ownership" of his or her job

The manager's scarcest resource may be his or her own time. Managers choose whether to do tasks themselves, delegate work to others, or not do the work (e.g., not respond to e-mails from other departments). Unfortunately, not responding often occurs, given the large number of claims on the HCO manager's time.

An effective manager meets his or her goals. Being effective includes helping the team and the HCO accomplish goals and exceed the expectations of key stakeholders. Some HCOs have ineffective managers who fail to adapt to changing circumstances, such as a new CEO, or shifting demographics or patient preferences. Sometimes managers achieve lowered performance due to external competitive pressures or new government regulations over which the managers have little control and to which they have not adequately prepared for or responded.

Goleman (1998) suggests that the most effective managers (whom he calls "leaders") have a high degree of "emotional intelligence," which is more important for managerial effectiveness than technical skills and general intelligence (IQ).

Goleman identifies five components of emotional intelligence: self-awareness, self-regulation (e.g., the ability to reflect before acting), motivation, empathy, and social skills.

Although effective managers vary in their backgrounds, experiences, emotional intelligence, styles, and the extent and nature of their formal education, researchers have tried, largely unsuccessfully, to identify underlying factors that lead to successful performance. Boyatzis (1995) developed a model that describes three set of managerial competencies (skills that are measurable):

- People skills such as efficiency orientation, planning, initiative, attention to detail, self-control, flexibility, empathy, persuasiveness, networking, negotiating, self-confidence, group management, developing others, and oral communication
- Use of concepts, systems thinking, pattern recognition, theory building, technology, quantitative analysis, and social objectivity
- Written communication and analytical reasoning

For an overview of the leadership competency approach, see Howard and colleagues (Howard, Healy, & Boyatzis, 2017).

> There should be a good fit between a manager's competencies and what the organization is seeking for a particular position.

Above all, there should be a good fit between a manager's competencies and what the organization is seeking for a particular position. A manager may be effective in one position and ineffective in another. When successive managers turn over in a particular position, this may indicate problems in the way the position has been designed rather than that the HCO has made a succession of bad hires. Joining a previously ineffective organization may be an excellent opportunity for a new, focused manager to remove obstacles that previously prevented team members from working together effectively.

An important trait of an effective manager is being able to work collaboratively with clinicians, understanding the needs of clinicians in delivering high-quality and efficient care. Although delivery organizations are more complex than they were 50 years ago, the traditional view lingers that the purpose of a hospital or clinic is to function as the work space of the clinical provider. It is still helpful for a manager to remember this culture and the unique and challenging day-to-day demands that busy doctors and other clinicians face in the workplace.

According to the Bureau of Labor Statistics (2015), there were 333,000 persons employed in the field as medical and health services managers in 2014. The median annual pay for medical and health service managers in 2016 was $96,540. This does not include the large number of people who spend only some of their time doing managerial tasks, such as clinicians chairing a quality committee or heading a clinical department. Managerial work increasingly requires data analysis and an ability to collect relevant information to guide practice. Such analysis is extensively used by senior management teams as well as by managers of clinical departments (Friedman & Kovner, 2018).

Managers contribute vitally to the functioning and health of an organization. A key responsibility of senior managers is to recruit, train, and develop the managers reporting to them. In well-run organizations, the process of recruiting and overseeing managers is facilitated by a rigorous approach to management effectiveness. Management objectives are set metrics used to assess performance, just as the board does for higher-level objectives of the HCO.

EVIDENCE-BASED MANAGEMENT

Management decisions should be based on the best evidence available. Managers generally make decisions based on evidence but it is shocking how frequently the evidence used is simplistic or poorly measured. Major decisions, such as merging two hospitals,

> **Management decisions should be based on the best evidence available.**

are sometimes made based on latest trends or gut instinct rather than on solid evidence that the merger will improve quality outcomes or financial viability. Day-to-day management interventions, such as increasing space in the emergency department waiting areas, are often based on anecdotal data rather than taking a systematic look at the pros and cons or at how other institutions design waiting areas.

A new field of inquiry, evidence-based management, is emerging to bring systematic data and information together to guide organizational improvements. **Evidence-based management** is defined as "the systematic application of the best available evidence to the evaluation of management strategies for improving organizational performance" (Hsu et al., 2006). Steps in the evidence-based management process include translating a specific management challenge into research questions; acquiring relevant research findings and other evidence; assessing the validity, quality, applicability, and adequacy of the evidence; presenting the evidence in a way that will be useful; and including all important stakeholders in the decision-making process (Barends, Rousseau, & Briner in Kovner & D'Aunno, 2017).

Traditionally, HCOs have not invested substantially in management research, seeing this as the responsibility of government or philanthropy. Many health systems have invested in analytical capacity to assess financial and reimbursement decisions but have tended to ignore analysis to improve day-to-day operations. Of course, there are exceptions to this, such as the Mayo Clinic and Intermountain Healthcare, which have developed staff capacity and data retrieval systems that allow for sophisticated analysis to develop evidence about best practices in organizing service delivery.

Examples of the type of questions management research can address include:

- How can hospital emergency services be best organized to reduce patient waiting time?
- How can hospital administrators be organized to facilitate working better as teams?

- What are financially viable approaches to expanding hours at ambulatory care clinics?
- How can transport services be best organized to minimize wait times in moving patients from patient to procedure rooms?

Deciding whether to invest and how much to invest on management research involves similar considerations as deciding how much to invest in management training and development. The returns on improved information for decision-making must be compared with the costs of obtaining the information. Managers need to determine when analysis to support evidence-based management should be done within a specific HCO or health system and whether this should be carried out alone or as part of a consortium. The National Science Foundation sponsors consortia of HCOs and universities to conduct this kind of research, called the Center for Healthcare Organizational Transformation (https://chotnsf.org/).

Managers who do not follow a process of evidence-based management often fail to investigate a sufficiently broad range of strategic alternatives or to sufficiently test assumptions upon which alternatives are based. This type of management failure is rarely found in other complex product sectors like banking, manufacturing, or food service delivery.

HCOs are more likely to practice evidence-based management when: external incentives for performance are strong, such as when payers pay for better performance with penalties for bad performance; when an HCO has a "hard-wired" questioning management culture rather than a more hierarchical culture; when there is focused accountability for decision making linked to the quality and timeliness of the process; and, when managers participate actively in the management research.

CHALLENGES MANAGERS FACE

HCO managers face many important challenges to which some managers are not responding adequately. External challenges include obtaining sufficient resources to support clinicians and satisfy customers. More directly under the manager's control are internal challenges such as:

- Measuring processes and outcomes to facilitate continual improvement
- Creating a culture that supports excellent clinical care
- Motivating and supporting employees

Stakeholders agree it is the manager's job to measure the operational processes, supply needed support to clinicians given the resources available, and communicate with staff. Much of the work today in HCOs is done in teams with different disciplines and often in different locations. This makes coordination of care and employee engagement difficult.

Delivering services effectively depends on agreement about standards of performance. High-performing HCOs seek benchmarks, or examples of other organizations that perform well, and set their performance as a standard or goal. See Exhibit 13.4 for a discussion of benchmarks for measuring performance at Mercy Health System (MHS).

For example, what is and what should be the waiting time for patients? This includes waiting time to contact an access point to the HCO, waiting time for an appointment with a clinician, waiting time in the clinician's office, and waiting time for treatment and discharge. These data should be collected routinely, sorted and analyzed, and discussed with staff providing the services so that continuous improvement can be implemented and results compared with those of HCOs providing similar services. This approach to monitoring and improving waiting time can be repeated for each task and administrative process that is the responsibility of the manager. A proactive attitude and a continuous improvement perspective are two key attributes of an effective management team.

Providing a supportive environment for clinicians often will only be successful if managers systematically learn what factors help create a supportive environment for the delivery of high-quality services. This involves observations of working conditions at high-performing peer organizations, communicating with clinicians about their views and feelings, and learning from managerial peers and the research literature about what works and doesn't work—and under what conditions.

> Providing a supportive environment for clinicians often will only be successful if managers systematically learn what factors help create a supportive environment for the delivery of high-quality services.

Managers have limited time and must focus on priorities. Obstacles to adopting recommended interventions to improve care processes and outcomes are many, including (a) insufficiently developed care delivery teams, (b) ineffective performance evaluation systems, and (c) lack of human resources capabilities. A workforce that has not been trained to work together cannot be expected to function

---

EXHIBIT 13.4   BENCHMARKS AT MERCY HEALTH SYSTEMS

Mercy Health Systems is an integrated health care organization providing health care services in southern Wisconsin and northeastern Illinois.

MHS was establishing goals and measures for its House of Mercy, a 25-bed homeless shelter that provides short-term emergency shelter and access to housing, job placement, and child care services. At first, MHS leaders were unsuccessful in locating available measures of "benchmark" or "best practice" for homeless shelters. The CEO insisted, however, that benchmarks be found.

House of Mercy staff held meetings with clients and volunteers and determined that other industries could supply proxy measures of performance. Stretch goals were set from benchmarks in the hotel industry, including volume of services, demand (wait list), facility conditions (cleanliness, comfort), client satisfaction, and availability of services needed by their clients.

as a team. Creating, leading, and motivating teams are critical activities for every manager. While it may be most efficient to hire staff with the required skills and experience who have already demonstrated key aspects of the HCO's culture, this is not always possible. Unfortunately, HCO managers often spend most of their time removing obstacles for new hires instead of spending time and energy motivating and directing new team members. A popular book on leadership emphasizes that one of the most important tasks of the leader is to "get the right people on the bus." Once the manager has hired the right staff, supervision and motivation are easier (Collins, 2001).

A related managerial challenge is effectively communicating with team members. There is a big distinction between waiting to talk and hearing what the other person is saying. A fundamental aspect of human nature is that we often hear what we want to hear rather than what is said (and not voiced). Communication involves connecting with a colleague and making sure he or she understands what is said and what behavior needs to follow. Often, repeating back what the other person has said is a useful approach to effective communication. And giving a complete message—even when some of it is not good news to the employee—can be critical to successful communication.

CONCLUSION

Donald Berwick, a health care visionary, sees the coming era as one that will combine the professional pride of clinicians from his father's generation with transparency and accountability required today. He calls this the era of "return to purpose," which he says has nine elements: avoid excess measurement, abandon complex incentives, get off the billing treadmill (stop focusing so much on the money), be part of a team, commit to quality science, promote transparency, protect civility, believe in the power of the patient, and reject greed. These elements seem like a good guide for achieving better health at reasonable cost and with high-quality services.

The current drivers of the health care enterprise are demand for improved outcomes and increased value. Consolidation has occurred within the health sector—both vertically, in terms of integrated health systems, and horizontally, in terms of mergers. Larger HCOs are better able to standardize work processes, adapt new measurement systems, and develop transparent processes of communication with key stakeholders, including clinicians and other workers, about performance and expectations for results.

Under these conditions, the role and importance of managers trained in the necessary skills and provided with the necessary experience increases. Emerging health systems require more sophistication from managers who understand how to work in teams, how to manage various types of workers, and how to use the best available evidence to make better decisions.

▶ CASE EXERCISE—STRATEGIC PLAN REPORT

What follows is a summary of an academic medical center's strategic plan:

- Mission: To care, cure, teach, and advance the health of the communities served
- Vision: To be a premier academic medical center that transforms and enriches lives
- Values: Humanity, innovation, teamwork, diversity, and quality
- Strategic goals:
  - Advance the partnership with the university college of medicine
  - Create notable centers of excellence in heart and cancer care
  - Build specialty care broadly
  - Develop an effective delivery system with superior access, quality, safety, and patient satisfaction
  - Maximize the effects of community service
- Organizational goals
  - Create a culture of high performance, motivation, and fulfilment
  - Sustain strong financial health
  - Invest in state-of-the-art facilities and technology
  - Build an aligned and interconnected organization
  - Forster supportive partnerships and alliances

The board of directors engages you as a consultant and asks that you prepare a report addressing the following questions:

1. How should organizational performance at academic medical center be measured?
2. How can top management be held accountable for accomplishing the plan?
3. How should the board of directors be involved in implementing the plan?

DISCUSSION QUESTIONS

1. How is performance measured in HCOs? How effective are these measurements?
2. What are the differences among public, nonprofit, and for-profit HCOs?
3. What skills and experience are required to govern and manage HCOs?
4. How should HCO performance be evaluated?
5. What measures of accountability are most effective for nonprofit HCOs?
6. What are emerging issues facing HCO boards? HCO managers?

REFERENCES

Bowen, W. G. (2008). *The board book*. New York, NY: W.W. Norton.
Boyatzis, R. E. (1995). Cornerstones of change: Building the path to self-directed learning. In R. E. Boyatzis, S. S. Cowan, & D. A. Kolb (Eds.), *Innovation in professional education* (pp. 50–94). San Francisco, CA: Jossey-Bass.

Bureau of Labor Statistics, U.S. Department of Labor. (2015). Medical and health services managers. In *Occupational Outlook Handbook: 2016–2017*. Retrieved from https://www.bls.gov/ooh/management-and-health-services-managers.htm

Collins, J. (2001). *Good to great: why some companies make the leap and others don't*. New York, NY: Harper Business. www.chotnsf.org.

Figueroa, J., Feyman, Y., Blumenthal, D., & Jha, A. (2017). Do the stars align? Distribution of high-quality ratings of healthcare sectors across U.S. markets. *BMJ Quality & Safety*, *27*(4), 287–292. doi: 10.1136/bmjqs-2017-006801

Friedman, L., & Kovner, A. R. (2018). *101 careers in healthcare management* (2nd ed.). New York, NY: Springer Publishing.

Goleman, D. (1998). What makes a leader? *Harvard Business Review*, *76*(6), 93–102. Retrieved from https://hbr.org/2004/01/what-makes-a-leader

Howard, A. R., Healy, S. L., & Boyatzis, R. E. (2017). Using leadership competencies as a framework for career readiness. *New Directions for Student Leadership*, 2017(156), 59–71. doi:10.1002/yd.20271

Hsu, J. L., Arroyo, I., Graetz, E., Neuwirth, E. B., Schmittdiel, J., Rundall, T. G., … Curtis, P. (2006). Methods for developing actionable evidence for consumers of health services research. In A. R. Kovner, D. J. Fine, & R. D'Aquila (Eds.), *Evidence-based management in healthcare*. Chicago, IL: Health Administration Press.

Kovner, A. R., & D'Aunno T. (Eds.). (2017). *Evidence-based management in healthcare: Principles, cases and perspectives* (2nd ed.). Chicago, IL: Health Administration Press.

Lemak, C. H., Paris, N. M., & McDonagh, K. J. (2017). Essential values for population health improvement. *Population Health Management*, *20*(4), 249–251. doi:10.1089/pop.2016.0126

Livingston, S. (2018). Racism in health care: Challenging the unspoken rules. *Modern Healthcare*, 12–14.

Longest, B. B. (1990). *Management practices for the health professional* (4th ed.). Norwalk, CT: Appleton & Lange.

Tsai, T. C., Jha, A. K., Gawande, A. A., Huckman, R. S., Bloom, N., & Sadun, R. (2015). Hospital board and management practices are strongly related to hospital performance on clinical quality metrics. *Health Affairs*, *34*(8), 1304–1311. doi:10.1377/hlthaff.2014.1282

14

Health Information Technology

Karen B. DeSalvo and Y. Claire Wang

LEARNING OBJECTIVES

▶ Define health information technology (HIT)

▶ Describe government's role in spurring HIT adoption and setting expectations for the market

▶ Demonstrate how HIT and health data have improved patient care and reduced health care costs

▶ Discuss how HIT and health data can improve population health

▶ Examine the role of HIT in the nation's evolving health care system and value-based care

▶ Introduce and explore examples of successful HIT adoption and use and public health

▶ Discuss what is needed in the future as HIT takes on a bigger role in health care and health improvement, including technology advancements and policy challenges

KEY TERMS

▶ clinical decision support

▶ computerized provider order entry (CPOE)

▶ consumer decision support

▶ cybersecurity

▶ electronic health records (EHRs)

▶ e-prescriptions

▶ health information exchange (HIE)

▶ interoperability

▶ patient portals

- ▶ remote patient monitoring (RPM)
- ▶ telehealth

TOPICAL OUTLINE

- ▶ Health data needs and HIT use cases
- ▶ HIT interoperability and standards
- ▶ Driving forces shaping the use of data and HIT
- ▶ Challenges to the more effective use of information and data
- ▶ Privacy and security
- ▶ Current marketplace and emerging opportunities

INTRODUCTION

The digital health revolution is well under way and provides an exciting and necessary underpinning for a highly efficient, effective, and modernized health care system. This chapter will explore the current health information technology (HIT) landscape in the United States, examine the importance of HIT in the nation's evolving health care system and its shift to value-based care, and discuss ways that HIT will continue to change the health system.

Health IT can enable health care professionals to improve the processing of insurance claims, accurately track patterns of disease outbreaks, study social determinants of health like access to public housing or food assistance, and even identify restaurants with health violations.*

HIT includes—but is not limited to—the use of **electronic health records** (EHRs) instead of paper medical records to document and maintain health information. At its core, HIT refers to the tools and systems used to electronically store, organize, manage, disseminate, and make meaning from health data. HIT makes it possible for health care providers to improve patient care through secure use and sharing of health information.

Health information technology (HIT) makes it possible for health care providers to improve patient care through secure use and sharing of health information.

In addition to EHRs, other organized data can be leveraged with clinical information from EHRs. These types of data include insurance claims, records about vital statistics, information about restaurants with health violations, disease outbreak pattern information, and data documenting issues related to the social determinants of health such as access to public housing or SNAP (Supplemental Nutrition Assistance Program) benefits.

Health informatics—the interdisciplinary study of the design, development, adoption, and application of IT-based innovations in health care services delivery, management, and planning—has its origins in the 1960s, as advancements

---

*To hear the podcast, go to https://bcove.video/2QyAa8v or access the ebook on Springer Publishing Connect™.

in computer engineering allowed for more practical application of computing technology in fields beyond computer science (National Information Center on Health Services Research and Health Care Technology: Informatics, 2018). Early notable efforts to apply IT solutions to health care delivery include Lockheed Corporation's Eclipsys system for computerized physician order entry and home-grown IT systems at Massachusetts General Hospital, the Regenstrief Institute, and the Department of Veterans Affairs (Tripathi, 2012). Commercial systems started to proliferate in the 1990s, but adoption of these systems was mainly limited to large health care delivery organizations, or health systems. Evidence from these major health systems demonstrated the value of HIT for reducing cost and improving care—especially in improving patient safety (Chen, Garrido, Chock, Okawa, & Liang, 2009; Jha, Perlin, Kizer, & Dudley, 2003; Lee, & Forbes, 2009; Walker, Pan, Johnston, Adler-Milstein, Bates, & Middleton, 2005). Seminal reports by the National Academy of Medicine in the early 2000s, *To Err Is Human* and *Crossing the Quality Chasm*, highlighted how tens of thousands of Americans die each year from preventable medical errors, and called for widespread use of HIT to help prevent some of these errors (Institute of Medicine, 2001; Kohn, Corrigan, Donaldson, eds., 2000). In 2005, the RAND Corporation estimated that the United States could save $81 billion per year through greater efficiency and improved safety by adopting electronic medical records (Hillestad, 2005).

Despite these early efforts and supporting evidence, the health care industry has been slower than other industries to embrace IT. Barriers to adopting HIT included the high costs of initial acquisition, implementation and ongoing maintenance, lack of business incentives to digitize data and share data outside one's system, and the lack of interoperability. Policy initiatives at the federal and state levels, as well as industry-led efforts in the United States, have been instrumental in addressing these challenges, resulting in exponential growth in HIT adoption and utilization in the past decade.

In 2009, fewer than one in five hospitals and physician offices used HIT but by 2016, 96% of hospitals and 78% of physician offices used EHR technology (Hillestad, 2005). Though health care continues to play catch-up with other industries, the wide adoption of EHRs and the digitization of the care experience now offers opportunities to harness the power of big data to continuously improve care quality, access, efficiency, and health outcomes for all. However, usability and workflow integration remain a challenge for many providers. The cost of acquiring, maintaining, and managing HIT systems also increasingly represent substantial investment for health care providers.

HEALTH DATA NEEDS AND IT USE CASES

The health care industry comprises a complex fabric of various stakeholders, and each sector has its own unique data needs and capabilities to translate that data into meaningful information. Providers, patients, insurers, and governmental entities are increasingly using a variety of HIT tools to support patient care and population health management.

Health Care Providers

The central HIT tool in the health care system is the EHR, which is—at its core—a digital versions of patients' paper charts. Authorized providers and staff across health care organizations can use EHRs to record, manage, and share patient information. EHRs can bring together information from current and past interactions with doctors, emergency facilities, school and workplace clinics, pharmacies, laboratories, and medical imaging facilities. Specifically, EHRs can:

- Contain electronic information about a patient's medical history, diagnoses, medications, immunization dates, allergies, radiology images, and lab and test results
- Archive and share this information digitally at various points of care
- Offer access portals to clinical decision support (CDS) tools that providers can use in managing and coordinating a patient's care
- Automate and streamline providers' workflow
- Increase organization and accuracy of patient information
- Support analyses based on aggregated patient data for quality improvement and population health management
- Support key market changes in payer requirements and consumer expectations
- Make possible a range of public health, health services, and medical research focused on improving individual and population health outcomes and the efficiency of care delivery

EHRs support electronic transmission of information that encompasses all aspects of patient care. For example, EHRs improve delivery at the point of care through a variety of **clinical decision support** tools. CDS utilizes clinical guidelines, patient-specific data, and algorithm-guided reasoning to generate alerts and offer information to providers as part of the regular workflow. Potential benefits of CDS include avoidance of errors such as adverse drug-drug interactions and dosing errors, increased quality of care, and improved efficiency (HealthIT.gov, 2018).

For example, providers use **computerized provider order entry (CPOE)** to submit orders for medications, lab tests, and imaging and to share instructions for patient care with other parts of the system. Prescriptions can be submitted electronically via the EHR and eliminate the hassle and potential errors of physical paper copies, with almost all retail pharmacies (98%) now accepting **e-prescriptions**.

Further, in contrast to traditional quality measures based on manual chart review or claims, electronic clinical quality measures (eCQMs) are calculated directly from patient EHR data. The development and adoption of eCQMs avoid manual data extraction from paper charts, which is both resource intense and error prone (eCQI Resource Center, 2018). Digitized health records and aggregated eCQMs can be analyzed to drive continuous process and quality improvement in health care delivery (Institute of Medicine, 2013).

Health information exchange (HIE) supports the secure electronic exchange of patient data among authorized health care providers and patients to ensure appropriate patient information is available at the point of care. HIE can also refer to discrete public and private networks that allow providers and patients to share medical information electronically across different EHRs and disparate HIT systems. For example, MyHealth Access Network is an HIE that connects more than 2,000 providers in Oklahoma so they can share patient data regardless of the local EHR product (MyHealth Access Network, 2018). The primary modes of HIE include directed exchange, query-based exchange, and con-

> Health information exchange supports the secure electronic exchange of patient data among authorized health care providers and patients to ensure appropriate patient information is available at the point of care.

sumer-mediated exchange. Directed exchange describes point-to-point sending of health data from one user to a trusted and authorized end recipient (which could be another IT system) to support referrals and care coordination. Query-based exchange supports unplanned care episodes and refers to providers exchanging information based on a request for patient data (i.e., a query) from existing data sources. Consumer-mediated exchange allows patients to access and share electronic records from and with their care providers.

Consumers and Individuals

Individuals have the right to review and obtain a copy their protected health information (PHI) as granted by the Health Insurance Portability and Accountability Act of 1996 (HIPAA). Individuals can receive electronic copies of their health record upon request. Some existing efforts to provide this access to electronic health information came in the form of **patient portals**. These portals offer people direct access to their PHI stored in the provider's EHR or by the health insurance benefits manager. They also allow streamlined electronic communications between patients and their physicians as well as allowing both to manage their administrative and care records. The patient is the central and constant factor across all providers he or she interacts with as well as the HIT systems containing the patient's PHI. For this reason, one key form of HIE is consumer-directed exchange (CDEx), also referred to as consumer-mediated exchange. Through trusted CDEx platforms, patients can request health data in a format to be shared with third-party or other entities as designated by the consumer. A 2010 study funded by the Robert Wood Johnson Foundation invited 105 primary care doctors to share their office visit notes with patients and found that patients reported clinically relevant benefits (e.g., feeling more "in control" of their own care), and the providers involved reported minimal impact on workflow (Delbanco, et al., 2012). Since then, participation in the OpenNotes initiative has grown, and an estimated 20 million patients in the United States had access to their doctors' notes in 2017 (OpenNotes, 2017).

In 2010, the Veterans Health Administration (VHA) launched the Blue Button initiative to give veterans the ability to download their health data on the MyHealtheVet portal; following successful deployment, this function was expanded to other federal programs and commercial insurers (Turvey, Klein, Fix, et al., 2014). At the request of the U.S. Government Accountability Office, the Department of Defense and Veterans Administration have also been working to improve interoperability

Consumer-mediated exchange can support patient self-management and clinician awareness, especially when both consumers and clinicians are trained to use the information effectively.

and achieve lifelong medical records for active duty and retired military members (U.S. Government Accountability Office, 2014). The federal government is also involved in certifying and regulating HIT use across the various health care programs, which is discussed in more detail later in this chapter.

Consumer-mediated exchange can support patient self-management and clinician awareness, especially when both consumers and clinicians are trained to use the information effectively. The Department of Veterans Affairs (VA) trained veterans to access and use the patient portal to share information with non-VA providers. The majority of participating veterans reported that the information would help them be more involved in their health care (78%) and planned to share it with non-VA providers (86%). As a result, 90% of the participating providers reported improved ability to make medication decisions, and 50% reported avoiding ordering an unnecessary laboratory test or procedure based on the information shared (Klein, 2017). Consumer-facing IT applications can also allow for providers to monitor symptoms remotely—such as home glucose monitoring for diabetic patients—and involve patients in managing and adhering to their care plan.

In addition to patients using data to support self-management, with the rising prevalence of high-deductible health plans leaving many insured patients responsible for their first-dollar health care spending, patients are increasingly demanding more transparent data on the price and quality of health care services. The Dartmouth Atlas of Health Care, first produced in 1996, was one early effort to analyze and compare health care utilization and expenditures and, in many ways, led to a growing interest in greater price transparency. Using Medicare claims data, the Atlas revealed dramatic variation in health care spending by hospital referral region (regional health care market) (The Trustees of Dartmouth College, 2018).

Insurer claims can provide insight into the total costs and use of care across all providers and settings. With the use of IT-supported data aggregation across multiple insurers, new **consumer decision support** tools can help consumers compare health insurance products and providers and aid patients in making informed decisions about spending their health care dollar. Some private insurers have started to integrate tools that aggregate pricing data and offer consumers with cost estimates for common health care services into consumer-facing benefits portals, along with patient self-management tools that can assist patients and their families in setting health behavior goals and adhering to treatment plans.

Public and private health insurers use HIT to receive and process claims, evaluate quality of care provided, and manage care for patients covered under their plans.

Health Insurers

Public and private health insurers use HIT to receive and process claims, evaluate quality of care provided, and manage care for patients covered under their plans. Administrative claims submitted by providers to insurers to receive reimbursement is an important source of data to evaluate patterns of care utilization and the quality of care. Insurers can use claims data to determine if appropriate care is delivered to a subset of patients, for example, by assessing the rate of colorectal cancer screenings for patients within a designated age range. Analysis of aggregated claims data can reveal variations in overall costs and quality across groups of providers.

Insurers use these analyses to manage preferred provider networks and incentivize improvements through value-based payment arrangements (Mehrotra, Adams, Thomas, & McGlynn, 2010). As one example, insurers will look to historical claims data to establish expected expenditure amounts and target prices for providers participating in episode- and population-based payment arrangements. In these models, insurers such as Medicare will incentivize providers to reduce spending below an anticipated financial benchmark; insurers use claims to determine whether providers have met the mark to earn value-based payment incentives (Centers for Medicare and Medicaid Services, 2016). Claims-based research can also support evidence-based management in provider operations, such as evaluation of workforce productivity and reallocation of resources to most appropriately meet demand and reduce inefficient use of clinician resources.

The government is a major health insurer across seven major health care programs: Medicare, Medicaid, the Children's Health Insurance Program (CHIP), Indian Health Services (IHS), TRICARE, the VHA, and the Federal Employee Health Benefits (FEHB) program. Despite serving different patient populations that in some cases utilize distinct provider systems, the federal programs coordinate on important initiatives to advance interoperability and patient accessibility to their electronic health data. As described later in this chapter, the U.S. Department of Health and Human Services has played a major role in incentivizing and subsidizing provider adoption of certified EHR technology for Medicare and Medicaid providers.

Governmental Public Health Entities

Governmental public health agencies have long used data to support the 10 essential public health services, which include monitoring health status to identify and solve community health problems (Centers for Disease Control and Prevention, 2018). Electronic health information systems present an opportunity for state and local health departments to harness the power of big data and more effectively serve as chief health strategists for their communities (DeSalvo, & Wang, 2016). For example, state health departments have traditionally tracked prevalence of chronic health conditions and related health risk behaviors through surveys such as the Behavioral Risk Factor Surveillance System. EHR-based surveillance systems can augment such information on population-level disease and risk factor incidence and prevalence with the added benefit of producing timelier data with less administrative burden (Klompas, et al., 2017).

Better integration and data-sharing between health care and public health can help to address the social determinants of health—factors such as income, education, and the environmental context in which people live, work, learn, and play that drive health outcomes, especially for vulnerable populations. Shared EHR data can support targeted public health interventions by recording patients' demographic data, including race, employment status, and zip code. State and federal government agencies also use electronic health data in the same manner as other health care insurers in administering Medicare, Medicaid, CHIP, and TRICARE and as a provider through operation of the VHA, IHS, Military Health System, and other public health services like sexually transmitted infection (STI) screenings and vaccination programs.

Researchers

Large-scale aggregation and analysis of digitized health records allows for researchers and developers to answer some of medicine's most pressing questions about the effectiveness, safety, and real-world outcomes of many therapies. The Patient-Centered Outcomes Research Institute (PCORI) launched the PCORnet initiative in 2013 to support research networks and enable complex analyses and queries across distributed virtual datasets (Fleurence, Curtis, Califf, Platt, Selby, & Brown, 2014). Clinical researchers can also utilize larger datasets to identify effective individualized prevention and disease treatments, or precision medicine. Precision medicine accounts for individual variabilities in genetics, environmental exposure, and lifestyle factors to inform the development of customized care plans (NIH / U.S. National Library of Medicine, 2015). As one example, the All of Us research program at the National Institutes of Health gathers health data from millions of people who voluntarily contribute information about their lifestyle and medical history to advance innovations in medicine (All of Us website, 2018).

▶ CASE EXERCISE 14.1—*NYC MACROSCOPE*

Dr. Shah is a primary care physician in New York City (NYC). She practices medicine in a small clinic with five other clinicians and a small practice staff. A few years ago, the group decided to adopt an electronic health record (EHR) system, but with their limited resources, they were unable to bring on a technical expert to help the team fully optimize EHR use. Luckily, the public health department in NYC launched a "Primary Care Information Project," which supported Dr. Shah's practice in using the electronic health information to make improvements in her patient care and participate in federal and local priorities initiatives. One of the initiatives her group participates in is the NYC Macroscope. The Macroscope uses aggregated and de-identified patient data from a virtual network of 700 distributed, practice-based EHRs, including Dr. Shah's, to monitor the prevalence of chronic conditions and risk factors for disease in more than 1.5 million patients.

Matt is an epidemiologist with the NYC Department of Health and Mental Hygiene (DOHMH). Matt and his team of public health professionals use the NYC Macroscope platform to support virtual public health surveillance. Many key indicators of interest to Matt's team and other public health researchers reside in the EHR, including smoking status, obesity, depression, and diabetes prevalence.

Prior to the implementation of Macroscope in 2012, Matt and his team used the NYC Health and Nutrition Examination Survey and the NYC Community Health Survey to track these same indicators; these reference surveys required in-person and telephonic survey administration, respectively, which were costly to administer and produced less timely data than Matt is now able to obtain from the Macroscope system. However, the NYC DOHMH continues to administer the surveillance surveys because the validity of the NYC Macroscope data in predicting population-level prevalence of disease and risk factors is still under evaluation.

1. What kind of health indicators would be of interest to both Dr. Shah for care delivery improvement and Matt for public health surveillance?

2. How should NYC DOHMH evaluate the validity of the NYC Macroscope data compared to traditional surveillance surveys?

3. What might be some of the key concerns for staff in both the practice and public health department to participate in this new effort and how might they be addressed?

Source: Data from Perlman, S.E., [Other Authors]. (2017). Innovations in population health surveillance: Using electronic health records for chronic disease surveillance. *American Journal of Public Health, 107*(6), 853–857.

HIT INTEROPERABILITY

Despite widespread gains in the adoption of EHRs among hospitals and providers, the U.S. health care system has not achieved widespread interoperability. The availability of health data via EHRs and health information networks has enabled more data-driven, team-based approaches to care coordination and targeted case management, but more progress is necessary. While most hospitals (82%) exchange health information with other hospitals and ambulatory care providers outside the system, HIE among physicians remains a challenge. Most hospitals and providers and hospitals do not have necessary patient information electronically available at the point of care, and less than one-third of providers (31%) are able to transfer electronic patient data from other providers into their EHRs (Jamoom, & Yang, 2016; Patel, Henry, Pylypchuk, & Searcy, 2016).

Interoperability is defined as "health IT that enables the secure exchange of electronic health information with, and use of electronic health information from, other health IT without special effort on the part of the user; allows for complete access, exchange, and use of all electronically accessible health information for authorized use under applicable State or Federal law; and does not constitute information blocking" (21st Century Cures Act of 2016, 2016b). There are several aspects of interoperability:

- *Syntactic interoperability:* Syntactic interoperability is achieved if two or more systems are capable of communicating and exchanging data. Syntactic interoperability is a

FIGURE 14.1   LEVELS OF HEALTH INFORMATION TECHNOLOGY INTEROPERABILITY

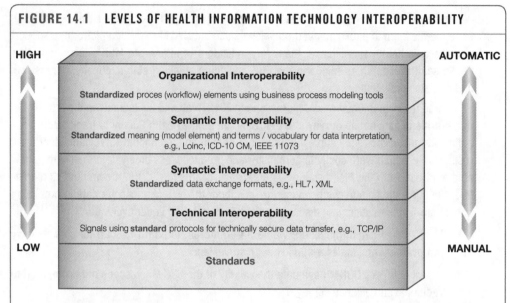

HIGH   AUTOMATIC

Organizational Interoperability

Standardized proces (workflow) elements using business process modeling tools

Semantic Interoperability

Standardized meaning (model element) and terms / vocabulary for data interpretation, e.g., Loinc, ICD-10 CM, IEEE 11073

Syntactic Interoperability

Standardized data exchange formats, e.g., HL7, XML

Technical Interoperability

Signals using **standard** protocols for technically secure data transfer, e.g., TCP/IP

LOW   MANUAL

Standards

Data exchanges on the low technical level require more manual intervention in order to achieve the desired communication of meaning; data exchanges on the higher levels use more sophisticated standardization, are more automatic and require less manual intervention.

Source: Oemig, F., & Snelick, R. (2016). *Healthcare interoperability standards compliance handbook* (p. 13, Fig. 1.3). Cham, Switzerland: Springer International Publishing.

prerequisite for semantic interoperability (HL7.org). An everyday example of syntactic interoperability is the ability of an electronic file in PDF format to be opened across multiple platforms without changing format, regardless of whether the end user opens the file on a Mac laptop, Dell desktop, or mobile phone. Syntactically interoperable HIT systems similarly use a standard set of file formats, such as the Clinical Data Architecture standard, to ensure medical records retain a consistent structure across various HIT components and products.

- *Semantic interoperability:* The clinical vocabularies and coding systems used to represent clinical information in HIT systems are often referred to as data "semantics." Semantic interoperability is the "ability to automatically interpret the information exchanged meaningfully and accurately in order to produce useful results as defined by the end users of both systems" (The Office of the National Coordinator for Health Information Technology, 2015). One standard that supports semantic interoperability is the *International Statistical Classification of Diseases and Related Health Problems*, currently in its 10th edition, or ICD-10. Providers use ICD-10 codes to describe patient diagnoses and symptoms in a consistent manner, which prevents miscommunication. For example, a patient presenting with symptoms of a heart attack may be diagnosed as having an acute myocardial infarction, or AMI. The ICD-10 offers a classification system for providers to distinguish among the various types of myocardial infarctions and communicate effectively among the care team in order to provide accurate treatment.

STANDARDS

Data exchange standards are required for interoperability in any industry. When different entities agree on and adopt a set of standards, information can be easily shared or understood, and hardware or software products from different vendors can work together. For example, standards allow websites to be seen by different web browsers, store-bought printers from different brands to connect to your Mac computer or PC, and cable channels to transmit their programs to any television in the home. These standards can include vocabulary, coding, and terminology standards (i.e., laboratory test results, clinical measurements, test orders, medical problems, and drug names), content and structure standards (i.e., data provenance), implementation specifications (i.e., infrastructure components to ensure consistency with standard implementation), and administrative standards (i.e., benefits and claims, nonclinical needs).

In health care, major standards development organizations such as Integrating the Healthcare Enterprise (IHE) and Health Level 7 (HL7) and regulatory bodies like National Institute of Technology (NIST) work to promote standards that increase the effectiveness and efficiency of HIT. The development of standards like LOINC (Logical Observation Identifiers Names and Codes) and ICD-10 (see Figure 14.1) over the past several decades significantly drives interoperability. To advance interoperability further, HIT developers and standard development organizations are currently investing resources into HL7's Fast Healthcare Interoperability Resources (FHIR, 2018), an emerging data standard that specifies an application programming interface (API) for exchanging health data in order to connect third-party apps to HIT systems (Fast Healthcare Interoperability Resources, 2018). A popular example of how APIs can work in practice is Google Maps. Many popular apps use or have used the Google Maps API, including Uber, Yelp, and Open Table, among others. However, meaningful interoperability requires much more than existence of standards: marketplace incentives, regulatory guidance and push-pull, and more important, a cultural change in how businesses compete and how they perceive data as an asset.

DRIVING FORCES SHAPING THE USE OF DATA AND HIT

The federal government has had strong influence in the HIT marketplace over the past two decades. In 2004, President George W. Bush established the Office of the National Coordinator for Health IT (ONC) to help bring the U.S. health system into the computer age. In 2009, Congress passed the Health Information Technology for Economic and Clinical Health (HITECH) Act, part of the American Recover and Reinvestment Act of 2009, which legislatively authorized ONC in statute and funded key programs and incentives for HIT adoption.

ONC is the principal federal entity charged with coordination of nationwide efforts to implement and use HIT and accelerate the electronic exchange of health information. ONC is organizationally located within the Office of the Secretary at the U.S. Department of Health and Human Services (DHHS). One of ONC's key activities is administration of the Health IT Certification Program, a voluntary certification program to provide for the certification of HIT standards, implementation specifications, and certification criteria adopted by the DHHS Secretary. ONC's overarching goal for electronic health information exchange is for information to follow a patient where and when it is needed, across organizations, IT systems, and geographic boundaries, and to make patients' medical records available to them in electronic format.

The HITECH Act of 2009 stimulated unprecedented growth in the adoption of EHRs through a combination of policies, programs, incentives, and penalties. In 2009, fewer than one in five hospitals and physician offices used HIT. As of 2016, 96% of hospitals and 78% of physician's offices use EHR technology (Fast Healthcare Interoperability Resources, 2018). A primary driver in the adoption of EHRs was the Medicare and Medicaid EHR Incentive Programs (commonly referred to as Meaningful Use), which was authorized by the HITECH Act. These programs administered by the Centers for Medicare & Medicaid Services (CMS) set aside approximately $30 billion to support eligible hospitals and providers to adopt and use EHRs certified by ONC's Health IT Certification Program. Eligible providers and hospitals that did not adopt certified EHRs and attest to criteria set by CMS would be subject to payment adjustments in the following years.

In addition to the EHR Incentive Programs, the HITECH Act provided ONC with $2 billion in discretionary funds to establish programs designed to reduce common barriers for adopting and using HIT. These programs included the Regional Extension Center Program, a program that funded 62 extension centers to provide small provider practices, public and critical access hospitals, and community health centers with technical assistance to adopt and use EHRs. Through the State Health Information Exchange Program, ONC funded each state and territory to accelerate data exchange within its jurisdiction. Recognizing the current workforce was not equipped for this transition from paper records to EHRs, ONC funded dozens of community colleges and universities, which collectively trained more than 20,000 HIT professionals between 2010 and 2013 (NORC at the University of Chicago, 2014). ONC also funded 17 communities through its Beacon Community Program to demonstrate how HIT could advance patient-centered care. ONC created the Strategic Health IT Advanced Research Projects (SHARP) program to support research to address well-documented problems that impede the adoption of HIT. One of the grants, SMART

The Office of the National Coordinator for Health IT is responsible for coordinating nationwide efforts to implement health information technology. This includes oversight of relevant efforts across the federal government's health programs administered by CMS, Veterans Health Administration, Defense Health Agency, as well as other relevant regulatory agencies such as the Federal Communications Commission and National Institute of Standards and Technology.

Health IT, funded Boston Children's Hospital and Harvard Medical School to create an open, standards-based technology platform that enables innovators to create apps that seamlessly and securely run across the health care system (SMART Health IT, 2018).

In late 2016, due to the lack of nationwide interoperability, a bipartisan majority in the U.S. Congress passed the 21st Century Cures Act, which includes several important provisions designed to accelerate interoperability. Key provisions in Title IV of the Cures Act focus on combating and penalizing information blocking, establishing or recognizing a trusted exchange framework and common agreement to promote the exchange of health data between health information networks, and requiring conditions and maintenance of certification by developers participating in the Health IT Certification Program. These conditions focus on ensuring that developers do not engage in information blocking; inhibit the appropriate exchange, access, and use of electronic health information; and do not prohibit or restrict communications regarding a product's usability, interoperability, security, user experience, business practices, and information on use.

The conditions of certification also require developers to publish APIs. APIs refer to technology that allows one software program to access the services provided by another software program. APIs can allow third-party developers to pull data from EHRs and build programs or apps on top of that data (JASON, 2013). These APIs must "allow health information from such technology to be accessed, exchanged, and used without special effort," and provide "access to all data elements of a patient's EHR to the extent permissible under applicable privacy laws."

HIT also represents a key strategy for curbing health care cost. With U.S. national health care expenditures accounting for 17.9% of GDP in 2016 (Cuckler, 2018) and medical price inflation exceeding overall economic inflation (HRSA, 2016), the federal government has made a concerted effort to adopt interoperable HIT systems as part of the supporting infrastructure for alternative payment models that reimburse providers based on the efficiency and quality of care provided.

CMS and private payers have introduced a variety of new value-based payment models that reimburse providers for quality of care and patient outcomes, moving away from a traditional fee-for-service structure. Value-based care models such as the accountable care organization (ACO)—in which a group of providers agree to take financial responsibility for the total cost of care, quality, and outcomes for a designated population of patients—require HIT to manage population health and better coordinate across systems of patient care. Held accountable for total patient costs, providers are investing in population health management systems, which use health data from the EHR and administrative data such as claims to identify patients who may be at risk for costly hospital admissions or have otherwise uncontrolled or complex health conditions. Care managers can use risk-stratified patient lists and disease registries to implement patient outreach and care coordination. Ultimately, HIT interoperability is central to transforming the

▶ CASE EXERCISE 14.2—AVERA HEALTH

The executive leadership team of Avera Health is used to dealing with complexity. The integrated delivery system based in Sioux Falls, South Dakota, includes more than 200 outpatient clinics and 33 hospitals, as well as home health, hospice care, and senior living facilities. The more than 300 provider locations that make up Avera are spread across five states in the upper Midwest and serve a population of nearly 1 million (About Avera, 2018). In addition to geographic spread, the individual Avera provider sites have been operating on a variety of EHR platforms that are not interoperable.

To address this interoperability gap, Avera Health established a single health information exchange (HIE) platform for the five-state area serviced by the organization. Patients are automatically enrolled in the HIE under an opt-out policy, and the function to exchange Consolidated-Clinical Document Architecture (C-CDA) is embedded into the clinician's EHR workflow. The high rate of patient and provider participation in the HIE has resulted in better patient care coordination, a decrease in redundant testing, and improvements in providers' ability to use up-to-date clinical information at the point of care at Avera Health (EHRA, 2017).

1. How might the leadership team evaluate the return on investment of the HIE platform?

2. What are some of the remaining barriers to providers regularly using the HIE to exchange patient data?

3. How should Avera Health communicate with patients about the inclusion of their health data in the HIE?

health care delivery system into one that provides better care, smarter spending, and healthier people (Burwell, 2015).

The Medicare and CHIP Reauthorization Act of 2015 (MACRA) changed the way Medicare pays providers by streamlining several quality payment programs into the Merit-based Incentive Payment System (MIPS) and introducing more enticing incentives for providers to join Advanced Alternative Payment Models (Medicare and CHIP Reauthorization Act of 2015, 2015). Collectively named the Quality Payment Program, Medicare's new reimbursement structure builds on the meaningful use requirements for provider use of certified EHR technology. Further, the quality performance, practice improvement, and resource-use components of the Quality Payment Program demands more advanced use of EHRs and data analytics for providers to be successful (Morrissey, 2017).

CHALLENGES TO MORE EFFECTIVE USE OF INFORMATION AND DATA

Despite the rapid uptake of EHRs and more advanced HIT systems across the health care industry, in many ways, the early promise of interoperable EHRs driving immediate and dramatic annual health care savings and care improvements seems overblown in retrospect. Systematic reviews of evidence regarding

HIE usage and effect have found little generalizable impact on overall costs, outcomes, or quality (Rahurkar, et al., 2015). Significant barriers to interoperability include technical limitations, policy challenges, and the lack of business drivers and incentives to share information with other health care providers. Most providers are still paid on a fee-for-service structure, in which reimbursement is based on the volume of services and patients served; a hospital under this reimbursement model may lack economic incentives to share a patient's care record with a competing hospital.

Providers struggle with effectively integrating the EHR into workflow, with common complaints including decreased time for face-to-face patient interactions and increased demands for timely data entry. A 2013 study by RAND Corporation found that EHR use negatively impacted physicians' overall job satisfaction (Friedberg, et al., 2013). Providers unsatisfied with the functionality or usability of their current EHR system feel stuck due to administrative challenges and costs associated with transitioning away from the current system. Data integration across providers, payers, and public health and other key stakeholders is also hindered by willful information blocking, when developers knowingly and unreasonably interfere with electronic health information exchange (Adler-Milstein, & Pfeifer, 2017). These challenges may inhibit providers from effectively harnessing the capability of electronic data systems for evidence-based management and organizational quality improvement.

PRIVACY AND SECURITY

Beyond the technical challenges, issues of privacy and security are a significant barrier to more ubiquitous availability and exchange of health information. Coordinated attention at the federal, state, and regional levels is needed both to develop and implement appropriate privacy and security policies and trusted exchange frameworks to ensure all data-sharing participants are following the same technical standards and procedures to protect health information. There is work under way at the federal level to fulfill the 21st Century Cures Act's requirement for ONC to "develop or support a trusted exchange framework, including a common agreement among health information networks nationally." Only by engaging all stakeholders, particularly consumers, can health information be protected and electronically exchanged in a manner that respects variations in individuals' views on privacy and access. If individuals and other participants in a network lack trust in electronic exchange of information because of perceived or actual risks, this distrust may affect their willingness to disclose necessary health information.

> Coordinated attention at the federal, state, and regional levels is needed both to develop and implement appropriate privacy and security policies and trusted exchange frameworks to ensure all data-sharing participants are following the same technical standards and procedures to protect health information.

EXHIBIT 14.1   SIX IMPERATIVES FOR IMPROVING CYBERSECURITY IN THE HEALTH CARE INDUSTRY

1. Define and streamline leadership, governance, and expectations for health care industry cybersecurity.
2. Increase the security and resilience of medical devices and HIT.
3. Develop the health care workforce capacity necessary to prioritize and ensure cybersecurity awareness and technical capabilities.
4. Increase health care industry readiness through improved cybersecurity awareness and education.
5. Identify mechanisms to protect research and development efforts and intellectual property from attacks or exposure.
6. Improve information sharing of industry threats, weaknesses, and mitigations.

Source: Health Care Industry Cybersecurity Task Force. (2017). Report on improving cybersecurity in the health care industry. Retrieved from https://www.phe.gov/Preparedness/planning/CyberTF/Documents/report2017.pdf.

Cybersecurity threats are a growing and constant concern for health care systems as more patient care operations and functions are transitioned to electronic systems. Without proper controls, HIT systems can be susceptible to hacking, identify theft, service disruption, and malicious software (malware). Large-scale cyberattacks are more frequently targeting health care providers with ransomware, whereby hackers take over valuable patient data and information management systems and demand a ransom from the providers before relinquishing control (Jarrett, 2017).

CURRENT MARKETPLACE AND EMERGING OPPORTUNITIES

There are many promising approaches to address the challenges of HIT. Widespread adoption of the HL7 FHIR standards and APIs could drive similar market-based innovation in consumer-facing health apps. These apps can have many different use cases, including population health analytics, integration of data from multiple devices that track fitness and activity, monitoring and improvement of medication adherence, chronic disease management, and identification of high-risk and high-cost patients and coordination of their care. Further, FHIR can facilitate consumer-directed exchange as more commonplace platforms give patients the ability to manage and aggregate their own electronic medical records from various providers via APIs, such as Apple's Health app. The largest public insurer CMS implemented "Blue Button 2.0," an API with claims data for more than 50 million Medicare beneficiaries, to encourage developers to innovate new value-added use cases for patients and providers around the standard (Centers for Medicare and Medicaid Services, 2018). CMS is also taking steps to prevent information blocking by requiring eligible clinicians to attest to following relevant standards and exchanging electronic health information with patients and other health care providers "regardless of the requestor's affiliation or technology vendor" as a condition of Medicare participation (Centers for Medicaid and Medicare Services, 2017).

Many other data sources relevant to patient care and population health management can be managed and integrated within the EHR. **Remote patient monitoring (RPM)** technologies collect health data and vital signs from patients when they are away from the point of care to support interventions when needed, such as remote glucose monitoring systems that send real-time glucose readings for diabetic patients and alert patients and their providers in case of uncontrolled blood sugar levels. RPM is one form of telehealth. **Telehealth** is defined as "the use of electronic information and telecommunication technologies to support and promote long-distance clinical health care, patient and professional health-related education, public health and health administration" (HRSA, 2018). mHealth—short for mobile health—refers to the use of mobile phones and other wireless technologies in medical care, including delivery of preventive services and health care education. In recognition of the expanded use of these now ubiquitous technologies in health care delivery, the 21st Century Cures Act clarified the Food and Drug Administration's jurisdiction over mobile medical software and devices that support clinical decision making (21st Century Cures Act of 2016, 2016a). Providers may also collect and use health-related data about a patient's social environment—such as housing status and food security—and administrative data, including health insurance enrollment and payment information as a part of the electronic medical record.

Other HIT products address specific pain points and blind spots in the current delivery system as providers transition to value-based payment. Providers in ACO arrangements are accountable for total health spending for a designated population of patients, but they have limited insight or control when patients seek care from providers outside the ACO. To solve for the problem of tracking patients' interactions with the larger health system, platforms such as PatientPing use administrative data available in admission, discharge, and transfer (ADT) feeds to provide more real-time clinical event notifications to accountable providers connected to the network (Patient Ping website, 2018).

Big data also presents an opportunity for advanced machine learning. Large technology companies have launched artificial intelligence tools that use advanced analytics and machine learning to optimize health care delivery. On a smaller scale, health systems now regularly use predictive algorithms to forecast everything from whether a patient is likely to pay a bill to whether a patient is at high risk of a costly hospitalization (Angraal, Krumholz, & Schulz, 2017).

Another emerging technology with the potential to positively disrupt the health care industry is blockchain. Initially used in the financial sector, blockchain technology utilizes distributed peer-to-peer networks to support secure, decentralized data management and validated transactions. Proposed applications of blockchain in health care include more automated transactions like prior authorizations and claims processing and greater patient insight into who can and has accessed their health data.

CONCLUSION

Electronic health information promises an array of potential benefits for individuals and the U.S. health care system at large through improved clinical care and smarter spending. Modern computer science presents opportunities for individuals, clinicians, and payers to have a fuller picture of a patient's health history and utilized informed decision making. No longer in paper form, health information is increasingly ready to be transmitted electronically and analyzed using sophisticated software. At the same time, this environment also poses new challenges and opportunities for protecting individually identifiable health information while encouraging greater interoperability and improved front-end usability. Eventually, the market will drive out technologies and approaches that fail to meet expectations. Yet, to make true advances toward shared accountability on health, innovators need to envision and explore new frontiers in data infrastructure and technologies that advance community-wide population health.

▶ CASE EXERCISE 14.3—ELECTRONIC HEALTH RECORDS

Dr. Ann Smith is a physician in rural New York, where she still keeps all of her patient records on paper, in folders, stored in file cabinets. Lately, she has been receiving a lot of information about HIT systems and is trying to decide what she should do about purchasing the software, how she can afford it, and when she will find the time to learn the program and train her staff.

Dr. Smith has a heavy workload and is the only physician within an 80-mile radius. She has three nurses on her staff. One of them also serves as the administrative assistant, who answers phone calls. She also has a part-time office manager who handles insurance claims and appeals. Dr. Smith is overwhelmed by the thought of switching to electronic records, and yet she knows she has to do it. She is 40 years old and plans to be in practice for many years to come. Money and time are both tight. With the exception of one nurse, her staff is older and was inherited by Dr. Smith from the previous doctor. Dr. Smith wonders how she will take care of her patients while trying to learn a new system. Yet, she knows, she is under pressure to adopt electronic records for her practice.

Keeping Dr. Smith's needs and concerns in mind, answer the following questions:

1. What should be Dr. Smith's first step toward adopting and implementing an EHR in her practice?

2. What are some ways she can work her own training into her schedule?

3. What are some of the key concerns for her staff, and how might they be addressed?

DISCUSSION QUESTIONS

1. Why has the health care sector been slower than other industries to adopt HIT?
2. What factors drove rapid growth in HIT adoption in the early 21st century?
3. What challenges do providers face in effectively using HIT within their practices? What are strategies to mitigate those barriers?

4. Why is interoperability important? What are the key approaches to driver interoperability?

5. How should the issue of patient privacy be addressed? What are some approaches you might suggest?

6. Provide an example of how HIT can be used to improve quality of care, reduce cost, and/or improve population health.

REFERENCES

21st Century Cures Act of 2016. (2016a). P.L. 114–146 §3060.

21st Century Cures Act of 2016. (2016b). P.L. 114–146 §4003.

About Avera. (2018). Retrieved from https://www.avera.org/about/

Adler-Milstein, J., & Pfeifer, E. (2017). Information blocking: Is it occurring and what policy strategies can address it? *The Milbank Quarterly, 95*(1), 117–135.

All of Us website. (2018). Retrieved from https://allofus.nih.gov

Angraal, S., Krumholz, H.M., & Schulz, W.L. (2017). Blockchain technology: Applications in health care. *Circulation: Cardiovascular Quality and Outcomes, 10*(9), e003800.

Burwell, S.M. (2015). Setting value-based payment goals—HHS efforts to improve U.S. health care. *New England Journal of Medicine, 372*(10), 897–899.

Centers for Disease Control and Prevention. (2018). The public health system & the 10 essential public health services. Retrieved from https://www.cdc.gov/stltpublichealth/publichealthservices/essentialhealthservices.html

Centers for Medicare and Medicaid Services. (2016). Medicare program; Medicare shared savings program; accountable care organizations—Revised benchmark rebasing methodology, facilitating transition to performance-based risk, and administrative finality of financial calculations. Final rule. *Federal Register, 81*(112).

Centers for Medicare and Medicaid Services. (2017). The merit-based incentive payment system advancing care information prevention of information blocking attestation: Making sure EHR information is shared. Retrieved from https://www.cms.gov/Medicare/Quality-Initiatives-Patient-Assessment-Instruments/Value-Based-Programs/MACRA-MIPS-and-APMs/ACI-Information-Blocking-fact-sheet.pdf

Centers for Medicare and Medicaid Services. (2018). Blue Button 2.0. Retrieved from https://www.bluebutton.cms.gov/

Chen, C., Garrido, T., Chock, D., Okawa, G., & Liang, L. (2009). The Kaiser Permanente electronic health record: Transforming and streamlining modalities of care. *Health Affairs, 28*, 323–333.

Cuckler, G.A. (2018). National health expenditure projections, 2017–26: Despite uncertainty, fundamentals primarily drive spending growth. *Health Affairs*. Retrieved from https://doi.org/10.1377/hlthaff.2017.1655

Delbanco, T., Walker, J., Bell, S. K., Darer, J. D., Elmore, J., & Faraq, N. (2012). Inviting patients to read their doctors' notes: A quasi-experimental study and look ahead. *Annals of Internal Medicine, 157*, 461–470.

DeSalvo, K., & Wang, Y. C. (2016). Health informatics in the public health 3.0 era: Intelligence for the chief health strategists. *Public Health Management and Practice, 22*, S1–S2.

eCQI Resource Center. (2018). What are electronic clinical quality measures (eCQMs)? Retrieved from https://ecqi.healthit.gov/ecqms

EHRA. (2017). Interoperability success stories: The journey continues. Retrieved from http://www.himss.org/sites/himssorg/files/EHRA-Interoperability-Success-Stories-june2017.pdf

Fast Healthcare Interoperability Resources. (2018). Welcome to FHIR®. Retrieved from https://www.hl7.org/fhir/

Fleurence, R., Curtis, L., Califf, R., Platt, R., Selby, J., & Brown, J. (2014). Launching PCOR-net, a national patient-centered clinical research network. *Journal of the American Medical Informatics Association, 21*(4), 578–582.

Friedberg, M. W., Chen, P. G., Van Busum, K. R., Aunon, F., Pham, C. et al. (2013). *Factors affecting physician professional satisfaction and their implications for patient care, health systems, and health policy.* Santa Monica, CA: RAND Corporation.

Health Care Industry Cybersecurity Task Force. (2017). Report on improving cybersecurity in the health care industry. Retrieved February 18, 2108, from https://www.phe.gov/Preparedness/planning/CyberTF/Documents/report2017.pdf

HealthIT.gov. (2018). Clinical decision support. Retrieved from https://www.healthit.gov/policy-researchers-implementers/clinical-decision-support-cds

Hillestad, R. (2005). Can electronic medical record systems transform health care? Potential health benefits, savings, and costs. *Health Affairs, 24*(5), 1103–1117.

HRSA. (2016). Consumer Price Index for medical care. Retrieved from https://www.hrsa.gov/get-health-care/affordable/hill-burton/cpi.html

HRSA. (2018). Telehealth Programs. Retrieved from https://www.hrsa.gov/rural-health/telehealth/ index.html

Institute of Medicine. (2001). *Crossing the quality chasm: A new health system for the 21st century.* Washington, DC: National Academies Press.

Institute of Medicine. (2013). *Digital data improvement priorities for continuous learning in health and health care: Workshop summary.* Washington, DC: National Academies Press.

Jamoom, E., & Yang, N. (2016). Table of electronic health record adoption and use among office-based physicians in the U.S. by state: 2015 National Electronic Health Records Survey. Retrieved from www.cdc.gov/nchs/data/ahcd/nehrs/2015nehrswebtable.pdf

Jarrett, M.P. (2017). Cybersecurity—A serious patient care concern. *Journal of the American Medical Association, 318*(14), 1319–1320.

JASON. (2013). *A robust health data infrastructure.* AHRQ Publication No. 14–0041-EF. Retrieved from https://www.healthit.gov/sites/default/files/ptp13-700hhs_white.pdf

Jha, A. K., Perlin, J. B., Kizer, K. W., Dudley, R. A. (2003). Effect of the transformation of the Veterans Affairs health care system on the quality of care. *New England Journal of Medicine, 348*, 2218–2227.

Klein, D. M. (2017). The veteran-initiated electronic care coordination: A multisite initiative to promote and evaluate consumer-mediated health information exchange. *Telemedicine Journal and E-Health, 23*(4), 264–272.

Klompas, M., Cocoros, N. M., Menchaca, J. T., Erani, D., Hafer, E., et al. (2017). State and local chronic disease surveillance using electronic health record systems. *American Journal of Public Health, 107(9)*, 1406–1412.

Kohn, L. T., Corrigan, J. M., Donaldson, M. S., (Eds.). (2000). *To err is human: Building a safer health system.* Washington, DC: National Academies Press.

Lee, B. J., & Forbes, K. (2009). The role of specialists in managing the health of populations with chronic illness: The example of chronic kidney disease. *BMJ, 39*, b2395.

Medicare and CHIP Reauthorization Act of 2015. (2015). H.R. 2, P.L. 114–10.

Mehrotra, A., Adams, J., Thomas, J., & McGlynn, E. (2010). The effect of different attribution rules on individual physician cost profiles. *Annals of Internal Medicine, 152*(10), 649–654.

Morrissey, J. (2017). MACRA success starts with IT. *Health Data Management, 25*(1)(02), 26–29.

MyHealth Access Network. (2018). What we do. Retrieved from https://myhealthaccess.net/what-we-do/

National Information Center on Health Services Research and Health Care Technology: Informatics. Retrieved from https://www.nlm.nih.gov/hsrinfo/informatics.html

NIH/U.S. National Library of Medicine. (2015). What is precision medicine? Retrieved from https://ghr.nlm.nih.gov/primer/precisionmedicine/definition

NORC at the University of Chicago. (2014). Evaluation of the information technology professionals in health care ("workforce") program: Summative report. Presented to the Office of the National Coordinator for Health IT. Retrieved from https://www.healthit.gov/sites/efault/files/workforceevaluationsummativereport.pdf

Open Notes. (2017). OpenNotes passes the 20 million mark. Retrieved from https://www.opennotes.org/news/opennotes-passes-the-20-million-mark/

Patel, V., Henry, J., Pylypchuk, Y., & Searcy, T. (2016). *Interoperability among U.S. non-federal acute care hospitals in 2015*. ONC Data Brief, no. 36. Washington, DC: Office of the National Coordinator for Health Information Technology.

PatientPing website. (2018). Retrieved from http://www.patientping.com/

Rahurkar, S., Vest, J. R., & Menachemi, N. (2015). Despite the spread of health information exchange, there is little evidence of its impact on cost, use, and quality of care. *Health Affairs, 34*(3), 477–483.

SMART Health IT. (2018). Retrieved from https://smarthealthit.org/

The Office of the National Coordinator for Health Information Technology. (2015). Connecting health and care for the nation: a shared nationwide interoperability roadmap, final version 1.0. Retrieved from https://www.healthit.gov/sites/default/files/hie-interoperability/nationwide-interoperability-roadmap-final-version-1.0.pdf

The Trustees of Dartmouth College. (2018). Dartmouth Atlas of Health Care. Retrieved from http:// www.dartmouthatlas.org/data/region/

Tripathi, M. (2012). EHR evolution: Policy and legislation forces changing the EHR. *Journal of AHIMA, 83*(10), 24–29.

Turvey, C., Klein, D., Fix, G. et al., (2014). Blue Button use by patients to access and share health record information using the Department of Veterans Affairs' online patient portal. *Journal of the American Medical Informatics Association, 21*(4), 657–663.

U.S. Government Accountability Office. (2014). VA and DOD need to support cost and schedule claims, develop interoperability plans, and improve collaboration. *GAO Reports*, i–42.

Walker, J., Pan, E., Johnston, D., Adler-Milstein, J., Bates, D. W., & Middleton, B. (2005). The value of health care information exchange and interoperability. *Health Affairs, Jan-Jun*: W5-10–W5-18.

IV

Future of U.S. Health Care

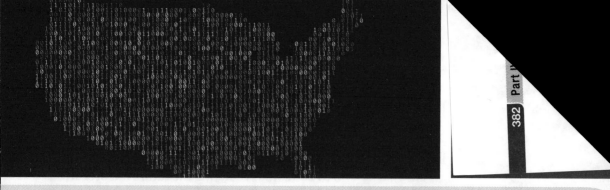

The Future of Health Care Delivery and Health Policy

James R. Knickman and Brian Elbel

LEARNING OBJECTIVES

► Explain why it is important to forecast the future
► Understand the forces in health care that shape change in the health system
► Describe the roles various stakeholders play in shaping the future
► Evaluate predictions about how the health system changed over the last five years
► Identify key challenges that will receive attention in the coming years

KEY TERMS

► outcomes
► predictive analytics
► stakeholders
► telehealth
► value

TOPICAL OUTLINE

► Why thinking about the future is important in health care planning
► Approaches to predicting the future
► Forces shaping change in the health system
► Key challenges that will receive attention in upcoming years
► Future prospects for different stakeholders in the health enterprise

INTRODUCTION

This final chapter focuses on the future of health and health care: Where is health care in America headed? What are the forces that will shape health care over the next 5 to 20 years? Predicting the future is a precarious undertaking. Fortunately for those who try to do it, most people forget what you predicted in the past when the future actually happens!

Integration and consolidation of services like long-term care, physician practices, outpatient surgery, and even insurance may well continue, and their impact on health outcomes is yet unknown.*

As authors, we will at least present our "self-evaluation" of predictions we made 5 years ago in the final chapter of the 11th edition of this text (Knickman and Kovner, 2015). In that chapter, Knickman and Kovner suggested to readers that the biggest changes over this recent period of time would focus on science and knowledge breakthroughs, major changes in payment approaches moving toward what has been called value-based payment systems in the above chapters, and marked movements toward integration of medical care with organizations merging and growing in both size and scope. Actually, these were rather accurate predictions, although the changes over the last 5 years have not been transformative but rather have involved steady small steps in the directions we suggested. In this chapter, we suggest that many of the changes we predicted earlier will continue to be major preoccupations of the health system in the next few years.

We dramatically missed one key thing that changed over recent years: the political dynamics in Washington, that have had sizable impacts on recent changes in the health system. As the 11th edition went to press, Barack Obama was serving a second term as president and was steadily steering the nation toward a more communal approach to financing health care (with large subsidies from the rich to poor and near-universal access to health insurance). He also was advancing approaches to public health and controversial services like abortion in directions favored by the more liberal parts of the American population. We never anticipated that voters would choose a stark change in leadership that is now moving health care and public health in very different directions. To say the least, this shows the precarious nature of forecasting the future.

However, it is worth the time and energy to think about the future and the forces that shape it. For an individual planning to work as a health professional, a sense of the future offers insight about what types of employment might be the most meaningful and the most viable. As a health care manager, making choices about how to ensure your hospital, medical practice, public health agency, or health care company is ready for the future requires a base of understanding about the dynamics shaping change. For a future policy maker, it is important to understand clearly how the system is evolving, what forces are shaping it, and how different changes in policy might affect future trends.

Even at the individual patient level, there is more and more attention on the issue of predicting the future. The concept of **predictive analytics** is the attempt to look at a patient's past utilization of services, past behavioral choices, and

---

*To hear the podcast, go to https://bcove.video/2DZA9E4 or access the ebook on Springer Publishing Connect™.

existing health needs to forecast the patient's use of health care in the future (Bates, Saria, Ohno-Machado, Shah, & Escobar, 2014). This field is getting increasingly sophisticated in using "big data" to make forecasts about a broad range of health issues such as whether a specific patient is at high risk of falling while in a hospital or whether a specific

> Having some sense of how the system is evolving at any point in history is useful for efforts to shape the system, no matter what one's role.

person is at high risk of becoming addicted to opioids if they are prescribed. This new type of forecast information shapes the delivery of both medical care and prevention-oriented interventions. We predict that this type of prediction will advance, though likely not as fast as many currently assume.

The predictions presented here are shaped by our vantage points as professors and active researchers working with a wide range of experts who actually shape the future of our health system. We also are fortunate to be able to base our forecasts on the analysis and insights presented by the accomplished and thoughtful authors in the 14 previous chapters of this text.

FORCES SHAPING CHANGE IN THE HEALTH SYSTEM

The preceding chapters present explanations of the forces that have shaped the health care system over the past 20 years or so and identify the challenges most important to address to improve the **value** and **outcomes** of health care. We think there are six key forces to keep in mind when developing forecasts for the future.

New Knowledge and Technology

By far, the key driver of potential change in the health system is emerging technology and medical know-how. It is possible that the rate of new breakthroughs in medicine and health promotion will be even faster than in the recent past.

One source of medical progress relates to the sequencing of the human genome at the start of the 21st century. It is now possible to map an individual's personal genome for less than $1,000; in the future, this information could act as the guide for identifying which new medical interventions (especially pharmaceutical interventions) work for a specific person and which ones will have terrible side effects or be ineffective. This knowledge will usher in an era of personalized medicine. Each cancer patient, for example, may have a treatment regimen most likely to work for that person based on his or her genome (Ginsburg & Phillips, 2018).

Current research efforts could lead to a better understanding of the risks facing each individual at birth related to contracting chronic diseases or specific categories of medical problems later in life. Potentially, preventive interventions will be able to alter the risk for specific conditions such as heart disease or Alzheimer's disease. Other advances also likely will occur, such as a universal vaccines for the flu or similar illnesses, which a person would need to take only once in his or her life. We hope this will also be the case for HIV.

Another major source of possible treatment improvements is stem-cell research. Stem-cell technologies could make it possible to grow tissue from a specific individual and for a specific organ. This tissue could be used to guide treatment interventions by seeing which interventions cause positive responses in the tissue where the disease is. Perhaps most dazzling, stem cells could grow new organs that would not be rejected by an individual when transplanted (Garakani & Saidi, 2017).

Somewhat related to the emerging knowledge from science and medical research is the likely emergence of new technologies to change the way medical providers manage our care. We already are experiencing the rapidly growing role of robotics in helping surgeons perform surgery with less invasive procedures.

The newest form of technology that could transform health care is artificial intelligence, or machine learning techniques (Beam & Kohane, 2018). Such methods can see patterns and connections in vast amounts of data in ways that are difficult for humans. These methods could make some of the personalized treatment above more common and assist doctors with diagnosis and management. It is becoming clearer how the digital revolution of the past 20 years will affect the ability of providers and patients to monitor health care problems remotely and have information relayed back and forth without the need for patients to visit doctors or go to a provider for testing and monitoring.

Some of these technologies could lower medical care costs and markedly expand the lifespan of individuals, and some will be quite expensive, especially when first introduced. What is new is that some interventions associated with applications of genome and stem-cell research and digital technologies will be prevention oriented. Lowering your risk of a heart attack or another life-threatening medical problem 20 years from now by undergoing some preventive intervention may become commonplace—but not necessarily affordable. Others could be very expensive but also not have a less dramatic influence on outcomes.

Such new medical interventions that could shape the future health system will be a challenge for the U.S. health care financing system. Will public and private payers be willing to fund these innovations? How much should we invest as a nation to fund the research to develop this new knowledge? What share of the research should be paid for by Americans and what share by residents of other countries? The changing world of medicine and science will raise many questions and challenges about the future—and our nation will need to address them all.

Income Disparities

It is an exciting prospect that new technologies and "know-how" will improve both medical care interventions and our ability to keep people healthy. A challenge will be whether disparities in income will make for difficult choices about adoptions of these technologies.

On the one hand, if we decide to make them available to every American, there will be further strains on government budgets (which would need to support these services for lower-income Americans). This will force choices about what other types of social investments would be foregone.

The other possibility is that we will let these technologies be used based on an individual's ability to pay for them. Since some are prevention oriented, unequal access to life-extending interventions may not be noticed for many years. It is unclear how the majority of Americans will react if life expectancies for the wealthy increase markedly while life expectancies for the bottom half or perhaps the bottom 65% of Americans remain unchanged. Life expectancies already are substantially higher for the wealthy than the poor. For example, in 2014, life expectancy was 87 years for men in the top income quartile compared to 77 years for men in the bottom income quartile, with similar differences found among women (Chetty et al., 2017). The reactions to the appropriateness of bigger spreads in life expectancy clearly will shape the future of the spread of the new approaches to promoting health and longevity being dreamed up these days.

The Potential of Creating a More Vibrant Culture of Health

More and more attention in the American health system is focused on the challenge of helping people live healthy lifestyles that will reduce their needs for medical care and improve the quality of life. This lifestyle change approach is the great new hope for reigning in our ever-increasing share of resources being devoted to medical care. The topic was covered in depth in Chapters 4 and 5.

One key shaper of this new focus on what sometimes is called "population health" has been a stream of research, starting with McGinnis and Foege (1993) in the United States and in the UK with work by Marmot and colleagues (1991), that shows how much social determinants of health, rather than medical care, influence life expectancy and the quality of life. As discussed frequently in the text, we now understand that well-being is not mainly due to medical care; it is due to how we lead our lives day to day.

In addition to research, the new focus on trying to keep people healthy has been influenced by the work of Donald Berwick (2008), initially while he headed the Institute for Health Improvement and then when he served as the head of the Centers for Medicare & Medicaid Services for the federal government between 2010 and 2011. Berwick developed the now well-known Triple Aim for the health system (discussed in Chapter 12) that explained in crisp terms the three goals we should have to improve the health of Americans:

- Improving the patient experience of care (including quality and satisfaction)
- Improving the health of populations (with a focus on prevention, lifestyle changes, and the social determinants of health)
- Reducing the per capita cost of health care (by focusing on delivering only care that has high value for the patient)

Health professionals have found these three aims compelling and logical, and the Triple Aim has motivated much more attention to both helping people lead healthy lives and considering how to eliminate health care that does not center on what patients want or need or that is not delivered in a high-quality, patient-centered manner.

Finally, philanthropies, especially the Robert Wood Johnson Foundation (RWJF), have become more and more focused on this population health challenge. RWJF has shaped its grant-making around the idea of creating a "culture of health" that will make healthy living the norm and the easy choice to make (Weil, 2016). A culture of health can happen by encouraging new norms that shape behavior and by using public policy to make it easier for people to make healthy choices: by building bike lanes, making healthy food more accessible, and taxing unhealthy things like cigarettes and sweetened beverages.

Most experts would say this culture of health goal is still more an aspiration than a reality. Many wealthy, younger Americans have embraced the idea, but it has not deeply penetrated less wealthy and less healthy parts of our population. However, we expect it will be a shaping force that could affect our health system in the years to come.

An Aging Population

The quiet but relentless demographic change affecting the health system is the aging of our population. In 1970, 10% of our population was over 65, but by 2030, more than 20% will be over 65 (U.S. Census Bureau, 2014). Our medical care system will become increasingly focused on the care of people over 75, who tend to have many chronic conditions and who frequently will require long-term care services, potentially expensive life-expanding services, and end-of-life services.

We do not really have a plan as a nation for how to meet the special needs of an aging population. There are not enough service providers trained in geriatrics or in how to deliver patient-centered care to people with complex medical conditions. While in past generations families have provided much of the supportive care for aging relatives, family structure changes, longer work hours for both sons and daughters, and residential mobility make family care giving more challenging.

Integration, Consolidation, and Other Changes in How Care Delivery Is Organized

Perhaps the biggest unknown in health care today is whether all of the current efforts to form integrated networks (see Chapter 11) will happen on a large scale and will improve health outcomes. Even in 2015, we noted this trend as important, and much consolidation has happened over the past 5 years. Federal grants to states during the Obama administration encouraged and supported integration in many states. Hospitals are merging into large, sometimes regional health systems involving not only hospitals but also long-term care facilities, physician practices, and diagnostic and outpatient surgery capacity. In some cases, health systems are even starting insurance companies to integrate the insurance/payment functions with delivery functions; value-based payment programs also are, in essence, encouraging hospitals to take responsibility for the total health of populations of people.

There is not strong evidence, however, that these integrated systems lead to better outcomes (Martin et al., 2016). There is a logic about integration as a strategy for improving efficiency of resource use and outcomes of care, but whether the wide array of provider types function well in this integrated environment and whether these systems are manageable remain open questions. Integrated networks have worked for systems such as the Kaiser-Permanente HMO, Intermountain Healthcare in Utah, the Geisinger Health System in Pennsylvania, Group Health of Puget Sound, and the Mayo Clinic in Minnesota. However, these systems have consistently been outliers in terms of their management and financing approaches. The challenge is whether the practices of these forward-thinking outliers can become the norm for the health industry.

The other question mark regarding the move toward integration is whether consolidation will weaken competition across providers, leading to price increases even if these networks are more efficient and effective. Economists generally postulate that, in most markets, market power drives prices more than efficiency (Glied & Altman, 2017; Scheffler, Shortell, & Wilensky, 2012). It will be a difficult balancing act for federal and state regulators to encourage the efficiency potentially associated with consolidation and to ameliorate the antitrust, anticompetitive side effects of consolidation.

Other organizational changes also will affect the delivery of health care across the country. Centers of excellence that develop great reputations for value and outcomes for specific types of surgeries and procedures may begin to draw patients from wider geographical areas. Insurers could contract with these centers of excellence and convince patients to travel longer distances to use them when they have a major health problem.

Disruptive Innovation

The final force shaping change in the health system is disruptive innovation from new health care players. We saw an initial example of this type of innovation in the rapid spread of the idea of urgent care centers. These centers were first built by entrepreneurs who saw opportunities to gain "market share" from emergency rooms and private physician practices.

Many other new ideas are being pursued by entrepreneurs working to make health care more accessible for patients and making the patient experience more attractive. New approaches to meeting the medical needs of patients include creating access to providers by e-mail or by telehealth tools, encouraging the use of apps that help people manage their chronic conditions, opening insurance companies that devote more resources than typical to prevention-oriented services, and starting new pharmaceutical companies that bring expensive drugs to market that address the needs of very small subsets of the population.

The number and scope of disruptive innovators are likely to expand quickly in the coming years. Consumers are very interested in care delivery approaches that offer easier access and more amenities: that is, more patient-focused services.

KEY CHALLENGES THAT WILL RECEIVE ATTENTION IN UPCOMING YEARS

Improving the Financing and Insurance Systems in Light of Ideological Differences

The approach to financing health care in America and the functioning of the insurance system clearly have evolved steadily over the past 5 to 10 years. However, these systems are still not working to ensure access to care for all Americans, and they are not yet encouraging efficient, value-oriented health care delivery in most communities. The insurance system, in particular, is in a precarious condition. More and more Americans work in settings where employers do not provide insurance coverage, and the price of insurance when purchased in the individual insurance market or through the Obamacare exchanges is often unaffordable for many working Americans.

Resolving the problems in the financing and insurance systems, however, is made quite complex given the stark differences in ideology among America about how the challenges should be addressed. Clearly, health care is a service where insurance is required because of the high costs of care and the variation in each person's risk of needing expensive services at any point in time. But, in order to design insurance systems that work, it is crucial that more consensus evolve about the roles government should play and about how much we should share the burden of health care needs across our population.

About half the American population currently believes that government needs to play crucial roles and that resources need to be redistributed from wealthy Americans to those who work but earn below median incomes. The other half of the population believes that anything the government does will be done poorly. In addition, a large share of Americans believe in the idea of rugged individualism where by each person needs to take care of him- or herself without redistribution of resources.

Even in the case of private insurance markets, many Americans do not think that healthier parts of the population (e.g., young people or people who do not have chronic health conditions) should pay more for insurance than might be necessary to protect their specific risk of needing care in order to subsidize the costs of insurance for parts of the population that have more expensive expected health care needs. Oher Americans feel that this is what insurance is about: spreading resources from the healthy to the less healthy with the presumption that, over the course of a lifetime, most individuals will have periods where they do face either chronic health conditions or relatively random acute conditions like cancer.

It will be a real challenge to design insurance systems that work efficiently without resolving these ideological differences. And it will be difficult to have stable markets for insurance if power shifts continually from faction to faction of the population.

Helping People Lead Healthy Lives

We clearly are attempting as a nation to increase attention on keeping people healthy, rather than thinking of the health system as totally focused on medical care that helps people when they get sick. We will increasingly try to move "upstream" in attempts to improve the health of Americans and avoid high costs of medical care.

However, we have a lot to learn about accomplishing this ambitious goal. It is easy to identify the problems but difficult to solve them. Poor access to affordable, healthy food and poor choices about what to eat are clear challenges, and we do not yet have evidence-based policies or interventions that result in people making better and consistent choices to eat healthy food. This is also true about behaviors such as keeping physically active or drinking, smoking, or using opioid drugs inappropriately.

Another challenge in creating a culture of health and making people healthier day by day is finding funds to pay for interventions that would transform population health. In theory, we would like to see some of our huge investments in medical care move to become investments in healthy living, but finding means to redirect this money from the health system has been difficult. Many of the investments needed to improve population health involve investments in social services that address people's social determinants of health. But there is no consensus about the logic of funding such social services because strong evidence about the effectiveness of specific types of social services often is lacking or not believed.

But energy is being directed at this challenge by the public sector, the health care sector, and private companies. Many communities are establishing the goal of creating a healthy community as a central commitment. Changing individuals' behaviors to encourage healthy choices, finding social and community interventions that work, and advancing the idea of a culture of health will take time and will be a challenge. It is difficult to predict when we will reach what Malcolm Gladwell (2002) has termed "the tipping point."

Addressing the Fundamental Cost Problem Related to Medical Care

A simple truth is that health care is just too expensive for the average American. As an example, consider the expenditures on health care for a typical 55-year-old covered by employer health insurance. The insurance for this person averaged $9,700 per year in 2015, and this person paid another $1,270 per year in out-of-pocket medical expenses (Health Care Cost Institute, 2016). For a married couple, this would add up to just under $22,000 per year. This is a lot of resources devoted to health care, especially since 50% of workers who are 55 earn less than $50,000 per year and 30% earn less than $30,000. The allocation of approximately $22,000 to health care for a married couple in this age group seems like a very large share of the total resources they have to pay for all of their needs. And, the burden of health care is even larger when a married couple is either not covered by employer insurance or when one of the two people has a job or a job that pays less than an average amount.

This large allocation of resources to health care might be worth the costs, but it is disturbing that a good share of the expenditures are due to potentially avoidable factors: (a) delivery of low value services that do not create much improved health, (b) high prices likely caused by using a market approach to setting prices in markets that do not work well, and (c) unhealthy lifestyles that many people lead as discussed earlier.

An ongoing challenge for the health system and a topic that will be front and center for health policy is attacking all three types of drivers of high expenditures for health care. It seems clear that federal and state governments either need to make markets work better or need to regulate more directly what services get delivered and what prices are paid for these services. And we need to accomplish the goal of creating a culture of health that leads to improved population health.

Markets could work better if we made sure that there is adequate competition among providers in every community and that these providers are competing by having to deliver valued services and by having to keep prices as low as possible. Markets also would work better if governments could negotiate the prices they paid for services. This type of negotiation works within many states that run Medicaid program but does not function at the federal level in establishing prices for devices, supplies, and pharmaceuticals for the Medicare program.

If lower prices and the elimination of low-value services is not possible, another alternative would be to at least ensure that every American has access to an affordable approach to medical care delivery. Other markets have created products that do not have every bell and whistle but that do represent viable low-cost options. One example is the automobile industry, where a person can spend $100,000 on a fancy car but also can purchase a car for $15,000 that does an effective job of getting the person safely from place to place. A challenge for the medical care system is to determine what an affordable choice for health care that leads to effective and safe care would look like. Disruptive entrepreneurs, such as Amazon, along with existing provider systems, such as Kaiser Permanente, are working on this type of option. The coming years will reveal whether such efforts are successful.

Improving Quality, Outcomes, and the Patient Experience When Receiving Care

The final challenge we predict will be addressed by the health system in the coming years is a push to improve quality, outcomes, and the patient care experience. Chapter 12 laid out the challenges facing quality improvement in our country. We expect big progress in this area driven by using electronic health records to drive quality (see Chapter 14) and by using big data to develop more evidence-based approaches to delivering care and managing the delivery of care. This improved quality of care should lead to better outcomes and perhaps lower need for extra care related to poor quality.

The lack of focus on improving the patient experience as medical care is being delivered as a shortcoming of our health system that has come into focus in recent years (Trzeciak & Mazzarelli, 2016). Too many patients are not given the chance for shared decision making regarding important choices about alternative treatment approaches. Too many patients do not even know what providers will charge for a given service. And often health care providers do not respect the time of patients or make services available when it is easy for patients to receive care.

Why is focused attention on consumer preferences not normal practice in health care as it is in almost every other service sector of our economy? Perhaps it is because providers too often see insurers as their customers, rather than patients. After all, it seems to a provider that the insurer is often paying the bill, rather than the patient.

Whatever the cause of less-than-ideal delivery practices and poor transparency that have been common in health care delivery, we think the demands for more patient-centered care will increase over the coming years. Again, disruptive innovators have noted this shortcoming in the health system and are designing ways to improve the patient experience in numerous ways. It is likely that the disruptors will force traditional providers to change their attentiveness to what patients expect when they need medical care services.

FUTURE PROSPECTS FOR DIFFERENT STAKEHOLDERS IN THE HEALTH ENTERPRISE

When looking toward the future, it is always useful to consider how different **stakeholders** could be affected. One constant in social interactions is that when a stakeholder is affected by a changing environment, the stakeholder reacts and tries to improve its position. How will key stakeholders be affected by the changes we predict, and how will they react? We consider the five key stakeholder groups identified in Chapter 1.

> One constant in social interactions is that when a stakeholder is affected by a changing environment, the stakeholder reacts and tries to improve its position.

Providers: Hospitals, Physicians, Nurses, and Other Caregivers

Each type of provider is affected by the technology of delivering service, the organizational environment affecting everyday work life, and financial arrangements. In many ways, the core practice of medicine will remain the same while continuing to evolve with emerging technology and know-how. However, organizational change likely will alter the day-to-day experience of some health care professionals. The new world of health care finance could either decrease incomes (as has happened for many types of physicians in recent years) or slow income growth.

How will physicians, hospitals, and other providers react? First, they will be politically active, looking to protect their personal interests affected by public policy. Second, they will seek more market power and more organizational power to control what happens to them. Finally, they will adapt and learn how to thrive in a changing health care world. This is what has happened in the past and what happens in most industries that undergo substantial change.

Employers

To date, employers have played a relatively passive role, accepting increases in the cost of the insurance they pay and working in small ways to shape insurance offerings that offer incentives to stay healthy and not to overuse health care. If employers continue to offer employees insurance coverage, they will continue to seek approaches that limit their medical care liabilities, and they will continue to encourage wellness activities that help to lower health costs and increase work-force productivity. They also will continue to add higher deductibles and copays to pass part of cost increases along to employees.

However, employers also could begin to exert active roles in health care, as described earlier. They will seek ways to limit increases in the health-related costs they have to pay. As the future evolves, this stakeholder will probably do well.

Insurers

The insurance system could face substantial changes as large health systems find it attractive to start their own insurance companies. However, the large insurance companies in the United States are increasingly diversified corporations that provide a wide range of services and expertise beyond managing risk and making payments. Most companies have sophisticated analytics capability, the ability to manage and use the very large data sets that are becoming important for managing health care systems, and the ability to use information technologies to manage the flow of dollars among players in the health system. Even if health systems start insurance companies, the major insurance corporations likely will provide services related to these insurance operations at health systems.

Public Policy Makers

Federal policy makers will be preoccupied with the difficult choices that must be made about the growing costs of the Medicare and Medicaid programs. In the case of Medicare, even if the growth of costs per enrollee slows (as occurred in 2013 and 2014), the aging of our population will increase total expenditures. The political dynamics in Washington also suggest that the grand debate about how much responsibility government should have to ensure access to health care for the poor and elderly will endure for the near future. There are sharp divisions between conservatives, who feel government should have as small a role as possible, and liberals, who think government should ensure access to health care services and is the logical entity to organize and fund insurance coverage for elders and the poor.

At the state level, we can continue to expect great differences in approaches to Medicaid services across states. Some states will try to limit the size of Medicaid programs as much as possible, whereas others will use Medicaid to expand services to state residents. Of course, all states will be interested in new organizational and reimbursement approaches that lower the per beneficiary costs of Medicaid. Trying to make this happen will be a major activity at the state government level.

Consumers

Finally, we get to what the possible changes will mean to users of the health system. In the current system, it is amazing that providers and payers and policy makers sometimes seem to view consumers as bystanders. Placing consumers at the center of every health care transaction and decision should be the goal of how the sector operates. It is possible that consumer advocacy groups could become more prominent in debates about how medical care is structured. It is also possible that consumer voices will more actively shape public policy if health issues become central concerns in political elections. Clearly, how consumers continue to react to experiences with the Patient Protection and Affordable Care Act (ACA) will have large ramifications for the initiative's future status.

Consumers will face many important personal decisions related to how they interact with the health system. They will need to decide whether they are willing to pay more money themselves for access to a wide panel of providers or whether they are willing to use a narrow network in order to lower their out-of-pocket spending. They will need to decide how much risk they want to take in the form of large deductibles and copays that will lower insurance premiums but increase their financial liability when illnesses occur. In addition, as described earlier, there likely will be many more medical interventions that become possible that are not covered by insurance. Consumers will need to determine how much of their wealth they will invest in interventions that could increase their chances of leading longer and healthier lives.

CONCLUSION

We began this text with a list of key stakeholders who shape the U.S. health care system: consumers; providers of care; insurance, pharmaceutical, and medical device companies; payers; and public policy makers. We ended with an assessment of likely effects of changes in our health system on each of these stakeholders.

These stakeholders all play a part in what will happen and in how it will happen. One of the most important requirements for an improved health system, however, is a cadre of motivated, well-trained, thoughtful leaders working throughout the health system. The earlier chapter on governance and management (Chapter 14) explains how good leadership is developed and emphasizes two important traits of effective leaders: (a) they are transparent, and (b) they hold themselves accountable. Leaders with these attributes are needed at the policy level and at the private-sector, corporate level. They are needed to organize the voices of consumers. Perhaps most important, leaders are needed throughout our health care service delivery system and our public health system.

Improvements come from the hard work and coordination of many individuals with knowledge and motivation. The readers of this book who are preparing for careers in the world of health care should be prepared for an exciting era of innovation and change in our health system. You should lead as health professionals, as consumers and patients, as citizens, and as payers of health care. The system will not improve without such leadership and the energy that comes from it.

▶ CASE EXERCISE—PAYMENTS AND BUDGET CAPS IN MEDICARE

Discuss what would have to take place in the United States for passage of either a single-payer system or budget caps in total payments to providers under the Medicare program. Address questions such as the following:

1. How will political ideology affect such a consideration?
2. How will out-of-pocket costs affect such a possible change?
3. What would be the transition challenges of making such a change?

DISCUSSION QUESTIONS

1. Why is it difficult to forecast the future of health care delivery in the United States?
2. Analyze a forecast about health care delivery. Do you agree or disagree with the forecast and why?
3. What forces do you think will drive the health care delivery system over the next 4 years?
4. What do you think are the most important ways the ACA will be changed in 2020?

REFERENCES

Bates, D. W., Saria, S., Ohno-Machado, L., Shah, A., & Escobar, G. (2014). Big data in health care: Using analytics to identify and manage high-risk and high-cost patients. *Health Affairs, 33*(7), 1123–1131. doi:10.1377/hlthaff.2014.0041

Beam, A. L., & Kohane, I. S. (2018). Big data and machine learning in health care. *Journal of the American Medical Association, 319*(13), 1317–1318. doi:10.1001/jama.2017.18391

Berwick, D., Nolan, T., Whittington, J. (2008). The triple aim: care, health, and cost. *Health Affairs, 27*(3). https://doi.org/10.1377/hlthaff.27.3.759.

Chetty, R., Stepner, M., Abraham, S., Lin, S., Scuderi, B., Turner, N., … Cutler, D. (2016). The association between income and life expectancy in the United States, 2001–2014. *Journal of the American Medical Association, 315*(16), 1750–1766. doi:10.1001/jama.2016.4226

Garakani, R., & Saidi, R. F. (2017). Recent progress in cell therapy in solid organ transplantation. *International Journal of Organ Transplantation Medicine, 8*(3), 125–131. PMCID: PMC5592099

Ginsburg, G. S., & Phillips, K. A. (2018). Precision medicine: From science to value. *Health Affairs, 37*(5), 694–701. doi:10.1377/hlthaff.2017.1624

Gladwell, M. (2002). *The tipping point: How little things can make a big difference*. Boston, MA: Back Bay Books.

Glied, S. A., & Altman, S. H. (2017). Beyond antitrust: Health care and health insurance market trends and the future of competition. *Health Affairs, 36*(9), 1572–1577. doi:10.1377/hlthaff.2017.0555

Health Care Cost Institute. (2016). *2015 Health care cost and utilization report*. Washington, DC: Health Care Cost Institute. Retrieved from http://www.healthcostinstitute.org

Knickman, J., and Kovner, A. (2015). *Jonas and Kovner's Health Care Delivery in the United States*, 11th ed. New York, NY: Springer Publishing Company, LLC.

Marmot, M. G., Stansfeld, S., Patel, C., North, F., Head, J., White, I., … Smith, G. D. (1991). Health inequalities among British civil servants: The Whitehall II study. *The Lancet, 337*(8754), 1387–1393. doi:10.1016/0140–6736(91)93068-K

Martin, L. T., Plough, A., Carman, K. G., Leviton, L., Bogdan, O., & Miller, C. E. (2016). Strengthening integration of health services and systems. *Health Affairs, 35*(11), 1976–1981. doi:10.1377/hlthaff.2016.0605

McGinnis, J. M., & Foege, W. H. (1993). Actual causes of death in the United States. *Journal of the American Medical Association, 270*(18), 2207–2212. doi:10.1001/jama.1993.03510180077038

Scheffler, R. M., Shortell, S. M., & Wilensky, G. R. (2012). Accountable care organizations and antitrust: Restructuring the health care market. *Journal of the American Medical Association, 307*(14), 1493–1494. doi:10.1001/jama.2012.451

Trzeciak, S., & Mazzarelli, A. J. (2016). Patient experience and health care quality. *Journal of the American Medical Association, 176*(10), 1575. doi:10.1001/jamainternmed.2016.5435

U.S. Census Bureau. (2014). *65+ in the United States: 2010*. pp. 23–212. Washington, DC: U.S. Government Printing Office.

Weil, A. R. (2016). Building a culture of health. *Health Affairs, 35*(11), 1953–1958. doi:10.1377/hlthaff.2016.0913

APPENDIX

U.S. GOVERNMENT PUBLIC HEALTH AGENCIES

The U.S. Department of Health and Human Services (DHHS) and the U.S. Department of Veterans Affairs (VA) are the pivotal instruments of public health in the United States. DHHS was first established in 1953 and is a Cabinet-level department. Its mission is to "enhance the health and well-being of all Americans, by providing for effective health and human services and by fostering sound, sustained advances in the sciences underlying medicine, public health, and social services." Its budget accounts for the majority of the federal budget and covers approximately a quarter of all federal spending. It also administers more grant funds than all other federal agencies combined. The U.S. Department of Veterans Affairs operates the largest integrated health care system in the United States, providing services to service members and veterans (see the last section in this appendix, the U.S. Department of Veterans Affairs). In 2016, it was the fifth highest-spending department in the federal government. Together, these two departments direct the majority of health prevention, treatment, innovation, and leadership in the United States.

DHHS Offices and Agencies
Agency for Healthcare Research and Quality

The Agency for Healthcare Research and Quality (AHRQ) promotes safety and quality in the national health care system. The Institute of Medicine report, "To Err Is Human," was the impetus for its establishment. Since the publication of that report in 1999, AHRQ's research has led to improved patient safety, error prevention, and a reduction in wasteful spending. Its mission is to "produce evidence to make health care safer, higher quality, more accessible, equitable, and affordable [...] and to make sure that the evidence is understood and used." To do so, the agency invests in research, creates materials and tools to put the results of that research into practice, and provides measures and data used by providers and policymakers. Some of its immediate concerns include antibiotic overuse and health care-associated infections, improved patient care for those with multiple chronic conditions, disseminating current research within electronic health records, and improving opioid addiction treatment services in rural communities. Website: https://www.ahrq.gov

Agency for Toxic Substances and Disease Registry

The Agency for Toxic Substances and Disease Registry (ATSDR) includes two divisions: the Division of Community Health Investigations and the Division of

Toxicology and Human Health Sciences. It uses an evidence-based approach to protect communities from environmental health threats in soil, water, and air due to natural disasters, chemical spills, and other emergencies. The agency was created by The Comprehensive Environmental Response, Compensation and Liability Act of 1980, and its mission is to "investigate environmental exposures to hazardous substances in communities and take action to reduce harmful exposures and their health consequences." It both works to prevent human exposure and to address exposure to harmful contaminants after the fact. Its priorities cover public health impact from exposures to harmful chemicals, protecting vulnerable populations from exposure, and advancing environmental science and medicine. The agency protects communities by assessing exposure within communities, offering the expertise needed to create action plans, and addressing community and health care provider questions. Website: https://www.atsdr.cdc.gov/

Centers for Disease Control and Prevention (CDC)

The goal of the Centers for Disease Control and Prevention (CDC) is to protect the health security of the United States. Its mission is to serve "as the national focus for developing and applying disease prevention and control, environmental health, and health promotion and health education activities designed to improve the health of the people of the United States." The CDC both conducts the science of epidemiology and disseminates public health education. The majority of its domestic funding is distributed directly to state and local entities. The CDC addresses three strategic priorities: (a) improve health security at home and around the world; (b) better prevent the leading causes of illness, injury, disability, and death; and (c) strengthen public health and health care collaboration. Website: https://www.cdc.gov/

Centers for Medicare & Medicaid Services

The original Medicare and Medicaid entities were established under President Lyndon B. Johnson in 1965. The Centers for Medicare & Medicaid Services (CMS) combined to form a single entity in 1977. It operates as a patient-first organization and includes Medicaid, Medicare, the Children's Health Insurance Program (CHIP), and the Health Insurance Exchanges. It comprises four consortia: (a) Consortium for Medicare Health Plans Operations; (b) Consortium for Financial Management and Fee for Service Operations; (c) Consortium for Medicaid and Children's Health Operations; and (d) the Consortium for Quality Improvement and Survey & Certification Operations. Eligibility for Medicare has increased to include the disabled, people with end-stage renal disease requiring dialysis or kidney transplant, and people 65 years or older that choose Medicare coverage. Medicaid covers low-income families, pregnant women, people of all ages with disabilities, and people who need long-term care. Medicaid programs are highly diverse and are dependent on state direction. Website: https://www.cms.gov/

Health Resources & Services Administration

The Health Resources & Services Administration (HRSA) comprises five bureaus and eleven offices. It addresses health equity for those who are geographically isolated or those who are economically or medically vulnerable. The HRSA's strategic plan includes five goals: (a) improve access to quality health care and services; (b) strengthen the health workforce; (c) build healthy communities; (d) improve health equity; and (e) strengthen HRSA program management and operations. The majority of its budget is distributed to community-based organizations; colleges and universities; hospitals; state, local, and tribal governments; and private entities. Its focus is on people living with HIV/AIDS, pregnant women, mothers and their families, and those unable to overcome barriers to high quality health care. Website: https://www.hrsa.gov/

Indian Health Service

The Indian Health Service (IHS) is a health care delivery system for federally recognized American Indian and Alaska Natives in the United States, ensuring comprehensive and culturally competent health care. The government-to-government relationship between the federal government and Indian Tribes was established in 1787 and is based on Article I, Section 8, of the Constitution. This relationship covers more than 550 federally recognized tribes in 35 states. The IHS was created in response to this relationship. Its mission is to "raise the physical, mental, social, and spiritual health of American Indians and Alaska Natives to the highest level." Website: https://www.ihs.gov/

National Institutes of Health

The National Institutes of Health (NIH) is a national medical research agency and is the largest public funder of biomedical research in the world. Some research is conducted directly within the NIH campus, but the majority of funded research is dispersed both domestically and internationally. The NIH comprises 27 different institutes and centers, each with its own unique agenda. NIH leadership oversees research planning, activities, and overall outlook for the agency. The mission of the NIH is to "seek fundamental knowledge about the nature and behavior of living systems and the application of that knowledge to enhance health, lengthen life, and reduce illness and disability." The NIH has had a direct and tangible impact on the national public health; under the leadership of the NIH, life expectancy in the United States has increased substantially, disability among people older than age 65 has decreased, and new diagnoses and deaths from all cancers combined have decreased. Website: https://www.nih.gov/

Office of the Assistant Secretary for Health

The Office of the Assistant Secretary for Health (ASH) operates under the leadership of the Assistant Secretary of Health, who advises the Secretary of the U.S.

Department for Health and Human Services on matters of public health and science. ASH manages twelve core public offices, including the Office of the Surgeon General and the U.S. Public Health Service Commissioned Corps. It also oversees ten regional health offices and ten presidential and secretarial advisory committees. The Assistant Secretary for Health develops policy recommendations for public health issues that encompass DHHS agencies. The DHHS Initiative on Multiple Chronic Conditions is a current key initiative. Website: https://www.hhs.gov/ash/index.html

Office of the Assistant Secretary for Preparedness and Response

The Office of the Assistant Secretary for Preparedness and Response (ASPR) leads national security initiatives to protect against and recover effectively from disasters and public health emergencies, including bioterrorism. In partnership with health care professionals, biotech firms, government offices, and the community, ASPR oversees readiness and response capabilities. Its mission is to "save lives and protect Americans from 21st century health security threats." The ASPR follows four priorities to achieve its mission: (a) provide strong leadership; (b) build a regional disaster health response system; (c) sustain robust and reliable public health security capabilities; and (d) advance an innovative medical countermeasure enterprise. Website: https://www.phe.gov/about/aspr/pages/default.aspx

Office of the Secretary

The U.S. Department of Health and Human Services (DHHS) is responsible for protecting the national health and providing essential human services. The Secretary is a member of the President's Cabinet, and the Office of the Secretary oversees more than 300 programs and 14 offices, including the Office of the Assistant Secretary for Health and the Office of the Assistant Secretary for Preparedness and Response. The current Office of the Secretary has four priorities: (a) the opioid crisis; (b) health insurance reform; (c) drug pricing; and (d) value-based care. Website: https://www.hhs.gov/about/leadership/secretary/index.html

Program Support Center

The Program Support Center (PSC) provides fee-for-service encompassing financial management and procurement; occupational health; and real estate, logistics, and operations support. It provides more than forty different services. The mission of the PSC is to "provide valuable, cost effective, and innovative mission support solutions to foster government efficiency." The center was created to reduce the DHHS' annual spending and to increase the quality of its administrative services. PSC also offers two products: Go!card®, which delivers transit subsidy fringe benefits to federal employees, and GovSpace, a scheduling system for conference rooms, offices, and other federal spaces. Website: https://www.psc.gov/

Substance Abuse and Mental Health Services Administration

In 1992, Congress created the Substance Abuse and Mental Health Services Administration (SAMHSA), which coordinates public health efforts to address behavioral health in the United States. Its mission is to "reduce the impact of substance abuse and mental illness on America's communities." SAMHSA operates using advisory councils or committees to obtain advice from mental health and substance use professionals. Those with mental health and/or substance use disorders comprise an especially vulnerable population in the United States, and SAMHSA works to make care more accessible while simultaneously minimizing costs to both individuals and government. It is on the frontlines of the opioid crisis, which was established as a public health emergency in 2017. SAMHSA also manages multiple 24/7 confidential helplines, including: *National Helpline* (also called the Treatment Referral Routing Service), which provides treatment referral for mental health and substance use disorders; *National Suicide Prevention Lifeline*, which provides prevention and crisis support to people in distress; and *Disaster Distress Helpline*, which provides crisis counseling for those experiencing disasters. Website: https://www.samhsa.gov/

U.S. Food and Drug Administration

The U.S. Food and Drug Administration (FDA) dates back to the establishment of the Agricultural Division in the Patent Office in 1848. The department was officially created by the 1906 Pure Food and Drugs Act. The FDA's mission is to protect public health by regulating foods, drugs, biologics, medical devices, electronic products that emit radiation, cosmetics, veterinary products, tobacco products, and many other products. Meat, poultry, and some egg products are not covered under the umbrella of "food" and are addressed separately by the U.S. Department of Agriculture. The organization's programs include program alignment, innovation, globalization, the Food Safety Modernization Act (FSMA), regulatory science, tobacco, transparency, medical countermeasures, sentinel initiative, and drug shortages. Its diverse goals also address counterterrorism by securing the national food supply and encouraging the development of new medical products. Website: https://www.fda.gov/

U.S. Department of Veterans Affairs

The mission of the U.S. Department of Veterans Affairs (VA) is "serving and honoring the men and women who are America's veterans." President Ronald Reagan established the VA as a Cabinet-level executive department in 1988. The department comprises three administrations: (a) the Veterans Benefits Administration (VBA); (b) the Veterans Health Administration (VHA); and (c) the National Cemetery Administration (NCA). The VA operates the largest integrated health care system in the United States and manages financial assistance, burial and memorial benefits, and other forms of support for eligible service members, veterans, and family members. There are twenty-two staff offices, including the

Board of Veterans' Appeals, the Office of Survivors Assistance, and the Office of the General Counsel. The VA also operates the 24/7 Veterans Crisis Line, which is a confidential crisis line available to all veterans, all service members, the United Stated National Guard and United States Army Reserve, and their family members and friends. Website: https://www.va.gov/

GLOSSARY

academic health center: An allopathic or osteopathic medical school, one or more health professions schools (e.g., allied health, dentistry, nursing, pharmacy, public health, veterinary medicine), and one or more owned or affiliated teaching hospitals or health systems.

academic medical centers: Hospitals and other types of providers that are affiliated with a medical school and play active roles in training new health care providers, especially physicians, and in clinical research in collaboration with a medical school.

access (to health care): An individual's ability to obtain medical services on a timely and financially acceptable basis. Factors determining ease of access also include availability of health care facilities, transportation to them, and reasonable hours of operation.

accountable care organizations (ACOs): An entity—usually a hospital or a physician group—that accepts responsibility for the medical care of a population of people. An insurer or government payer develops some form of financial incentives to motivate the ACO to ensure that health care cost patterns for the covered group are better than the patterns for comparable people not in the group. First initiated by the Medicare program, various versions of the ACO idea are being tried by a range of payers.

accountability: Being responsible for making informed and wise decisions that affect health outcomes and processes of care at a given level of quality and a given level of cost.

accreditation: A decision made by a recognized organization that an institution substantially meets appropriate standards.

activities of daily living (ADLs): Tasks required for a person's normal functioning. These include activities such as eating, bathing, and toileting.

acute care: Medical care of a limited duration, provided in a hospital or outpatient setting, to treat an injury or short-term illness.

administrative efficiency: Measuring whether the enormous bureaucracy required to operate health systems work smoothly and swiftly.

advanced practice nurse: Registered nurse, such as a clinical nurse specialist, nurse practitioner, nurse anesthetist, or nurse midwife, with a master's or doctoral degree concentrating on a specific area of practice.

adverse selection: A process that results in people who have more serious illnesses and health challenges ending up in one group while healthier people end up in another group. Often used to describe what can happen when the purchase of health insurance is voluntary rather than mandated.

advocacy: Actions taken by an individual or group aiming to influence public policy, resource allocation, and other decisions. Activities may include media campaigns, public speaking, funding and publishing research, conducting polls, and lobbying.

alliance: Organizational relationship for specific purposes.

ambulatory care: Health care services that patients receive when they are not an inpatient or home in bed.

ambulatory care sensitive conditions: Conditions for which patients are hospitalized that could have been handled on an outpatient basis.

appropriate care: Care for which expected health benefits exceed negative consequences.

assisted living: A living arrangement that is designed to help people who have problems performing activities of daily living. Generally, a place to live that has a lower level of services than a nursing home but more services than an independent living residence.

Association of State and Territorial Health Officials (ASTHO): An organization representing public health agencies and public health proffessionals in the United States.

attending physicians: Doctors who have "privileges" to use a particular hospital for inpatient care of their patients.

average daily census: The number of people who stay overnight in a hospital bed on a typical day at a specific hospital.

average length of stay (ALOS): The average number of days a patient admitted to a hospital stays there as a patient.

avoidable mortality: A count of unnecessary deaths from diseases for which effective public health and medical interventions are available.

Bayes theorem: A formula for determining conditional probability (the likelihood of an event occurring given that another event has occurred) that allows for revising existing predictions or theories given new evidence.

behavioral health services: Clinical and supportive activities intended to treat or manage mental illness and/or alcohol or substance abuse (chemical dependency).

behavioral risk factor: An element of personal behavior—such as unbalanced nutrition, use of tobacco products, leading a sedentary lifestyle, or the abuse of alcohol— that leads to an increased risk of developing one or more diseases or negative health conditions.

benchmark: The best-known value for a specific measure, from any source. **beneficiary:** Any person, either a subscriber or a dependent, eligible for service under a health plan contract.

benefits: Specific areas of plan coverage, such as outpatient visits, hospitalizations, or prescription drugs, that make up the range of medical services marketed under a health plan.

biotechnology: The use of living organisms and biological systems to develop medical products and medical treatments. Biotechnology also is used in fields such as agriculture, new fuel products, and plastics.

bundled payment: A payment arrangement whereby a provider is paid a fixed amount of money to address a specific medical problem, often for a specific period of time. For example, a surgeon could receive a bundled payment that covers his or her services, the cost of any medical assistants used, the cost of any devices required for the surgery, and perhaps the cost of the surgical suite itself.

capitation (capitated payments): A payment method in which a physician or hospital is paid a fixed amount per patient per year, regardless of the volume or cost of services each patient requires.

carrier: An insurer; an underwriter of risk that is engaged in providing, paying for, or reimbursing all or part of the cost of health services under group insurance policies or contracts, medical or hospital services agreements, membership or subscription contracts, or similar arrangements in exchange for premiums or other periodic charges.

case management: A broadly used term that could describe a range of services directed at coordinating the care a person receives, making sure the person gets the care needed, or making sure the person follows medical advice. Case management is performed by different types of caregiver, ranging from physicians and nurses to community health workers, who often focus on helping a patient get social services he or she needs in addition to medical services.

case manager: An individual who coordinates and oversees other health care workers in finding the most effective methods of caring for specific patients and arranges for necessary services.

cash (monetary) assistance programs: Previously referred to as welfare, provide financial support to qualifying low-income individuals or families. These programs include Temporary Assistance for Needy Families (TANF), Supplemental Security Income (SSI), and Unemployment Insurance (UI).

catastrophic coverage: A type of insurance that pays only for high-cost health care, usually associated with injuries and chronic conditions, such as cancer and AIDS.

census: In the United States, refers to the count of members of the national population and their demographic characteristics undertaken by the U.S. Census Bureau every 10 years; in the health care delivery system specifically, refers to the number of patients in a hospital or other health care institution at any one time.

centers of care: Facilities that provide outpatient rehabilitative services for patients with a particular, specific illness, such as multiple sclerosis, Parkinson's disease, or stroke.

Centers for Medicare & Medicaid Services (CMS): Administers Medicare, Medicaid, and the Children's Health Insurance Program (CHIP). Formerly called the Health Care Financing Administration (HCFA).

certificates of need: Approval for major new services and construction or renovation of hospitals or related facilities, as issued by states.

certification: Issued from the federal government for a hospital to receive reimbursement for services proved to Medicare and Medicaid patients.

charity care: Care given to needy patients without expectation of payment. Sometimes subsidized by the federal or state governments.

chronic care: Treatment or rehabilitative health services provided to individuals on a long-term basis (more than 30 days), in both inpatient and ambulatory settings.

chronic care model: Organizing care to be proactive and focused on keeping people as healthy as possible, instead of performing reactively when people are injured or sick. A critical aspect is the focus on patient self-management.

chronic illness: Ongoing medical conditions that can be treated but not cured.

clinical decision support: Utilizes clinical guidelines, patient-specific data, and algorithm-guided reasoning to generate alerts and offer information to providers as part of the regular workflow.

clinical nurse practitioner: Nurse with extra training who accepts additional clinical responsibility for medical diagnosis or treatment.

clinical trials: The testing on patients in a clinical setting of a diagnostic, preventive, or therapeutic intervention, using a study design that will provide for a valid estimation of safety and efficiency.

closed panel: A managed care plan that contracts with physicians on an exclusive basis for services and does not allow those physicians to see patients who are members of another managed care organization.

coinsurance: An insurance provision that limits the amount of plan coverage to a certain percentage, commonly 80%. Any additional costs are paid out-of-pocket by members.

community benefits: Programs and services offered by medical care providers and other health care organizations to improve health in communities and increase access to health care. Hospitals are required to spend money on community benefits based on their tax status and, often, on the public funds they received to build the hospital.

community health improvement: Focuses on collaboration among a wide array of organizations (e.g., public health departments, health care delivery organizations, social service agencies, government entities, etc.) to address issues impacting the health of a particular community.

community hospital: A hospital offering short-term general and other special services, owned by a corporation or agency other than the federal government. A term often used to distinguish a hospital from those that emphasize teaching and research in addition to service delivery.

community rating: The rating system by which a plan or an indemnity carrier uses the total experience of the subscribers or members within a given geographic area, or "community," to determine a reimbursement rate that is common for all groups, regardless of the individual claims experience of any one group.

comorbidity: One or more disorders or diseases occurring simultaneously or sequentially with a primary disorder or disease.

comparative effectiveness research: Studies that compare two or more health care technologies, products, or services against each other or against the conventional standard of care. Interventions are also compared for their costs relative to their benefits.

competency: The combination of knowledge, skills, personal characteristics, and individual and social behavior needed to perform a job effectively.

complementary and alternative medicine: Diagnostic and treatment interventions that fall outside the realm of state-licensed medical practice as it is defined by the privilege to use certain restricted diagnostic regimens, prescribe drugs, and practice surgery. Such disciplines include chiropractic, acupuncture, homeopathy, herbal medicine, naturopathy, and therapeutic touch.

comprehensive coverage: A health insurance system that pays for a broad range of services.

computerized physician order entry (CPOE): A process of electronically entering medical practitioner instructions for the treatment of hospitalized patients under a physician's care.

computerized provider order entry (CPOE): Used to submit orders for medications, lab tests, and imaging, and to share instructions for patient care with other parts of the system.

Consolidated Omnibus Budget Reconciliation Act of 1985 (COBRA): Federal law (P.L. 99–272) that requires all employer-sponsored health plans to offer certain employees and their families the opportunity to continue, at their personal expense, health insurance coverage under their group plan for up to 18, 24, or 36 months, depending on the qualifying event, after their coverage normally would have ceased (e.g., due to the death or retirement of the employee, divorce or legal separation, resignation or termination of employment, or bankruptcy of the employer).

consumer decision support: Tools that help consumers compare health insurance products and providers, and aid patients in making informed decisions about spending their health care dollar.

consumer-driven health care: Approaches to insurance that focus on making consumers sense price signals when they purchase health care.

consumers: The individuals purchasing and utilizing health care.

continuing care retirement community: Provides a full range of long-term care facilities and services—an assisted living facility and a skilled nursing facility.

continuity of care: Includes continuity of information (e.g., shared medical records), continuity across primary and secondary care (e.g., discharge planning from specialist to generalist care), and provider continuity (e.g., seeing the same provider each time).

continuous quality improvement (CQI): A systematic approach to improve processe of health care, such as admission to the hospital or delivery of patient medications.

continuum of care: Encompasses care from the cradle to the grave and includes services focused on both the prevention and the treatment of medical conditions and diseases as well as end-of-life care.

copayment: A specified amount that an insured individual must pay for a specified service or procedure (e.g., $8 for an office visit).

corporate practice of medicine (CPOM): Physician practices that are owned by business corporations or entities, rather than those owned by one practitioner or a partnership of practitioners.

cost-sharing: A provision that requires individuals to cover some part of their medical expenses (e.g., copayments, coinsurance, deductibles).

cost-shifting: Passing the excess costs of care for one group onto another group. For example, if the rate one group of health plan enrollees pays for services is less than the actual cost of those services, the difference can be made up through higher-than-cost charges to another group.

credentialing: The most common use of the term refers to obtaining and reviewing the documentation that a practitioner has the training and experience that is required for a job.

cross-sectoral collaborative approaches: Collaborative approaches essential to addressing underlying causes of poor health and therefore to improving health and health equity at the population level.

customer friendly: A practice that focuses on making the experience both useful and free of hassles for the patient as a consumer of healthcare.

cybersecurity: Keeping safe and secure patient data, generally in the electronic health record.

data: In health, an event, condition, or disease occurrence that is counted. In health services, an episode of care, costs of care, expenditures, quantification of human resources and facilities and their characteristics, and the like.

deductible: The amount insured individuals must pay out-of-pocket, usually annually on a calendar-year basis, before insurance will begin to cover their health care costs.

defensive medicine: The practice of physicians recommending a diagnostic test or treatment that is not necessarily optimal for the patient, but which serves to protect the physician against the patient's potentially bringing a lawsuit for insufficient care.

defined contribution plan: Benefits plan that gives employees a certain amount of total compensation to allocate among various benefits, rather than providing employees with the specific benefits, such as hospitalization coverage.

demographic characteristics: Such characteristics of an individual or population group (averages in the latter case) as age, sex, marital status, ethnicity, geographic location, occupation, and income.

denominator: For health care, the total number of people among whom numerator items are being counted.

determinants of health: The core factors or cause of health outcomes, usually at a very basic or core level.

diagnosis-related groups (DRGs): Groups of inpatient discharges with final diagnoses that are similar clinically and in resource consumption; used as a basis of payment by the Medicare program and, as a result, widely accepted by others.

discharge planning: A part of the patient management guidelines and the nursing care plan that identifies the expected discharge date and coordinates the various services necessary to achieve the target.

Disproportionate Share Hospitals (DSH) program: A hospital that provides a large amount (or disproportionate share) of uncompensated care and/or care to Medicaid and low income Medicare beneficiaries.

dose-response effect: Methodologically, a situation in which the change in dose (exposure) causes a proportionate change in outcome. Good evidence of a robust relationship between causal factor and outcome.

dual eligible: Describes the status of individuals in the United States who qualify to receive benefits from both the Medicare and Medicaid programs simultaneously.

electronic health records (EHRs): Digital records that contain a comprehensive patient medical history, combining information from multiple provider sources. Also called electronic medical records (EMRs).

emergency care: Designed to provide immediate care for sudden, serious illness or injury.

Emergency Medical Treatment and Labor Act (EMTALA): A portion of the COBRA law setting forth requirements for hospitals participating in Medicare to provide emergency care so that patients who cannot pay are not "dumped" to other hospitals.

emotional intelligence: A person's capacity to perceive, control, express, and evaluate emotions in interpersonal relationships.

Employee Retirement Income Security Act (ERISA): A 1974 federal law (P.L. 93–406) that set the standards of disclosure for employee benefit plans to ensure workers the right to at least part of their pensions. The law governs most private pensions and other employee benefits and overrides all state laws that concern employee benefits, including health benefits; therefore, ERISA preempts state laws in their application to self-funded, private employer–sponsored health insurance plans.

enabling factors: Skills or physical elements, such as availability and accessibility of resources, that make it either possible or easier for individuals or populations to change their behavior or environment. Examples include living conditions, social support, resources, and skills.

encounter: A patient visit to a provider.

end-of-life care: Care that helps people with advanced, progressive, incurable illnesses to live as well as possible until they die. Types of care include management of pain and other symptoms as well as psychological, spiritual, social, and practical support.

energy balance equation: The amount of energy (calories) expended versus the amount consumed.

enrollment: The process by which an individual and family become subscriber(s) for coverage in a health plan.

entitlements: Government benefits (e.g., Medicare, Medicaid, Social Security, food assistance programs) that are provided automatically to all qualified individuals and are therefore part of mandatory spending programs.

e-prescriptions: Prescriptions submitted electronically via the EHR which eliminate the hassle and potential errors of physical paper copies.

evidence-based management: The use of the best available evidence to make management decisions.

evidence-based medicine (EBM): That portion of medical practice, estimated at much less than 50%, that is based on established scientific findings.

experience rating: A method used to determine the cost of health insurance premiums, whereby the cost is based on the previous amount a certain group (e.g., all the employees of a particular business) paid for medical services.

Federal Employee Health Benefits Program (FEHBP): The health plans made available to federal employees as part of their employment benefits.

fee-for-service: A billing system in which a health care provider charges a patient a set amount for each individual service provided.

fee schedule: A listing of accepted fees or established allowances for specified medical procedures, as used in health plans.

fixed costs: Costs that do not change or vary with fluctuations in enrollment or in utilization of services.

food assistance programs: Previously referred to as food stamps, provide financial support to qualifying individuals or families who are food insecure. These programs include the Supplemental Nutrition Assistance Program (SNAP) and the Special Supplemental Nutrition Program for Women, Infants, and Children (WIC).

formulary: A listing of drugs prepared by, for example, a hospital or a managed care company, that a drug plan will pay for.

for-profit hospitals: Those owned by private corporations that declare dividends or otherwise distribute profits to individuals, also called investor-owned; many are also community hospitals.

fragmentation: Care that is delivered by different providers who are not co-located or within proximity of each other. Generally refers to care that is not coordinated carefully and that can lead to waste or mistakes in treatments.

full-time equivalent (FTE): A way of calibrating the workforce used when some employees work part time and some employees work full time. For example, a person who works 4 hours per day generally would be considered a .5 FTE worker.

gatekeeper: A health care practitioner who makes decisions regarding the type and volume of services to which a patient may have access; generally used by health maintenance organizations (HMOs) to control unnecessary utilization of services.

generic drug: A therapeutic drug, originally protected by a patent, the chemical composition of which meets the standards for that drug set by the Food and Drug Administration, usually manufactured by a different company than the branded drug.

governance: The activity of an organization that monitors the outside environment, selects appropriate alternatives, and negotiates the implementation of these alternatives with others inside and outside the organization.

governing board: A group of individuals who, under state law, own an organization, regardless of whether they can obtain any financial advantage through such ownership.

graduate medical education: The education and training of physicians beyond the 4 years of medical school, in positions that may be termed internships, residencies, fellowships, postgraduate Years 1, 2, 3, and so on. Although one can enter medical school with only an undergraduate degree, in the United States, the 4 years of medical school leading to the MD or DO (doctor of osteopathy) degrees are customarily referred to as "undergraduate medical education."

group model: An HMO that contracts with a medical group for the provision of health care services. The relationship between the HMO and the medical group is generally very close, although there are wide variations in the relative independence of the group from the HMO; a form of closed panel health plan.

group practice: Three or more physicians who deliver patient care, make joint use of equipment and personnel, and divide income by a prearranged formula.

handoff: The changeover of a patient's care from one provider to another, usually in the context of a hospital stay.

heath (World Health Organization definition): More than the absence of disease, rather "a state of complete mental, physical, and social well-being."

health care: Many factors that contribute to physical and mental health in a population or society.

health care delivery: The provision of preventive, treatment, or rehabilitative health services, from short term to long term, to individuals as well as groups of people, by individual practitioners, institutions, or public health agencies.

health care providers: Professional health service workers—physicians, dentists, psychologists—who are licensed to practice independently of any other health service worker; hospitals and other institutions offering health care services.

health care workforce: All of the people, professional and nonprofessional alike, who work in the health care services industry.

health exchange: A government-regulated marketplace of insurance plans with different levels of coverage offered to individuals and small businesses without health insurance.

health homes: Created by the ACA to give states an option for providing patient-centered, medical home–type services to Medicaid beneficiaries suffering from severe or multiple chronic conditions.

Health Impact Assessments (HIAs): Help policymakers and community stakeholders to identify the health impacts of decisions about non-health issues, such as economic development, housing or transportation plans.

health information exchange (HIE): The secure electronic exchange of patient data among authorized health care providers and patients to ensure appropriate patient information is available at the point of care.

Health Insurance Portability and Accountability Act of 1996 (HIPAA): Key provisions of this federal law improve health coverage for workers and their families when they change or lose jobs and establish privacy standards for medical information; overseen by the Department of Health and Human Services Office of Civil Rights.

health maintenance: Providing screening and prevention services that can keep people from becoming ill and identifying illnesses early when they might be easier to treat.

health maintenance organization (HMO): A managed care company that organizes and provides health care for its enrollees for a fixed, prepaid premium.

health need factor: Vulnerability in physical, mental and social health.

Health Plan Employer Data and Information Set (HEDIS): A standard set of performance measures of the quality and performance of health plans sponsored by the National Committee for Quality Assurance (NCQA).

health professionals: Generally refers to people who work in health delivery who have advanced training, focused education, or advanced academic degrees.

health promotion (personal): The science and art of helping people change their lifestyles to move toward a state of optimal health. Optimal health is defined as a balance of physical, emotional, social, spiritual, and intellectual health.

health status of entire populations: The incidence, prevalence, and distribution of health problems and differences by places and populations.

health systems: Organizations that operate multiple service units under single ownership.

healthy behavior: An action such as regular exercise, eating a balanced diet, or obtaining necessary vaccinations that people practice to maintain, attain, or regain good health and to prevent illness.

Healthy People 2020: Formal goals and objectives for the nation's health status that aim to be achieved by the year 2020. Th e Healthy People objectives are updated every 10 years by the federal government.

home health care: Health services provided in an individual's home.

horizontal integration: Affiliations among providers of the same type (e.g., a hospital forming relationships with other hospitals).

hospice care: Programs that operate in different settings to provide palliative care and comprehensive support services to dying patients, as well as counseling and bereavement support for their family members. Hospice care is reimbursable under Medicare and many state Medicaid programs, as well as by private insurers.

hospitalists: Physicians, usually hospital employees, who practice only in acute care settings to provide inpatient care otherwise provided by attending physicians.

hospitalization: The admission of a patient to a hospital.

hospitalization coverage: A type of insurance coverage for most inpatient hospital costs (e.g., room and board), diagnostic and therapeutic services, care for emergency illnesses or injuries, laboratory and x-ray services, and certain other specified procedures.

human genome: The human genetic code, involving billions of base pairs in the DNA sequence of 26,000 to 40,000 genes in the 23 human chromosomes.

incidence: The number of new events, disease cases, or conditions counted in a defined population during a defined period of time.

indemnity insurance: Benefits paid in a predetermined amount in the event of a covered loss; differs from reimbursement, which provides benefits based on actual expenses incurred. There are fewer restrictions on what a doctor may charge and what an insurer may pay for a treatment, and generally there are also fewer restrictions on a patient's ability to access specialty services.

independent living facility: Housing designed for seniors 55 years of age and older who do not require assistance with daily activities or round-the-clock skilled nursing, but who may benefit from convenient services, a senior-friendly environment, and social opportunities.

independent practice association (IPA): Association of independent physicians formed as a separate legal entity for contracting purposes with health plans.

infant mortality: The death of a child born alive before 1 year of age.

information technology (IT): Electronic systems that store, retrieve, manipulate, and communicate information. Health care organizations want information technology that is accessible—with privacy safeguards—to multiple users within an organization.

innovation: Developing new treatments, medical instruments, and drugs for the bewildering array of diseases and health conditions that beset us.

inpatient: A patient who requires an overnight stay in the hospital.

inputs: Resources needed to carry out a process or provide a service. In health care, these resources typically include finances, buildings, supplies, equipment, personnel, and clients.

instrumental activity of daily living (IADL): Everyday tasks, such as housework, taking medication, preparing meals, shopping, and responding to emergency alerts, among others. These tasks are considered less crucial than the type of tasks called *activities of daily living (ADLs)*.

insurance exchanges: Entities that link individuals to health insurance offerings. The 2010 Patient Protection and Affordable Care Act (ACA) relies extensively on state-specific insurance exchanges to manage the enrollment of individuals in subsidized and nonsubsidized insurance policies offered by private insurance companies. Private insurance exchanges also are emerging to assist people in enrolling in Medicare offerings and other types of insurance products.

integrated delivery system (IDS): A group of health care organizations that collectively provides a full range of health-related services in a coordinated fashion to those using the system.

international medical school graduate: A U.S. citizen or noncitizen physician who has graduated from a medical school not located in the United States that is also not accredited by the U.S. medical school accrediting body, the Liaison Committee on Medical Education.

interoperability: Health IT that enables the secure exchange of electronic health information with, and use of electronic health information from, other health IT without special effort on the part of the user; allows for complete access, exchange, and use of all electronically accessible health information for authorized use under applicable State or Federal law; and does not constitute information blocking.

interprofessional education: An approach to training different types of health professionals (e.g., physicians and nurses) together for part of the training period so that they get a better sense of the relative and overlapping roles of each type of professional. It is believed to make each type of clinician understand how to treat patients in a collaborative way.

investor-owned hospital: A hospital owned by one or more private parties or a corporation for the purpose of generating a profitable return on investment.

labor market: The interplay between people looking for jobs in the health sector (the supply side) and health care organizations looking to hire people qualified to do specific health-related jobs (the demand side). A labor market is working efficiently when supply and demand are about equal.

length of stay: The number of days spent by a specific person in a hospital during one episode of care.

licensure: A system established by a given state recognizing the achievement of a defined level of education, experience, and examination performance, which qualifies the person or organization meeting those standards to work or operate in a defined area of practice, which is prohibited to any person or organization that has not met those standards.

life expectancy: The predicted average number of years of life remaining for a person at a given age.

long-term care: A general term for a range of services provided to chronically ill, physically disabled, or mentally disabled patients in a nursing home or through long-term home health care.

loss ratio: A term used to describe the amount of money spent on health care. An insurance company with a loss ratio of 0.85, for instance, spends 85 cents of every premium dollar on health care and the remaining 15 cents on administrative costs, such as marketing and profits.

managed care: A system of health care delivery that influences or controls utilization of services and costs of services. The degree of influence depends on the model used. For example, a preferred provider organization (PPO) charges patients lower rates if they use the providers in its preferred network. HMOs, on the other hand, may choose not to reimburse for health services received from providers with whom the HMO does not contract.

management: The task of overseeing the operations of a complex set of processes and tasks as required for health care delivery or public health activities. Generally refers to what administrators do behind the scenes to assure that clinicians can deliver health services effectively.

mandated benefits: Benefits that a health plan is required to provide by law. This term generally refers to benefits above and beyond routine insurance-type benefits, and it generally applies at the state level (where there is high variability). Common examples include in vitro fertilization, defined days of inpatient mental health or substance abuse treatment, and other special condition treatments.

Medicaid: A joint federal-state program of health care coverage for low income individuals, under Title XIX of the federal Social Security Act. States set benefits and eligibility requirements and administer the program. Medicaid is the major source of payment for nursing home care of the elderly.

medical home: A physician-directed medical practice with a team of providers in which each patient has an ongoing relationship with a personal physician, who coordinates care. A medical home has an aim of reducing fragmentation in care delivery but it does not provide as comprehensive a set of services as what is termed a *Health Home*.

medical model: The set of procedures traditionally used by Western physicians to diagnose and treat illness: complaint, history, physical examination, ancillary tests if necessary, diagnosis, treatment, and prognosis with and without treatment.

medical savings account: Accounts similar to individual retirement accounts (IRAs) into which employers and employees can make tax-deferred contributions and from which employees may withdraw funds to pay covered health care expenses.

medically indigent: Those who do not have and cannot afford medical insurance coverage yet who are not eligible financially for Medicaid.

Medicare: A federal entitlement program of health care coverage for the elderly and disabled and people with end-stage renal disease, governed by Title XVIII of the federal Social Security Act and consisting of several parts: Part A for institutional and home care; Part B for physician care; a managed care component (informally called Part C); and Part D, covering prescription drugs.

Medicare Prescription Drug, Improvement, and Modernization Act (MMA): Federal law signed in 2004 that offers a discount card at a nominal fee to Medicare beneficiaries for drugs and a prescription drug benefit that started in 2006 for those on Medicare who enroll and pay a premium. This benefit often is called Part D of Medicare.

medigap: Also known as Medicare supplemental insurance, a type of private insurance coverage that may be purchased by an individual enrolled in Medicare to cover certain needed services that are not covered by Medicare Part A or B (i.e., that fall into "gaps").

moral hazard: An economics and actuarial term describing the expectation that people will use more of a service if it is free at the point of purchase. Most experts believe that health insurance creates moral hazard for many types of medical care, thus serving to increase total expenditures on services.

morbidity: An episode of sickness, as defined by a health professional. A morbidity rate is the number of such episodes occurring in a given population during a given period of time.

mortality: Death. A mortality rate is the number of deaths—either the crude rate, which is all deaths, or a specific rate, which is number of deaths by, for example, a specific cause, at a specific location, or within a specific age group—occurring during a given period of time.

multisectoral collaboration: The coming together of many part of a community to improve quality of life. In the health sector, it generally is used to describe partnerships involving, for example, medical care providers, public health providers, government leaders, business leaders, community based organizations, and community residents.

multiple determinants: A term that refers to the fact that what determines health outcomes arises from multiple places, including the social and economic environment, the physical environment, genetics, medical care, and health-related behaviors.

multispecialty group practice (MSGP): An MSGP employs primary and specialty care physicians who share common governance, infrastructure, and finances; refer patients for services offered within the group; and are typically affiliated with a particular hospital or hospitals.

natality: Technical term for birth rate. The combination of natality and mortality rates indicate a population's increase, decrease, or whether its size remains generally consistent.

National Association of County and City Health Officials (NACCHO): A professional association whose members are mostly public health leaders and professionals working at the county or city/community levels.

national health insurance (NHI): A system for paying for one or more categories of health care services that is organized on a nationwide basis, established by and usually operated by a government agency.

National Health Service (NHS): A comprehensive, government-funded and operated system, such as that found in Great Britain.

neighborhood effects: The interaction of social and physical environmental determinants; for example, the negative interaction between the physical environment (poor housing, presence of crime and violence, absence of stores with healthy foods) and social determinants related to poverty.

nongovernmental organizations: Generally used outside the United States to describe any organization that is not a government agency. In the United States, the terms used more generally for this sector are non-profit organizations.

nurse practitioner (NP): Registered nurses who have been trained at the master's level in providing primary care services, expanded health care evaluations, and decision making, and can write prescriptions, either independently or under a physician's supervision, depending on state law.

office visit: A formal, face-to-face contact between a physician and a patient in a health center, office, or hospital outpatient department.

on-the-job training: Training that takes place once an individual is hired.

open enrollment period: A period, often once per year, when new enrollees are accepted into an insurance plan. Insurers do not want to have enrollment open all year long because they fear people will only purchase insurance once they get sick.

out-of-pocket: Health care expenses paid by patients that are not reimbursed by health insurance companies, such as deductibles, copays, and coinsurance.

outcomes: Measures of treatments and effectiveness in terms of access, quality, and cost.

outlier: Under a DRG system of payment, additional per diem payments are made to hospitals for cases requiring extraordinary stays. Such cases are referred to as long-stay outliers.

outpatient: Not requiring an overnight hospital or health care facility stay.

overscreening: Screening or testing for diseases that may not be medically necessary, potentially also resulting in false-positive test results.

palliative care: Pain and symptom management and emotional and spiritual support for individuals facing a chronic, debilitating, or life-threatening illness.

patient-centered medical home (PCMH): A widely accepted philosophy (not a destination) of primary care that is patient centered, comprehensive, team based, coordinated, accessible, and focused on quality and safety.

patient engagement: The process of involving individuals in their health care, disease management, or preventive behaviors.

patient outcomes: What happens after a person receives health care or a health-related intervention. This term most frequently refers to whether or not the services or interventions eliminate the medical problem experienced by a person before receiving care. But outcomes also include a range of factors related to how well the patient is treated, such as wait times or clarity of explanations offered to a patient about the services received.

patient portals: Secure websites or applications that give patients access to personal health information and allow them to interact and communicate with their health care providers.

Patient Protection and Affordable Care Act (ACA): The 2010 health reform act that could extend insurance coverage to as many as 32 million Americans. The law also included regulations that affect the quality of coverage insurers must offer. Additionally, the law created a range of initiatives focused on encouraging reform in how medical care is organized and delivered, with a goal of reducing costs and improving quality and outcomes. Finally, other aspects of the law provided funding for expanded primary care capacity and a wide range of other health system improvements. This law is often referred to as *Obamacare*.

pay-for-performance (PFP): To reward hospitals, physicians, and others for achieving particular quality or efficiency goals.

payer mix: The distribution of payments/payers to a provider or health system, which determines financial viability.

per diem payment: Reimbursement rates that are paid to providers for each day of services provided to a patient, based on the patient's illness or condition.

performance management: The process of systematically assessing how well a health care organization is doing when it cares for people. Performance generally is rated based on specific outcomes, often suggested by national quality assurance agencies. Various dimensions of performance can be assessed at the individual staff level, the department level, or the total organization level.

performance measurement: Measuring, monitoring, and enhancing staff performance to improve overall organizational performance.

physician assistant (PA): A specially trained and licensed worker who performs certain medical procedures generally under the supervision of a physician. Physician assistants are usually not registered nurses.

point-of-service plan (POS): A managed care plan that offers enrollees the option of receiving services from participating or nonparticipating providers. The benefits package is designed to encourage the use of participating providers through higher deductibles or only partial reimbursement for services provided by nonparticipating providers.

policy development: To create and advocate for solutions to achieve public health goals.

policy issue: A social issue or problem (including one related to health) that might be addressed through a governmental law or initiative. Addressing a policy issue generally involves defining the problem, stating the goal, and creating and debating alternative approaches for resolving the problem to reach the goal. Debating policy issues is a key role of the political and governmental process.

population health: The health outcomes of a group of people and the distribution of outcomes within that group. The field of population health assesses how patterns of health determinants affect health outcomes and develops policies and interventions that link these areas.

practice ecology model: The need to address not just the behavior of individual providers, but also the powerful effects of the health care systems and environments in which providers practice.

predictive analytics: In the health care context, a data analytic method to use past data about a patient to predict the patient's future outcomes or needs.

predisposing factor: Preexisting characteristics of an individual or his or her context that may influence (encourage or inhibit) a health-related behavior. Some are amenable to change (e.g., knowledge, attitudes) whereas others are not (e.g., genetic or demographic characteristics).

preexisting condition: A physical and/or mental condition of an insured that first manifests itself prior to issuance of a policy or that exists before issuance and for which treatment was received.

preferred provider organization (PPO): A limited group (panel) of providers (doctors and/or hospitals) who agree to provide health care to subscribers for a negotiated and usually discounted fee and who agree to utilization review.

prehospital care: Includes medical services provided in the community, such as stabilization by emergency services before or during transportation to a health care facility.

premium: A periodic payment required to keep an insurance policy in force.

prepayment: A method of providing, in advance, for the cost of predetermined benefits for a population group through regular periodic payments in the form of premiums, dues, or contributions, including contributions that are made to a health and welfare fund by employers on behalf of their employees and payments to managed care organizations made by federal agencies for people who are Medicare eligible.

prescription: An order from a licensed physician or an authorized designee to a pharmacy, directing the latter to dispense a given drug with written instructions for its use.

prevalence: The total number of events, disease cases, or conditions existing in a defined population, counted during a defined period of time or at a given point in time (known as point-prevalence).

primary care: The general health care that people receive on a routine basis that is not associated with an acute or chronic illness or disability and may be provided by a physician, nurse practitioner, or physician assistant. Primary care also includes visits to physicians to develop an initial diagnosis of a possible medical problem.

primary care practitioners: Doctors in family practice, general internal medicine, obstetrics/gynecology, or pediatrics; nurse practitioners and midwives; and may also include psychiatrists and emergency care physicians.

primary prevention: Helping people avoid the onset of a health condition.

private practice: A solo or group physician practice that is not a corporate practice or a hospital-based practice or a publicly run practice. It is owned by some or all of the physicians in the practice.

privileges: Rights granted annually to physicians and affiliate staff members to perform specified kinds of care in the hospital.

professionalism: The conduct, aims, or qualities that characterize members of a given profession.

Public Health Accreditation Board (PHAB): Created national voluntary performance standards for public health agencies, with development, refinement, and review.

public health agencies: Official agencies established by state or local government that provide environmental health services, preventive medical services, and, sometimes, therapeutic services.

public hospital: A hospital operated by a government agency. In the United States, the most common are the federal Veterans Health Administration hospitals (restricted to certain categories of veterans), state mental hospitals, and county and city general hospitals.

quality assurance: A formal set of activities to measure the quality of services provided and to implement safeguards to make sure quality levels are consistently high.

quality improvement: Activities undertaken to improve quality relative to accepted standards of care.

quaternary care: An extension of tertiary care, entails providing the most complex medical and surgical care for highly specialized and unusual cases.

registered nurse (RN): A nurse who is a graduate of an approved education program leading to a diploma, an associate degree, or a bachelor's degree who also has met the requirements of experience and exam passage to be licensed in a given state.

rehabilitation clinics: Service organizations in which various types of trained professionals deliver services to people with a medical condition that causes physical problems, creating disabilities. The aim is to restore functional abilities to as high a level as possible.

reinsurance: Insurance purchased by a health plan to protect it against extremely high-cost cases.

remote patient monitoring (RPM): Technology designed to collect health data and vital signs from patients when they are away from the point of care to support interventions when needed.

reserves: A fiscal method of withholding a certain percentage of premiums to provide a fund for committed but undelivered health care and such uncertainties as higher hospital utilization levels than expected, overutilization of referrals, and catastrophes.

reverse causality: When two things are related to one another but the issue of which one causes the other can be unclear. For example, we observe that people with high income are healthier than people with low income and assume that this means income is a determinant of health. It may be the reverse, with good health leading to high incomes.

risk management: Identification, evaluation, and corrective action against organizational behavior that would otherwise result in financial loss or legal liability.

safety-net provider: A provider that delivers care for free or at a reduced cost to low-income and/or uninsured patients. Safety net providers can do this by being subsidized by governments or by raising charitable donations.

same-day surgery: Procedures that are done on an outpatient basis.

Sarbanes-Oxley Act (SOA): The 2002 federal legislation that affects corporate governance, financial disclosure, and the practice of public accounting.

scope of practice: The types of services that a person with a specific type of training is legally allowed to perform. As an example, nurses have different legal scopes of practice than physicians do.

secondary prevention: Efforts to help people who already have a medical condition ensure the problem does not get worse.

self-perpetuating governance boards: Boards in which existing board members appoint new board members as terms expire.

single specialty group practice: A practice with two or more physicians that have the same medical specialty.

skilled nursing facility (SNF): A facility in which people who are too frail to live alone or have very serious ongoing medical disabilities live and are taken care of.

social determinants: The circumstances in which people are born, grow up, live, work, and age, and the systems in place to address illness that are, in turn, shaped by larger forces, including economics, social policies, and politics.

social ecological models: Models that integrate behavioral science with clinical and public health approaches. They redefined what the targets of successful health interventions need to be—not just individuals but also the powerful social contexts in which they live and work. And they emphasized that a person's health behavior is affected by multiple levels of influence: interpersonal factors (e.g., physiologic factors, knowledge, skill, motivation), social factors (e.g., social–cultural norms, supports, and networks), organizational and community factors, broader environmental influences, and public policies.

social marketing strategies: The use of marketing to design and implement programs to promote socially beneficial behavior change.

socialized medicine: Organizing the delivery of medicine using government or some other group-based organization to assure that the overall medical needs of a population can be met. Generally, it involves sharing expenses and often involves the idea of government-run delivery organizations. The concept is based on the idea that health and access to health care are "rights" and not just "commodities."

solo practice: Individual practice of medicine by a physician who does not practice in a group or does not share personnel, facilities, or equipment with three or more physicians.

specialty care: Medical services delivered by a physician trained to be an expert in one specific area of medicine. It is the type of care that requires extensive knowledge about how to diagnose and treat one specific type of medical problem.

special hospital: Provide diagnostic and treatment services for patients who have specified medical conditions, both surgical and nonsurgical.

staff model: An HMO that employs providers who see members in their own facilities. A form of closed-panel HMO.

stakeholders: Persons with an interest in the performance of an organization. Examples of hospital stakeholders are physicians and nurses, payers, managers, patients, and government.

Stark legislation: Federal laws (named after their sponsor, California Representative Fortney "Pete" Stark) that place limits on physicians' referring patients to facilities in which they have a financial interest.

subacute care: A level of inpatient care needed by a patient immediately after or instead of hospitalization for an acute illness, injury, or exacerbation of a disease process.

surveillance: Generally, ongoing observation of a population for rapid and accurate detection of events, conditions, or emerging diseases.

telehealth: The use of electronic information and telecommunication technologies to support and promote long-distance clinical health care, patient and professional health-related education, public health and health administration.

tertiary care: Medical care or procedures performed by specialized physicians and teams in specially equipped hospitals. Advanced cancer care, burn treatment, and advanced surgeries are examples of tertiary care. Quaternary care is even more highly specialized, rarely used, and sometimes experimental.

The Joint Commission: Formerly the Joint Commission on Accreditation of Healthcare Organizations, The Joint Commission is a national organization of representatives of health care providers: the American College of Physicians, American College of Surgeons, American Hospital Association, American Medical Association, and consumer representatives. The Joint Commission inspects and accredits the quality of operations for hospitals and other health care organizations.

transparency: Operating in an accountable way by providing health care consumers cost and quality data before treatment so they can choose the best care at the best price.

Triple Aim: The concurrent pursuit of three objectives to improve the U.S. health care system: improving patients' health care experience, improving health outcomes, and reducing health care costs. This is a concept developed and advanced by an organization called the Institute for Health Improvement.

uninsured: In the United States, a person who has no third-party source of payment for health care services.

universal health insurance: A national health insurance system that provides for comprehensive coverage for all permanent residents of a country.

urgent care center: A health care center that offers walk-in access and extended hours to individuals with illnesses and injuries that do not require emergency care.

utilization: Quantity of services used by patients, such as hospital days, physician visits, or prescriptions.

utilization review: A system for measuring and evaluating how physicians utilize services for their patients against established standards.

value: Health care that is measured by the outcomes achieved instead of the amount of services delivered.

vertical integration: Affiliations among providers of different types (e.g., a hospital, clinic, and nursing home forming an affiliation).

vital statistics: Numbers and rates for items such as births, deaths, abortions, fetal deaths, fertility, life expectancy, marriages, and divorces.

volume-driven: Providers (such as hospitals, physicians, and health centers) gain increased revenue and profit by delivering more services to people.

vulnerable populations: Groups of people who are likely to be at greater risk for developing health problems because of challenges such as limited access to resources, poverty, marginalized sociocultural status, limited education, chronic mental illness, homelessness, incarceration, or age.

waste: System and organizational inefficiencies that lead to higher health care costs without improved outcomes.

workforce: The people engaged in or available for work in a particular industry, such as health care.

INDEX

Note: Page numbers followed by *t* and *f* refer to pages containing tables and figures, respectively.